The Art of Palpatory Diagnosis in Oriental Medicine

To my parents, who taught me
that love is touch

Skya Gardner-Abbate began her career as a medical
sociologist serving as a Peace Corps volunteer in Brazil,
then later taught in the Sociology Department of the
University of Rhode Island (1978–81).

In 1983 she graduated from the acupuncture program of
the Institute of Traditional Medicine (Santa Fe, New Mexico)
and has since undertaken two advanced clinical training
programs with the Academy of Traditional Chinese Medicine
in Beijing, China (1988 and 1989).

Skya is a licenced Doctor of Oriental Medicine in the
state of New Mexico, Executive Director of Southwest
Acupuncture College (with three campuses in Santa Fe and
Albuquerque, New Mexico, and Boulder, Colorado), where
she teaches needle technique, diagnosis and Japanese
acupuncture systems, and former President of the New
Mexico Association of Acupuncture and Oriental Medicine.
She also has a private practice integrating classical Chinese
diagnosis with her subspecialty in Japanese diagnosis. She
has served over 6 years as an educational expert and
Commissioner for the Accreditation Commission for
Acupuncture and Oriental Medicine, the national
organization which accredits professional degree programs
in Oriental medicine.

Skya is the author of *Beijing: the new forbidden city*
(1991) and *Holding the tiger's tail: an acupuncture
techniques manual in the treatment of disease* (1996) and is
a regular contributor to the *American Journal of
Acupuncture*.

For Churchill Livingstone:

Publishing Manager: Inta Ozols
Project Manager: Jane Dingwall
Design Direction: George Ajayi

The Art of Palpatory Diagnosis in Oriental Medicine

Skya Gardner-Abbate MA DOM DiplAc DiplCH
Department of Clinical Medicine, Southwest Acupuncture College, Santa Fe/Albuquerque/Boulder, USA

Foreword by

Mark D Seem PhD LAc
President, Tri-State College of Acupuncture, New York, USA

Research by **Miguel Viddo**

Illustrations by **Christine R Oagley**

Photographs by **Jill Fineberg** and **Natasha Lane**

Cover calligraphy by **Siu-Leung Lee**

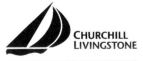
CHURCHILL
LIVINGSTONE

EDINBURGH LONDON NEW YORK PHILADELPHIA ST LOUIS SYDNEY TORONTO 2001

CHURCHILL LIVINGSTONE
An imprint of Harcourt Publishers Limited

© Harcourt Publishers Limited 2001

 is a registered trademark of Harcourt Publishers Limited

First published 2001
 Reprinted 2001

ISBN 0 443 07058 X

British Library Cataloguing in Publication Data
A catalogue record for this book is available from the British Library.

Library of Congress Cataloging in Publication Data
A catalog record for this book is available from the Library of Congress.

Note
Medical knowledge is constantly changing. As new information becomes available, changes in treatment, procedures, equipment and the use of drugs become necessary. The author and the publishers have taken care to ensure that the information given in this text is accurate and up to date. However, readers are strongly advised to confirm that the information, especially with regard to drug usage, complies with latest legislation and standards of practice.

The
publisher's
policy is to use
paper manufactured
from sustainable forests

Transferred to digital printing 2006
Printed and bound by CPI Antony Rowe, Eastbourne

Contents

Foreword

The Art of Palpatory Diagnosis in Oriental Medicine by Skya Gardner-Abbate shows how the infusion of Japanese acupuncture into North America over the past two decades is beginning to reshape how this wonderful medicine might be practiced – as an *art of palpation*.

In this comprehensive text, the author presents palpation not just as assessment and diagnosis, not just as treatment, but as an avenue through which client and practitioner might share something profound of the experience of illness that unites them.

Skya Gardner-Abbate bases her exploration of palpation in acupuncture not only on a poetic feel for Japanese-style treatment as a palpatory practice, but also on her hands-on feel derived from a decade and a half of practice and teaching aimed at integrating Japanese acupuncture into Chinese acupuncture and Traditional Chinese Medicine approaches.

In this ambitious textbook, the author provides English-speaking practitioners of acupuncture, Oriental bodywork and physical medicine with a step-by-step approach for coming to grips with the basics of Japanese acupuncture in such a way as to integrate them into their own practices.

These basics begin with an evaluation of the abdomen as a starting point for treatment and the author moves from a review of the key abdominal maps to her own simplified approach to abdominal evaluation. From this beginning in the *root*, she moves to the palpation and release of key areas of the body as stressed by the renowned Kiiko Matsumoto, namely the sinuses, the neck and SCM, the navel, the rectus abdominis and scars. She covers key points in Japanese acupuncture for clearing these areas, Japanese needle techniques and the role of the Eight Curious Vessels in this style of treatment according to various Japanese practitioners.

Whether readers use this text as an introductory glimpse at the role of palpation in Japanese acupuncture or as a course in the basics of this approach, they are sure to come away with a more vibrant, dynamic feel for what lies beneath the acupuncture meridians and points and how this might all be accessed through informed touch.

New York 2000   Mark D Seem

Preface

To write a book on palpation is not an easy task; palpation needs to be done, demonstrated and practiced. However, it is not impossible and the written word is an important guide and reference for any practitioner.

A Chinese proverb states, 'Give me a fish and I will eat for a day. Teach me to fish, and I will eat for a lifetime'. With this thought in mind, this book has been conceived. The purpose of this illustrative manual is not to provide all the answers (or the fish) as to why one uses palpation as a primary diagnostic and treatment modality but rather to explain how to seek the answers to diagnosis and treatment. It emphasizes a thinking approach, not the solutions to what must be the individuality of every treatment. In this work it will be seen that palpation can be used for every condition, be it internal or musculoskeletal, because it is a way of thinking, fishing, if you will, for the proper diagnosis and treatment of each patient. It is a method derived from immediate sensory experience and traditional clinical theory.

The book has several interrelated goals.

1. To share with students and practitioners the system of palpation, an ancient Chinese art which has lost its footing in modern-day China yet has its basis in classical Chinese medicine. It is the heart of diagnosis and treatment in modern-day Japanese acupuncture. It is an important diagnostic tool that allows us to supplement patient complaint with verifiable bodily evidence. Thus the role of palpation as a method of diagnosis and treatment in both Chinese and Japanese orientations is stressed.

2. To illustrate the integration of Chinese and Japanese medical thought; that is, to see them as interrelated, classically based systems.

3. To illustrate that abdominal diagnosis can be used for the diagnosis and treatment of virtually every condition.

4. To show practitioners how to perform it and integrate it into their existing practices.

5. To explain how other modalities can be combined into these treatment plans.

6. To share clinical information derived from 16 years of teaching and practical experience with these systems.

7. And finally, to enhance practitioners' awareness with the skills and diagnostic frameworks that will enable them to view the body as a system instead of perceiving the patient from a more fragmented 'treatment of disease' approach.

If the aforementioned objectives are accomplished, practitioners, after reading this book, should know more about palpation than they did previously. Assisted by the simple forms that I have developed and the tables, illustrations and photos, practitioners can learn how to organize their data into a new way of perceiving them. Readers should be able to attain the following competencies if they assiduously practice the techniques presented herein.

1. Professionally palpate the Hara (abdomen) and pretest other diagnostically significant

points so as to collect data that will aid the formation of a diagnostic pattern.

2. Gather further pathological data by inspection, auscultation, olfaction and inquiry.

3. Integrate traditional Chinese methods of diagnosis with the Japanese diagnostic and therapeutic system.

4. Effectively clear energetic blockages and redress those imbalances with the corresponding tools and a minimum use of needles.

5. Learn how to use all these tools in a safe and appropriate manner.

Features of this book that guide the reader towards these goals include the following.

1. Each chapter presents a new topic that builds upon the previous chapter's material. Hence the book is meant to be read as a whole.

2. Every chapter introduces relevant words and concepts. For easy reference they are reiterated at the end of each chapter.

3. A question section at the end of each chapter tests the subjects covered in that chapter so that readers can test their grasp of the material before moving on to subsequent chapters. Individually, the reader can benefit by answering the questions, thereby actively assimilating the text. Additionally, if used as a textbook by teachers, the questions offer good opportunities for class discussion to share different insights on the text material. Multiple choice answers are listed in the 'Answers' section of the book (p. 279).

4. Several chapters are devoted to the clarification of complex theoretical material not found in other texts to enhance the infrastructure of the reader's understanding of this approach.

5. Interesting supplemental literature is incorporated into specific chapters so that the reader can see the connection between the material expounded and other supportive literature.

6. Illustrative figures and photos are generously included to portray diagnostic concepts and demonstrate needle techniques and palpatory exams. A special segment on navel diagnosis, never before seen in other books, is included here.

7. Ample tables summarizing differential diagnosis or other useful clinical data are included for assimilation of material, quick reference and easy implementation.

8. Actual cases derived from personal clinical experience are integrated whenever the concepts covered need further elaboration. In this way practitioners can study patient progress and get a sense of how to use the material.

9. Forms outlining procedures, diagnoses and possible treatment strategies supplement the theoretical material in each chapter so that the practitioner is assisted in organizing and performing the palpatory exams. The forms are provided again in the 'Form' section of the book (p. 235) for clinical use. They may be copied to assist in treating patients.

A poetic rendition of the Chinese concept of palpation has been offered as 'The magic hand returns spring'. This means that through the tremendous inherent power of touch, the resilient, resurrected, sprout-like energy of spring in our lives can be accessed and attained. With this view in mind, I invite you to let this book, like a magic hand, guide you in breathing new life into your clinical practice and your patients' lives. You will find that the prodromes of our patients' 'dis-ease' are frequently hidden just below the threshold of touch, the gateway to the connection with our social, emotional, spiritual, physical, 'spring-like' selves.

New Mexico 2000   Skya Gardner-Abbate

Acknowledgments

In grateful acknowledgment to Dr Nyugen Van Nghi, the practitioner who first pointed out to me the power of palpation and reshaped my conceptions about the power of point energetics and Oriental medicine in general.

To Kiiko Matsumoto for challenging me to cultivate my clinical skills in every area from diagnosis, to palpation, through to treatment.

To the students of Southwest Acupuncture College, Santa Fe and Albuquerque, from 1991 to 1999, for allowing me to teach them this potent system of medicine and supporting me as I grappled with understanding and presenting this material.

The theoretical and clinical basis of palpation

1

Touch as therapy

Humans have a fundamental need to be touched. Numerous studies in the area of psychology have pointed to the critical effects of loving and appropriate touch on the social and emotional development of the person (Ackerman 1990, pp. 67–123, Ornstein 1989, pp. 37–45). They have convincingly and dramatically demonstrated how lack of touch affects the development of the mind and the body.

Studies in the field of medicine have also suggested that touch is indeed correlated with some aspects of social, emotional and physical well-being (Center for Positive Living 1990, pp. 330–331, Gagne 1994, Keller & Bzdek 1986, Verrees 1996).

Being touched and cuddled is essential to healthy human development. During the early 19th century, if a child was separated from its parents it was sent to a foundling institution. This was in effect a death sentence. A study of 10 such institutions in 1915 revealed that in all but one, every single baby under the age of 2 died. The reasons for this tragedy were unknown. Nutrition appeared sufficient. Sanitation was adequate, if not overzealous. But the fear of germs and transmission of infectious disease led to no-touch policies. As a result, the infants were seldom touched or handled (Ornstein 1989, p. 42).

Adults who are deprived of physical stroking in childhood often adopt compulsive, destructive habits such as nail biting, overeating or smoking. There is some speculation that violent behavior too may be a result of touch deprivation in early childhood (Ryan & Travis 1991, p. 58).

A 1975 clinical study, later published by the *Journal of Nursing*, showed that hemoglobin levels rose significantly higher in patients after a session of therapeutic touch than they did in a control group. Hemoglobin, of course, is the component of the red Blood corpuscle that carries oxygen to the cells (Center for Positive Living 1990, p. 3).

Further beneficial results include faster growth rate in premature babies, slower heart rate, lowered muscular tension, lower stress, increased vitality, decrease in pain, improved breathing, reduction in anxiety and depression, increase in emotional affect and overall immune enhancement. The lesson of such studies is that touch can bestow a therapeutic effectiveness that is both within our ability to give and perhaps far outlasts the effects of chemical, surgical or mechanical therapies.

Palpation, as a method of determining that the body might be ill or that something might be wrong, however subtle, goes back to prehistory, as does the attempt to make that area better by touch. Diseases are not only reflected at points but may also be treated by acupuncture or massage therapy at the sensitive spots.

HISTORICAL ROOTS OF PALPATION

In the annals of Chinese medicine, palpation of specific body parts had a long but crude history. It was largely derived from trial and error, observation over the centuries or serendipitous events. For most of Chinese history it was considered indecent to touch the body of a person of the opposite sex except for the pulse. When examining the patient's body became prohibited in the late Qing period (19th century), reading the pulse became almost the sole diagnostic technique available to the Chinese physician. It is still the king of diagnostic techniques in modern Chinese medicine (Alphen & Aris 1995, p. 179).

For whatever reasons – the coldness of the climate in areas where most of the medical theory originated, cultural modesty or a penchant for intellectual methods of diagnosis – bodily palpation suffered in comparison with the continued development of the other methods of diagnosis: inspection, auscultation, olfaction, inquiry and pulse palpation. Despite this, palpation did and does have a rightful place in the repertoire of Chinese therapeutics.

American practitioner and author Mark Seem offers us an important historical perspective when he states, 'For the truth of the matter, throughout the long history of Chinese acupuncture, there has never been a single, unified system of diagnosis and treatment but rather an appreciation for the multiplicity of approaches possible in any given situation' (Seem 1992).

He continues:

…What differentiates various schools of thought in Chinese Medicine is which of the frameworks is predominant. Yin/Yang, Five Phases; Qi, Blood, Fluids, Essence; Zang-Fu; Pathogenic Factors; Channels and Collaterals. In TCM (modern day, communist sanctioned medicine) the main frameworks or filters through which a patient complaint is approached is Yin/Yang (as Eight principles); Qi, Blood, Fluid, Essence; Zang-Fu (the heavyweight in this approach), and pathogenic factors. The Five Phases are glaringly absent, as are the Channels and Collaterals. (Seem 1989a)

Interestingly, Channels and Collaterals (or meridian theory) and Five Phase theory are the underpinnings of palpatory diagnosis.

The 'herbalization' of Chinese medicine, a term used to describe an acupuncture point selection approach akin to adding herbs to a formula, utilized Zang-Fu theory in preference to other diagnostic paradigms. This movement further contributed to making most of the therapeutics more cerebral and divorced from patient contact. This historical development, coupled with the advent of communism when the spiritualism of Chinese philosophy was removed from medicine, transformed its delivery. It became less individualistic, less energetic, more symptomatic and more mechanistic. These two major historical events synergistically combined to reduce the use of body palpation as a method of diagnosis and treatment within the cultural schema.

Clinical practice in modern China has increasingly divorced itself from the opportunity to palpate the patient. Patients who would normally see a private doctor in the United States are treated as outpatients in hospitals in China because there is limited privatization of business. The need for medical care is enormous and doctors are in great demand. Bureaucratic regulations in hospitals set quotas for overworked doctors but classically trained* doctors of Chinese medicine strive to meet these daily quotas without sacrificing their theoretical outlook on how the patient should be treated. Whether because of time constraints or previous cultural predilection, bodily palpation as a method of diagnosis is glaringly absent in the Chinese system of therapeutics in China.

In contrast to China, Japan distinguished itself by taking the art of palpation and developing it into not only a primary tool with which to determine the health of the individual but the identical mechanism by which to correct the pathologies identified. In his *Illustrated guide to the Asian arts of healing*, Alphen notes that the assimilation of Chinese medicine adapted to the needs and circumstances of the Japanese. 'Japanised' Chinese medicine took shape. Uniquely Japanese is the practice of measuring the abdominal palpation in addition to regular pulse palpation when evaluating the patient's physical and psychic condition according to the four methods (Alphen & Aris 1995, p. 233).

Japanese practitioner Shudo Denmei concurs when he notes that unlike the rest of Oriental medicine, abdominal diagnosis developed very little in China. Instead, it became popular in Japan from the 17th century when it began to develop into a unique diagnostic system in its own right. It seems that tongue diagnosis took the place of abdominal diagnosis in China, so carefully do they examine the shape, color and coating of the tongue. Very few texts of Chinese medicine have anything to say about abdominal diagnosis. Some scholars in Japan have suggested that this is because the Chinese have been more reluctant than the Japanese to expose their abdomens. He concludes by saying, 'I am not so sure diagnosis developed because the Japanese were more willing to bare their bellies, but it is true that his-

torically Japanese society has had less inhibitions about nudity' (Denmei 1990, p. 88).

Denmei continues to extrapolate: 'The development of abdominal diagnosis in meridian therapy was, without a doubt, based upon *The Classic of Difficulties*. In Chapter 16, the findings of pulsation, induration, and tenderness on the abdomen are mentioned in reference to diagnosis' (Denmei 1990, p. 91).

Japanese practitioner Mubunsai, in the late 1600s, maintained that examining and treating the abdomen directly is sufficient to cure nine out of 10 diseases. Yoshimasu Todo, the most influential figure in the neoclassical school of Japanese acupuncture in the 1700s, claimed that, 'The abdomen is the source of life, and therefore the myriad diseases have their root here. The abdomen must always be examined in order to diagnose disease' (Denmei 1990, p. 89).

Kiiko Matsumoto, the talented modern acupuncturist who is promoting a system of Japanese therapeutics within the United States, provides another historical summary on palpation. She writes:

Abdominal diagnosis is an idea that has appeared in the famous texts of internal medicine and acupuncture through the entire history of Oriental medicine. It has played a greater or lesser role in the systems of diagnosis used at different times by different practitioners, gaining or losing prestige and acceptance based on a variety of trends and cultural conditions, few of which have been clearly identified or studied. Abdominal diagnosis through palpation was used in the Ming dynasty in China, but does not seem to have played a large role in the practice of internal medicine or acupuncture. However in Japan, at the same time, the classics had been absorbed and were being applied in practice. The art and practice of palpation was beginning to become generally known. Todo Yoshimasu's work concerning abdominal palpation had become very important. In the field of acupuncture, Waichi Sugiyama refined and developed palpation to a very fine art. Sugiyama, a blind acupuncturist who lived from 1610–1695, was the inventor of the insertion tube. In Japan he is often seen as the father of acupuncture. Developing extraordinary sensitivity and skill with his hands, he became a great healer, and contributed a significant body of information regarding palpation. The core of information that Sugiyama taught is still of great utility, providing an excellent theoretical foundation for much of modern practice. (Matsumoto & Birch 1988, p. 29)

---

* 'Classically trained' is an epithet many of the doctors I studied with in China used to distinguish themselves from physicians of barefoot doctor lineage or others with a preponderance of training in Western medicine or those who followed the TCM herbal orientation, based upon syndromes of the Zang-Fu, Eight Categories and Qi and Blood. Classically trained refers to the fact that their practice methods stem primarily from the *Neijing, Nanjing* time, the classical period.

So we see that as the Zang-Fu orientation took precedence over meridian acupuncture in China, meridian acupuncture in Japan retained a role in the Japanese therapeutic system and progressed through a series of refinements which has brought it to the art it is today in modern-day Japanese medicine. As in the case of China, a combination of cultural experience and theoretical outlook led to the cultivation of palpation – in the latter country, its preeminence. While TCM acupuncturists focus on Zang-Fu, it must be remembered, says Seem, that one always treats along meridians and at acupuncture points. A meridian perspective will therefore add depth to a TCM acupuncture practice and viewpoint (Seem 1990, p. 100). Palpation after all contacts the meridians and the Qi of the meridians.

A review of Japanese classical theory and history then shows that the origins of palpatory diagnosis and the diagnostic significance of those findings have their roots and meaning in Chinese medicine. The tendency to ignore history has contributed to the myopic view of Japanese palpation as being a system separate from Traditional Chinese Medicine and hence foreign and extraneous to an acupuncture education or practice. Yet palpation is one of the four methods of diagnosis in Oriental medicine – it is integral to its practice. As the *Nanjing* shows us, it is necessary to the education of practitioners of the human condition (Unschuld 1986, pp. 212–220).

THE FUTURE

Looking at the current state of affairs in today's healthcare models reinforces further support for the value of palpation as a diagnostic modality. A repeated source of dissatisfaction reported by patients treated by allopathic medicine is the lack of appropriate therapeutic physical contact. The somatized symptoms of patient complaint are as frequently ignored and dismissed by medical doctors as are the patient's psychological ones. For whatever reason – fear of sexually inappropriate behavior, threats of lawsuits, lack of training or, more likely, the absence of a medical paradigm in which to place and interpret those complaints – the allopathic doctor of the 21st

century does not 'touch' the patient on many levels. The longest clinical relationship with a body in medical school may indeed be the cadaver that was dissected in the first year of anatomy class.

Considering the fact that most American acupuncturists received their training from Chinese books, Chinese teachers or American teachers trained in the Chinese system, it is not surprising that the average American acupuncturist uses very little palpation as a diagnostic modality. The fact that the American healthcare model does not stress touch creates a setting in which palpation may play little to no role in one's practice.

As the American public becomes increasingly alienated from the Western healthcare system because of the lack of attentiveness to the individual, the lack of touch and the lack of individuation in the mass-oriented model, the Oriental medical practitioner stands at the threshold of public awareness and acceptance. Clinicians of whatever system of therapeutics must recognize that the needs of the public are the needs of the person. They will not be able to sustain a practice if it is modeled on the shortcomings of the allopathic system. They must look at the uniqueness of each person in order to both get results in treatment and to become the medicine of the future. As the classics remind us, the principle of medicine is the principle of humaneness (Unschuld 1979, p. 99). One of the ways of practicing humaneness is therapeutic touch. The uniqueness of the patient can be appreciated from the information gained from palpatory diagnosis.

CLINICAL UTILITY

A primary aim of this book is to explore palpatory diagnosis and to explain it within the philosophical infrastructure of Chinese medicine. With this understanding, a greater appreciation of palpation as a direct way in which bodies can describe their disharmonies can be attained by the patient and the practitioner instead of disproportionately relying upon verbal reports obtained through inquiry or the intricacies of pulse diagnosis. The simple art of palpation provides an immediate, visceral and verifiable clue, to both the patient and the practitioner, as to the subtle energetic imbalances that may be slowly forming and which later could lead to more serious bodily illness.

Palpation is an interactive process. Mark Seem, in his pivotal book *Acupuncture imaging*, reminds us that in the therapeutic process both sender and receiver are essential. Seem says:

> The practitioner who works to be attuned to the event before him, and the patient in his actual living energetic state, form an intimate union in the phenomenological bodymind energetic approach, leaving no room for an elitist stance, still present in some Oriental medical herbal approaches, where the doctor coldly palpates the radial artery, looks at the tongue, asks a few questions, then makes a diagnostic pronouncement and writes orders to be followed by the compliant patient. (Seem 1990, p. 71)

The point Seem is making is that some Oriental medical approaches do not incorporate a form of therapy that is meaningful to the patient. Tongue and pulse diagnosis in and of themselves do not evoke a bodily awareness for the patient in the way that palpation does. As a result, patients do not receive reinforcement from the diagnostic process about their health.

My personal experience with palpation has been the most satisfying aspect of my clinical experience. Before discovering this art, as much as I enjoyed clinical practice, I felt that I was largely making intellectual diagnoses about my patients. Even though these were sound diagnoses that lead to good clinical results, I believed the results could be better and that both the patient and I needed to connect on a more concrete level. I wanted to somehow impress upon them an awareness of their condition, not just treat it.

Patient education has always been an operating principle of mine because I believe that the body heals itself that and, as the *Neijing* reminds us, the superior physician is a teacher. I wanted to empower my patients, to give them the tools for their diseases' redirection, and generally it was out of the question for the patient to learn how to use needles. As acupuncturist Stephen Howard so astutely puts it, 'Every practitioner, in all traditions, has the potential to treat at every level, depending on how the practitioner and the patient choose to frame the healing work they embark on together' (Howard 1995, p. 6). My discovery of palpation met many of these criteria and offered the context within which I preferred to treat.

Simultaneously, I discovered another side of myself, one that assimilated knowledge through touch. My sensory powers were at least put on par with my analytical ones, not subjugated to them, as a Zang-Fu approach would dictate. Secondly, the patients and I enjoyed it. Even though the palpation could hurt, patients and I would laugh and communicate as I probed the points. These reactions were therapeutic in themselves. The laughs and cries and 'oohs' and 'ahs' the patients expressed dramatically put us both in contact with the degree of their bodily disharmony.

There is no doubt in my mind of the truth of the old adage that laughter is the best medicine. Clinical research by Dr Lee Beck from the Loma Linda School of Public Health has suggested that laughter lowers levels of stress hormones and strengthens the immune system. This is further supported by an article in the *Journal of the National Cancer Institute* (Ziegler 1995). And an older text, the *Neijing*, reminds us that acupuncture has to move the patient's spirit to be successful; it is not merely mechanical (Larree & Rochat de la Vallee 1990–91). Certainly palpation does that through the laughter and eye contact that are part and parcel of the palpatory process.

Invariably the patients would inquire, 'Why does it hurt so much?', 'What does this point do?' and 'Why doesn't that point hurt?'. And I would offer my explanations to establish that body–mind connection. Week by week, the patients would find that certain points became less tender and new ones occasionally surfaced, depending upon what they were experiencing. There was both an objective as well as a subjective feeling of accomplishment that acted as a verifiable index to the patients and myself that their condition was changing, if not actually improving. I always taught patients the clinical significance of the tender points and when the points got better, the patients could always correlate the improvement in the points with a positive change in their symptoms. I would teach them point locations, palpation methods, clinical energetics and organ interrelationships so that they would better understand their bodies.

Patients always left the acupuncture clinic more aware of how their problems came about and how they could try to treat them. Between visits the patients had points to work on to accelerate the healing process; thus they were involved in their own healing. When I saw them it was my job to perceive the patterns of disharmony and redirect the energy. This partnership enhanced the therapeutic relationship and the rate of recovery.

What was occurring, as Mark Seem recognizes; was that:

...the palpation/evaluation/imaging process often evokes changes in and of itself, with no needling. Palpating the affected zone while providing an energetic description of the zone leads the client into a bodymind energetic image. Such awareness, which we all carry deep inside, is a preverbal, organic and visceral, largely unconscious, right brain way of processing the world. While the client might retort that this sort of pressure would hurt anyone at those points, that the pain at the top of his foot is insignificant, and what, anyway, does it have to do with his major problem, he knows, at some deeper, older, earlier (even prenatal in some instances) level, that these zones where he is reactive are all part of a whole, connected, patterned response that forms a single unit. (Seem 1990, p. 59)

The idea of palpation releasing even prenatal feelings is very profound. It is certainly a tenet that massage therapists have long maintained – that emotional history can have a somatic organization. Therefore work on the tissues can release this stored memory. An instance that rather dramatically illustrates this point and what can ensue during palpation is described later in Case 11.3.

Palpation is a very efficient paradigm not only because it is the vehicle for diagnosis but also because it is a major part of the treatment modality. Diagnosis and treatment are accomplished simultaneously. Another reason for the speed of healing centers around the fact that treatment of the root of the illness is more likely to be addressed with meridian-style acupuncture because the Hara is a reflection of the root. This root treatment is the fundamental orientation to Japanese meridian therapy. As Fratkin so aptly extracts from his studies with Fukushima, Shudo, Manaka and Serizawa (leading meridian acupuncturists), root treatment is a whole-body treatment, based on evaluating fundamental meridian imbalances and restoring them to harmony. Root balancing allows the energetic network to return to its most efficient posture, facilitating and accelerating healing (Fratkin 1995).

Palpation is a therapeutic process that brings about a strong connection between the patient and the practitioner. It is almost unsurpassed in establishing mutual rapport and trust, stimulating the inherent vital Qi of the body and reminding it of the way it is supposed to be. Touch, eye contact and laughter are powerful ways to establish a connection with the patient's spirit, truly the essential Oriental medical treatment plan.

In summary, palpation is a simple, elegant, effective method of diagnosis and treatment, so dramatic in its results that there is a tendency for the observer or the uninitiated to misunderstand it. If it appears simplistic it is only because the system has been refined through practice on thousands of patients by the ancients and because of a confidence in its clinical efficacy on the part of the practitioner. It is the ultimate enigma; an enjoyable and challenging way to cluster the unique energetic configurations of each person and systematically apply a way of thinking to the responses it elicits. It is classically inspired and time-tested medicine, where the root cause of a disease is treated and prevention and health maintenance is practiced by the clinician and the patient. It is the magic hand.

NEW WORDS AND CONCEPTS

Meridian acupuncture – classical acupuncture based upon the Five Elements in which the complex interaction of all the meridians, both main and secondary, and their patterns of disharmony are stressed as a basis of constructing treatment plans. Palpation utilizes the Qi of the Channels and Collaterals.

The 'four methods' – the four traditional Chinese methods of diagnosis used to gather information about the patient. They are inspection, auscultation, olfaction (the character for auscultation and olfaction is the same, hence four versus five methods of diagnosis), palpation and inquiry.

Therapeutic touch – a method of healing in which practitioners attempt to influence the patient's bioelectrical field by using their intent to heal in order to direct the life energy to flow through the patient.

Zang-Fu diagnosis – a diagnostic approach central to the core of Traditional Chinese Medicine which emphasizes the organs and their interrelationships.

QUESTIONS

1. Why isn't Japanese-style acupuncture really a separate system of acupuncture unrelated to Chinese medicine?

2. How do you think palpation would establish patients' awareness of their body–mind connection to aid in healing?

3. What factors may have caused palpation to play a less significant part in modern Chinese medical treatment and diagnosis?

4. In Japan medical practitioners were often blind persons (up to 25% are so today). From this, we can infer a lot about the importance of our sensory powers. As a practitioner, compare the current use of your sensory abilities with your intellectual skills in diagnosing and treating patients. Which do you rely on more and why?

2

Traditional Chinese medicine and Japanese acupuncture: similarities and differences

As we have seen in Chapter 1, in meridian-style acupuncture, the information derived from palpation is the primary basis for determining the treatment strategy. It is considered to be the most important method of diagnosis (Denmei 1990, p. 36). A detailed examination of the patient by touch is what enables Japanese practitioners to determine the appropriate treatment for each patient. Alphen points out that, 'Uniquely Japanese is the practice of measuring abdominal palpation in addition to regular pulse palpation when evaluating the patient's physical and psychic condition according to the four methods' (Alphen & Aris 1995, p. 233).

In my understanding of both Chinese and Japanese medical systems, Japanese acupuncture is a development of Chinese meridian-style acupuncture. By this, I mean that Japanese acupuncture represents a development in classical Chinese medicine because it has its roots in the ancient Chinese texts. Japanese acupuncture has continued to elaborate and refine these ancient ideas, specifically palpation, over the centuries. Although palpation may be the least sophisticated means of examination according to the classics, it is nevertheless the most crucial stage of diagnosis in meridian therapy. The findings from all other phases of examination are used primarily to confirm what is felt at our fingertip (Denmei 1990, pp. 36, 44–45).

Like all diagnostic frameworks, Japanese acupuncture, with its emphasis on meridian energetics, emphasizes the perception of the body as energy organized in a particular way. It is a very simple model that puts more importance on the big pictures of Qi, Blood, Yin and Yang, instead of on the details of organ dysfunction. It is my experience that any disorder can be treated through this approach.

A fundamental premise of the great bodywork therapist Ida Rolf, founder of the Rolfing technique, was that the body could be reshaped through the skillful use of touch just as it can be reshaped, albeit negatively, through injury or habitual misuse. Palpation is a tool that can both diagnose and reshape the energetic and physical manifestations of the Zang-Fu organs and the vital Qi that they regulate. This reality is consonant with the Oriental viewpoint, as expressed through the Law of the Unity of Opposites (Yin/Yang theory), that has always asserted the inseparable relationship between energy and matter. Seem also agrees with this when he states, 'The palpation/evaluation/imaging process often provokes changes in and of itself with no needling' (Seem 1989b p. 67). Touch studies and clinical practice confirm this.

Matsumoto shows that palpation is useful both diagnostically and therapeutically. She writes:

Scientifically it produces profound changes in the body. Because connective tissues have piezoelectric properties, the application of pressure anywhere in the body will generate small electric currents. These currents will have numerous physiological effects, just as they do in acupuncture. This is aside from the effects of mechanical stimulation of muscular tissues, blood vessels, and nervous tissues that are known to have beneficial effects on stress and blood circulation.

Pressure applied to living tissue can actually transform the tissues. Work done on organic gels, part of the cytoplasm of cells, shows that pressure will cause the gel to become a sol (solution). Thus particle accumulations trapped in the gel state may become released at the same time that the gel is hydrated. Hydration makes the gel more energetically conductive.

These effects will also show to some degree in the process of diagnosis by palpation. The diagnosis itself can often have therapeutic value and is often relaxing to the patient. It will also, to some degree, prepare the tissues that are treated, making them in their temporary sol state, more energetically active. This can only enhance the effects of acupuncture and moxibustion. This in part may explain why the classical texts discuss the application of pressure to a point before needling. (Matsumoto & Birch 1988)

As mentioned in Chapter 1, as far as we can tell, the Chinese never cultivated the art of bodily palpation to the extent that they did other methods of diagnosis. While various Japanese schools of thought did engage in its cultivation, and history is obscure in assigning a definitive claim to this development, what is known is that both the Japanese acupuncturists and herbalists used it as a fundamental theoretical orientation in the 17th century and that the basis of their paradigm was the *Nanjing, The classic of difficult questions* or the *Five Element classic*, one of the two fundamental Chinese classics. Since that time, numerous practitioners, including myself, have produced abdominal maps and differential diagnosis findings based upon the classics and verified by clinical experience. Thus we can see that classical and contemporary Japanese acupuncture has a firm historical basis in the Chinese classics even though the Chinese did not continue to develop this recognized method of diagnosis.

As modern-day practitioners, especially in America but also worldwide, we have the opportunity to reunite the Chinese and Japanese systems with their classical roots, thus building on the proven value of the classical material with clinical advances that have arisen from over four centuries of use by the Japanese. This is because Chinese medicine, which is already firmly established in America and other countries, is experiencing the new trend in Japanese therapeutics due to the introduction of Japanese practitioners, books and study groups in the US and abroad. Classical Chinese medicine is coming to the fore again, being rediscovered. But this is also happening against the backdrop of each particular culture's view of medicine. It is that uniqueness that will ultimately create a world medicine based upon proven theory.

Apart from the differences between the primary methods of diagnosis and treatment modalities employed by Chinese and Japanese practitioners, there are other differences as well. Some of the tools for restoring balance to the patient are different for the Chinese and Japanese practitioner. Table 2.1 summarizes these treatment differences for quick comparison and clini-

Table 2.1   Chinese and Japanese treatment style differences

Tool	Chinese	Japanese
Size of needles	Large gauge (e.g. #28, 30)	Small gauge (#36)
Number of needles	Generally many	As few as possible
Depth of insertions	Deep to meridian level	Superficial, only contacting tendinomuscular meridians or Minute and Blood Luos
Da qi sensation	Strong	None to little
Methods of tonification and dispersion	Many methods	Basically achieved through angle of insertion. Dispersion achieved through palpation. Tonification reinforced with needles
Types of patient	Normal and strong constitutional types or Excess conditions	Normal and delicate, needle-sensitive patients
Moxa use	Contraindicated in Hot conditions	Not contraindicated in Hot conditions, only true Excess conditions
Moxa size	Large size	Rice size or with Tiger Thermie warmer
Concept of points	Small, discrete areas	Large areas
Theories and treatment plans	Classical diagnostic frameworks, for example, Zang-Fu, Six Divisions, etc. Treatment plan emphasizes treating the branch and the root most of the time unless condition is acute	Broad general diagnosis, westernized names or none at all. Treatment plan emphasizes treating the root

cal usage. Let us compare and contrast some of the more salient features.

NEEDLES

While the Chinese in modern China tend to use many large-gauge needles, insert them deeply to the standard text depths and look for a strong sensation of 'Da qi' (or Qi arrival), the Japanese have invented superfine needles. Japanese needle technique tends to be extremely shallow and no sensation of Qi arrival is typically elicited. The Qi is not always sought at the meridian level as the Chinese do, but usually superficially in the region of the Minute, Blood and Luo meridians. There is even a style of Japanese acupuncture called contact needling where needles are not even inserted into the skin but simply placed directly above the skin.

In Japanese acupuncture tonification and dispersion with needles are fundamentally accomplished by angling the needle with or against the flow of the meridian, instead of the relatively more vigorous needle manipulation which characterizes the Chinese technique. The Chinese, however, sometimes use this technique as well.

The Japanese style is an ideal method of treatment for young people, elderly patients, those with weakened conditions such as Essence Deficiency diseases or for those who fear needles. In contrast, a more vigorous needling style is perhaps better suited for strong constitutional types, Excess conditions or Wei syndromes. These two different styles of needle technique are depicted in Figure 2.1.

MOXA

Moxa use is widespread in both traditions; the basic difference is the method and amount of application. The Chinese tend to use moxa in large quantities because of its undeniable, unsurpassed effects in regulating the Qi and Blood. The Japanese favor moxa as well but in smaller quantities such as rice grain size pieces.

Acupuncturist Shudo Denmei suggests that the use of moxa became contraindicated in Chinese practice for 'Hot' conditions because in herbal medicine Hot herbs were contraindicated for these conditions. This faulty equation then carried over into the contraindication of moxa for Hot conditions. The Japanese did not make this

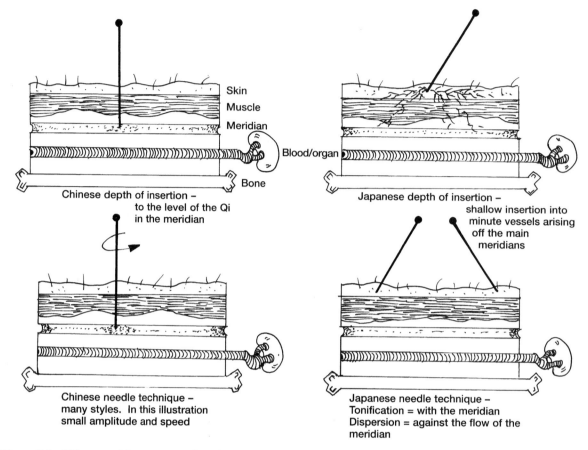

Chinese depth of insertion –
to the level of the Qi
in the meridian

Japanese depth of insertion –
shallow insertion into
minute vessels arising
off the main
meridians

Chinese needle technique –
many styles. In this illustration
small amplitude and speed

Japanese needle technique –
Tonification = with the meridian
Dispersion = against the flow of the
meridian

Figure 2.1 Chinese and Japanese needle techniques.

analogy, hence much of their moxa use has a broader range of applicability even on points such as 'Water' points or for conditions that normally would not be heated. It is only if the person's entire energetic configuration is characterized as an Excess Heat condition that moxa would not be used.

The Japanese sometimes administer the moxa in tools called the Tiger Thermie warmer and the Lion Thermie warmer (Fig. 2.2). The tremendous advantage of these implements is that they allow the therapeutic properties of the moxa's mild heat to penetrate to the meridian level but simultaneously mechanical pressure can be applied to the patient. This mechanical pressure is useful in breaking up blockages as well as bringing energy to an affected area. Also, the heat is soothing and

mild and not as noxious as large amounts of moxa smoke may be.

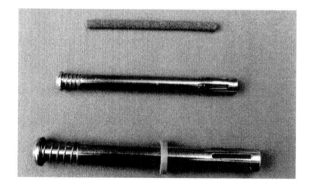

Figure 2.2 The Tiger Thermie and Lion Thermie moxa warmers.

POINTS

The Japanese concept of an acupuncture point tends to be bigger than the current Chinese definitions. This development largely arose from the need to teach thousands of Chinese physicians point location in a standardized manner. Teaching large numbers did not facilitate learning point location from an experiential perspective, as was the traditional method.

In the Japanese system, points are frequently referred to as 'areas'. Because of their larger size, the areas lend themselves well to palpation.

DIAGNOSIS

Finally there is some difference between the diagnostic frameworks used in the two traditions. The Chinese will tend to name a patient's condition based upon one of many diagnostic frameworks such as Liver Qi Stagnation (Zang-Fu) or Wood overacting on Earth (Five Elements). The Japanese tend to name problems either in very broad general terms, such as Qi or Blood Deficiency, in Western terms (such as neurovascular compression) or not at all. In the latter case, treatment is contingent upon the 'pattern' of presentation; that is, not solely an intellectual diagnosis but a picture of what the root pathologies, the most fundamental underlying imbalances relayed by palpation, are. It is a whole-body pattern that summarizes the core energy of the person and is not confined to organ syndromes. It is determined by palpating the Hara, rather than through a less somatic modality.

Both the specificity of the westernization of the disease and the vagueness of the patterns of presentation can be a source of confusion to the practitioner of Chinese medicine who may like to categorize all the signs and symptoms into a neat syndrome. However, the ability to see both of these as an added dimension to the understanding of the patient may ultimately prove more beneficial.

Naming a disorder is not as important as knowing how to treat it and within any system of therapeutics, treatment is the bottom line. Try to integrate your Chinese understandings into the broader Japanese picture. In this book, whenever possible, I will attempt to explain what is going on from my combined training and perspectives in Chinese and Japanese acupuncture so that readers can build upon their education and practice instead of disregarding it.

In looking at these differences, which appear to be directly antithetical to each other, it is interesting to note that each works. Some are better for certain conditions and certain patients and these will be discussed in subsequent chapters. Other treatment styles that are divergent in both systems will be covered as they come up in particular chapters.

NEW WORDS AND CONCEPTS

Essence Deficiency syndromes – illnesses due to Jing Deficiency which are essentially characterized by early aging or an autoimmune response; that is, the body degenerating by turning on itself.

Minute and Blood Luos – numerous small pathways, similar to capillaries, which provide passage for Qi and Blood from the main meridians that go to every part of the body.

Tiger Thermie and Lion Thermie warmers – metal moxa instruments. The Lion Thermie warmer is larger than the Tiger Thermie warmer. See Appendix 4 for suppliers. Their use will be described in later chapters.

Wei syndromes – a constellation of symptoms that involve paralysis, such as stroke sequelae and polio.

QUESTIONS

1. For each of the tools listed in Table 2.1, think of some clinical examples of when it would be advantageous for you as a practitioner to have knowledge of both treatment styles.

2. What are the major differences between Chinese and Japanese diagnostic techniques and patterns (frameworks)?

3. Discuss/support the view of Japanese acupuncture as the classical practice of Chinese medicine.

4. Using the Chinese theory of meridians, explain how a superficial needling technique can contact Qi.

3

Why use abdominal diagnosis?

Why is the abdomen such an important and comprehensive site for diagnosis? Looking back at the fundamental theories of Yin and Yang, we know that the front of the body is Yin. Because of its Yin nature, the abdomen allows itself to be more readily evaluated, more so than the back of the body, because it is relatively soft and unprotected. It houses the internal organs and it is through this surface that they are easily palpated and percussed. The abdomen, or the Hara as the Japanese call it, is the cavity where the living Qi of the Zang-Fu organs, the life force, resides. It is requisite and sacred to palpate it.

The Front Mu points of the Zang-Fu organs are located on the front of the body in the abdominal and thoracic regions. Front Mu points, also referred to as Alarm points or Front Collecting points, are diagnostic of the fundamental, basic energy of the body, that is, the Yin and Yang. They are particularly reactive to pathological changes in the body. When their corresponding Zang-Fu organs are diseased, the state of the Yin and Yang of the organs can be determined by palpating the Front Mu points.*

As far as traditional categories of points that have been palpated are concerned, the Front Mu points represent a major division, along with Back Shu points, Yuan (source) points, Xi (cleft) points, clinically effective points and, of course,

---

* Remember that the purest concept of the Zang-Fu organs pertains not only to the organ but its meridian network of internal and external pathways and all the Five Element correspondences.

any area that is part of the patient's major complaint.[†] Palpation – the feeling of a point or an area to detect disease – is a viable method of diagnosis that fills several important functions in the diagnostic and treatment process. Its benefits are outlined below and summarized in Box 3.1.

Palpation is obviously a physical method of diagnosis. As such, it is an objective, dependable and more easily learned diagnostic modality than intellectual systems such as the pulse that may take years to feel properly. It is a direct way of determining the condition of the Zang-Fu organs without relying upon patients' verbal perception of their major complaint. Instead, practitioners rely upon what they feel when palpating and the patient's experience of that palpation. In

this way, patients are given the opportunity to comment on their experience of their body.

Interestingly, in another sense, palpation has the unique ability to address what we could call the even more energetic, formless energies of Yin, Yang, Qi and Blood and the Zang-Fu organs – the roots of disease – even before there are any symptoms. Because palpation touches the tissues, it can release muscular rigidity. In doing so, the surface (or Wei or muscular level) is freed up so that the energy of the organ or meridian complex can be reached. This is what could be called the preclinical, preprodromal or energetic signs that appear before there are any physical complaints. As a result of the ability to perceive 'dis-ease' on this level, the clinician has the capacity to clarify the root of illness. This assists in directing treatment. Preventive medicine is thus made possible. This concept is developed further in Chapter 8.

Because of this ability to pick up the early signs of illness, palpation is excellent for what could be termed difficult-to-diagnose conditions. Such conditions include mixed Excess/Deficiency syndromes, where the symptoms are often confusing due to the dual nature of the condition.

CATEGORIES OF ILLNESS

Abdominal palpation is good for diagnosing all types of illness. It is especially clinically effective for three troublesome categories of illness that are not only complicated to treat but are also on the increase throughout the world: Essence Deficiency illnesses, Fire syndromes and Blood Stasis diseases.

Essence Deficiency illnesses are those disorders associated with Essence or Jing deficiency. They can be treated with unprecedented effectiveness when palpation is used because palpation can reach the root or the core, i.e. the Jing level. These illnesses include premature menopause, chronic progressive degenerative diseases like multiple sclerosis, AIDS, Epstein–Barr virus and fibromyalgia. Additionally, illnesses caused by removal of organs or organs damaged by radiation, diseases due to long-term stress, viruses, toxic chemicals or chronic bacterial infection, dietary imbalances and emotional disturbances can also be treated.

> **Box 3.1 The benefits of abdominal diagnosis**
>
> 1. In a sense, more physical, palpable, visible, subject to 'the four methods of diagnosis' than a more intellectual energetic system such as the pulse that takes years to cultivate.
> 2. In a sense, more energetic, accessing the formless energy, the roots of disease, even if there are no symptoms. It is prodromal, preceding physical complaints, therefore making root treatment possible.
> 3. Good for difficult-to-diagnose conditions (mixed Excess/Deficiency syndromes) where symptoms may be confusing.
> 4. Useful for all conditions and clinically effective for such difficult diseases as:
>   ‣ Essence Deficiency syndromes
>   ‣ Fire syndromes
>   ‣ Blood Stasis illnesses.
> 5. Patients like it, both those who are deficient and don't like needles and those who are robust and like touch.
> 6. Provides a dramatic and clear indicator of the treatment accomplished to both the patient and the practitioner. Puts patients in contact with their body and their health. Patients can learn it and do it daily, thereby restoring health maintenance to the individual. It returns to the spirit of Chinese medicine; that is, prevention.
> 7. It clears excesses and simultaneously supports the root.

[†] As a reminder, differentially Back Shu points are diagnostic of the condition of the Qi and Blood. Yuan (source) points detect the condition of the Yuan Qi, Xi (cleft) points are for accumulations and blockage and clinically effective points for certain organ–meridian pathology.

The reason why these three categories of illness can be treated through palpation is because the Master and Coupled points of the Eight Extraordinary Meridians are the foundation of the palpation schema and treatment plan. As we know, their use is closely connected with Jing problems.

As Seem says, 'The complex dynamics of the regular meridians, secondary vessels and 8 extraordinary channels are crucial to erecting an appropriate treatment plan' (Seem 1989a). Dr Tran Viet Dzung states, 'The Curious Meridians are supraphysiologic channels, and they play a very important part in reinforcing the Yin-Yang system of the Principal Channels' (Dzung 1989). Furthermore, Giovanni Maciocia, quoting from *The study of the Eight Extraordinary Vessels*, by Li Shi Zhen, writes, 'If the doctor understands the extraordinary vessels he or she can master the 12 channels and the 15 Connecting vessels. If the Daoist sage understands the extraordinary vessels he or she can practice Qi Gong, the windows of the Spirit are open and the way of the Dao is open' (Maciocia 1993). And finally Nguyen Van Nghi asserts that an acupuncturist's education is severely deficient if he does not have an understanding of the energetics and trajectories of the Eight Curious Vessels. Herbalists, on the other hand, do not need to know this information (Van Nghi 1987). For a more comprehensive explanation on the use of the Curious Vessels, see Chapter 9.

Related illnesses called immunodeficiency diseases can also be addressed through palpation. Immunodeficiency disorders can be inherited, acquired through infection or produced unintentionally by drugs such as those used to treat cancer or transplant patients.

Diseases that fall into the category of Fire syndromes are also well treated through the palpatory process. These illnesses include chronic inflammatory diseases such as joint pain, colitis, sore throat, night sweats, hot flashes, pent-up anger and burning sensations. In short, any inflammation is well treated through this modality. Inflammatory diseases are designated by a disease name ending in 'itis'.

Finally, Blood Stasis diseases, diseases characterized by sharp pains, injuries, surgeries, trauma, chronic inflammation and abdominal congestion and other signs and symptoms of Blood Stasis are efficaciously addressed through the system of palpation.

BENEFITS FOR PATIENTS

An important property of palpation is that patients like it. In particular, patients who are Deficient tend to like the touch as well as the attention paid to their bodily condition. Those who don't like needles, or those whose conditions don't lend themselves to many needles such as children, the elderly or weakened patients suffering from Deficiency illnesses, enjoy this form of treatment which, though certainly felt, is still non-invasive. Even robust patients and those in good health seem to enjoy the bodily awareness that comes from palpation.

In my experience, this technique is not suitable for patients whose conditions could be called excessive in general or Excess from an Eight Principle perspective. I believe that very few patients fall into this category, perhaps 5% of the population. Excessive patients exhibit excessive symptoms such as full heat, thirst, red face, a strong forceful pulse, a red tongue with a thick yellow coat. There is usually an emotional component as a manifestation of this excessiveness which is generally anger. The patient may have high Blood pressure of the Excess type, drink alcohol and be under stress. Concomitantly these patients' Qi creates a bodily armor that tends to be unresponsive to palpation. They seem to dislike touch and needles. They are better treated with herbs or deep bodywork although lifestyle factors are usually at the root and need to be addressed. As we all know, such behaviors are difficult to change. Subsequent chapters discuss such patients further as well as how to work with them.

Another benefit for patients with the palpatory system is that it provides a dramatic and clear indicator of what the treatment has accomplished to both the patient and the practitioner. The areas being palpated are prodded, physically but also verbally and humorously; that is, the patient is touched as a whole. Patients are put in contact with their bodies in an even deeper way than with just the needles. The practitioner should point out to patients through supportive language what the palpatory findings suggest so as to educate them about their health. Patients can then learn many of the treatment techniques that are accomplished through palpation. The practitioner thereby puts health maintenance into the hands of the individual and the preventive spirit of Chinese medicine is thus brought back to preeminence.

In terms of a treatment strategy, palpation performs the dual function of clearing Excess and then tonifying any underlying Deficiency. As Shudo Denmei believes and Mark Seem supports:

> ...yang tends towards excess and Yin towards deficiency. Yang excess usually corresponds with Yang excess symptoms while Yin deficiency does not. Dispersing the Yang excess therefore, always requires careful attention to signs of local excess and relieving associated symptoms through the activation of this excess. In such a case, tender, painful, tight points will be deactivated thereby freeing up the blockage and promoting smooth flow of Qi through the area. The dispersal of excess not only relieves local symptoms but also restores normal circulation thereby supporting Yin (internal circulation and function). (Seem 1992)

That is, clearing the surface supports the root. Palpation is the tool to disperse the Excess and support the root.

As I established in the Preface, there are no exact answers on how to perform palpation, only a thinking process which inspires it. Hopefully this will become evident as you continue with this book.

NEW WORDS AND CONCEPTS

Blood Stasis illnesses – illnesses due to Blood Stagnation exhibiting the characteristic manifestations of Blood Stagnation in Chinese medicine.

Chronic inflammatory diseases – illnesses of long duration with the characteristic signs of inflammation.

Chronic progressive degenerative diseases – long-term diseases in which the body loses its integrity and is breaking down.

Fire syndromes – illnesses characterized by Heat of the Excess or Deficient variety. They generally have inflammation and its characteristic symptoms of pain, redness, fever and swelling as part of their presentation.

Hara – the abdomen which houses the internal organs.

Palpation – the process of examining the surface of the body by touch to detect the presence of disease and to observe the patient's reaction to pressure. It is also a method of treatment.

QUESTIONS

1. Certain categories of points traditionally palpated in Chinese medicine are diagnostic of particular conditions. Do you know the difference? We will see that all these points represent the main points that are palpated in the Japanese system.

Front Mu points	Indicate the condition of the Yin and Yang of the organs
Back Shu points	Diagnostic of the Qi and the Blood of the associated organ
Xi (cleft) points	Points of accumulation or blockage in the organ–meridian complex
Yuan (source) points	Contain the original Qi of the organs
Clinically effective points	Points either on one of the 14 meridians or in the extra point system that have known clinical efficacy in the treatment of certain illness

2. How is abdominal palpation preventive and what is the mechanism by which it treats and supports the root?

3. What three troublesome categories of illnesses is abdominal palpation especially good for?

4. What are the functions of palpation in the diagnostic process? Compare abdominal palpation to pulse palpation, to the other 'four methods', plus

any other diagnostic styles in terms of their ability to access the 'formless energy' of the body.

5. List three Fire syndromes that can be treated with abdominal clearing.

6. Name three Essence Deficiency syndromes that can be treated with abdominal palpation.

7. Name three Blood Stasis diseases that can be treated with abdominal palpation.

4

Abdominal maps in history

Many cultures throughout the ages have attempted to understand what they could not see in the human body. In ancient times, many cultures drew maps depicting where they believed the internal organs resided. Without the benefit of magnetic resonance imaging or CAT scans, they not only succeeded in producing many colorful and illustrative ones but also in many cases more accurate energetic ones than those that heat sensing and modern-day dyes reveal (Denmei 1990, p. 90, Matsumoto & Birch 1988, p. 342, Alphen & Aris 1995, pp. 18, 31, 44, 121).

CLASSICAL ABDOMINAL MAPS

The first abdominal maps that are relevant to this book come from the *Nanjing*. In analyzing them, an internal consistency can be noted between the correspondences of the Elements such as the directions, the seasons and the organs on the abdomen, as Five Element theory maintains. While these abdominal maps may at first glance appear rudimentary and simple, they have been tested by time. There is a profound amount of information within the apparent simplicity of these maps that will serve practitioners well if they pay attention to the palpatory as well as observational findings as interpreted through these correspondences. This information is discussed below and illustrated in Figures 4.1–4.5.

The Elements

According to the *Nanjing*, each of the Five Elements is represented on the abdomen. All the

23

associations pertaining to the Five Elements are pertinent to the abdomen. For instance, relatively speaking, pathology found in the Wood area of the abdomen is less significant than that found in the Metal area because Wood energy is more 'sproutlike' than 'metal-ish'. The key words here are 'relatively speaking'. Likewise, the healthy Wood area should feel more resilient than the Metal area and the Metal area should feel firmer, because of their elemental nature.

For instance, tightness in the Wood area is less significant than tightness in the Metal area because the nature of Wood is more adaptable than Metal. The relevant clinical diagnoses pertaining to these findings are discussed later in this book, specifically in Chapter 8.

The Elements on the abdomen are depicted in Figure 4.1. Various emotions may be stored in the abdomen at the corresponding elemental site; for instance, grief may be lodged in the Metal area.

The directions

Figure 4.2 superimposes the cardinal directions on the abdomen. The directions are obviously a subset of the Five Element correspondences. This drawing illustrates that the area above the navel pertains to Yang, that is, the South. The Fire element is found above this area and correspondingly, the organs of the Heart and the Pericardium. Below the navel are Yin, the North, the Water element and the organs of the Bladder and principally the Kidney. To the right of the navel (the patient's right) is the West, corresponding to the Metal element and to the organs of the Lung and the Large Intestine. The left side of the navel (patient's left) is the East which is the spring and the organs of the Liver and the Gall Bladder. Finally, the center, the navel itself, is the Earth element, with its corresponding organ of the Spleen.

An interesting interpretation of clinical findings on the abdomen centers on the directions. Remember that the right side is Yin and the left side is Yang; below is Yin and above is Yang. While Yin and Yang are always relative depending upon the issue under consideration, in the case of abdominal findings pathology found on

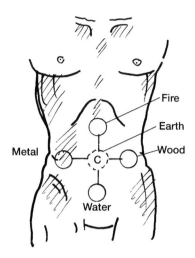

Figure 4.1 The Elements on the abdomen.

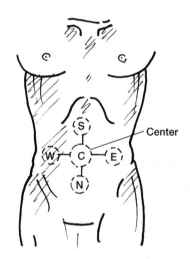

Figure 4.2 The directions on the abdomen.

the right (West) and below (North) will be more significant and generally more serious than that found on the left or in other areas because Yin is more deep and structive than Yang.

The organs

Classical literature made correspondences between areas of the abdomen and the organs based upon the proximity of these organs to the surface and their energetic functions. Hence, in terms of anatomical proximity and energetic function, the lateral costal region pertains to the Liver and Gall Bladder, the umbilical region to the Spleen, Stomach and Intestines, and the lower abdomen to the Lung, Liver, Bladder and Kidney.* Consequently, correlations can be made between the symptoms presented in these areas and the palpatory findings.

Some organ physiology can be diagnosed by consulting the organ map presented here. However, remember that in Chinese medicine the concept of an organ is not just the literal discrete material physical organ but rather encompasses the entire constellation of energetics, functions, associations and internal pathways that are subsumed under the Chinese definition of Zang-Fu organ. To stress this, when talking about organs in the Chinese sense, I will usually refer to the organ as an organ–meridian complex.

Due to Five Element associations, it is very interesting to see that for palpation purposes, the condition of the Lung is initially assessed to the right of the navel, that of the Liver to the left of the navel, of the Heart in the epigastric region, of the Kidney below the umbilicus, and of the Spleen just around the immediate area of the umbilicus. This is not to say that other significant data cannot be obtained from various palpatory techniques performed in close proximity to the anatomical organ. However, the energetic site is the first region we look to in the palpatory exam. The energetic model of organ pathology is in Figure 4.3.

In the Five Element system as it pertains to the abdominal map, as well as in many other diagnostic paradigms, the Yin organs are stressed over the Yang organs. While the Yang organs per se are not drawn on the abdomen, the Five Element diagnostic paradigm has always implied that each set of Five Element organs is an integrated system that cannot be separated, a couple bound for life. The Yang organs are just that; that is, they are the Yang functional counterpart to the Yin organs. The Yin organs represent a deeper energetic level. This is not to say that there are no Fu

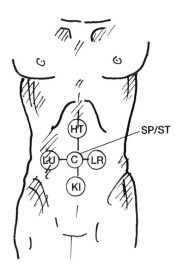

Figure 4.3 The organ map.

organ pathologies; there will be ways to account for any Yang disharmonies but their pathologies generally involve their Yin counterparts.

Note that by using this microsystem of the abdomen upon which to focus the diagnosis, the vitality of the organs can be ascertained. Later more areas and points will be palpated to offer more specific clinical data about various aspects of the organs.

Just like tongue diagnosis maps or various pulse systems which are also guides of where to read the energy of an organ–meridian complex, so too palpation maps can furnish the practitioner with a very accurate index of the condition of the undifferentiated living Qi of the body.

The seasons

The seasonal use of the abdominal map is quite illustrative in explaining etiology, pathophysiology and prognosis. Other parameters will undoubtedly enter into this assessment but there is a tremendous richness to this simple seasonal map whose use might not seem relevant or obvious at first glance.

In the unending cycle of Five Phase dynamics Water is the first element, the source of all energy, the root of Qi and the root of life as well as the source to which it all returns. It pertains to the

---

* The reason why the Lung is detected in the lower abdomen is discussed in later chapters.

season of winter. Certain palpatory findings garnered in this area will point to the early, formless, preclinical, preprodromal signs of an illness, the roots of an illness before it has developed. However, it is also the final stage of a disease. Wood, the second element, pertains to spring. The 'spring' of a disorder represents the early stages of illness. It may be an acute, temporary disharmony or an illness that is developing. Fire corresponds to summer. The 'summer' of a disorder, followed by its 'late summer' (Earth), 'fall' (Metal) and finally the 'winter' (Water) again are correlated with manifestations that are the possible scenarios for the evolution of an illness, with each in turn becoming more problematic.

In each stage the disease is becoming more chronic, more concretized, generally more physical and more serious. Spring disorders may occur in the spring as well as have Wind associated with them, such as with conjunctivitis or allergies. Summer disorders include gastrointestinal illness and redness, heat, fever, inflammation and skin problems. Late summer diseases tend to have Fullness and Damp as clinical manifestations, as in the case of arthritis. Fall disorders, like the common cold and other respiratory problems, generally have Lung and energy symptoms connected with them. Winter disorders signify a more chronic or advanced disorder or even the terminal stages of pathology or its early roots, as was discussed previously.

The significance of the seasonal analogies to a disease will depend upon the discrete pathology that is discerned. The use of the seasonal map of the abdomen is akin to the seasonal use of Five Element points to treat various diseases (see Table 4.1 on the seasonal use of acupuncture points and Figure 4.4 on the seasons and the abdominal map).

In summary, these abdominal maps are clinically useful in the diagnosis of the fundamental energy of the patient. All these areas are palpated and, contingent upon the area of the abdomen, certain findings are expected because of the Elements, organs, directions and seasons that are represented in that area. This information is collated in Figure 4.5. Their interpretation is outlined in Chapter 6 on the components, characteristics and clinical significance of the healthy Hara and in Chapter 8 on the clinical significance and differential diagnosis of the abdominal diagnosis points.

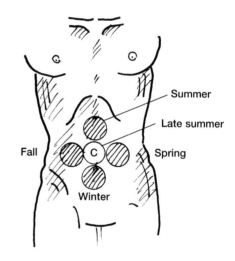

Figure 4.4 The seasons and the abdominal map.

Table 4.1 The seasonal use of acupuncture points

Shu point	Jing (well)	Ying (spring)	Shu (stream)	Jing (river)	He (sea)
Seasonal usage	The season of spring as well as the *spring* of a disease	Summer or the *summer* of a disease	Late summer or the *late summer* of a disease	Fall or the *fall* of a disease	Winter or the *winter* of a disease
Clinical manifestations	Mental disorders, chest disorders, coma, unconsciousness, stifling sensation in chest, acute problems, apparent fullness, first aid	Fevers, febrile diseases	Painful joints caused by pathogenic Heat and Damp	Asthma, throat and cough disorders, alternating chills and fever	Disorders of the Fu organs, bleeding stomach, diarrhea. (Tends not to affect the meridian at this level)

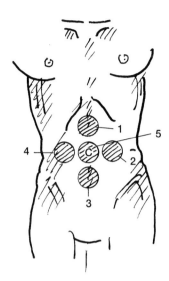

1 = Fire–South–Heart–Summer
2 = Wood–East–Liver–Spring
3 = Water–North–Kidney–Winter
4 = Metal–West–Lung–Fall
5 = Earth–Center–Spleen–Late Summer

Figure 4.5   The integrated map of the Elements, directions, organs and seasons.

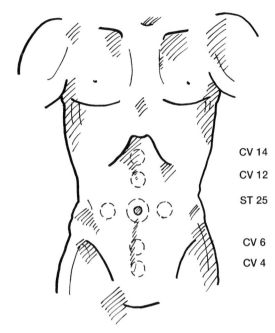

Figure 4.6   The modified abdominal map.

Other abdominal maps can be found by consulting the references cited earlier and readers are encouraged to do so to add to their appreciation of the medicine. For the purposes of explaining the material presented in this book, the integrated map which provides a synthesis of the others summarizes the clinical information that will be most valuable to the practitioner. From each separate map we can glean a sense of the basic configurational and elemental structive energies involved (Fig. 4.1), relevant organs (Fig. 4.3) and prognosis (Figs 4.2 and 4.4).

MODIFIED ABDOMINAL MAP

The first abdominal examination that is conducted is what I call the healthy Hara examination. This examination offers the big picture of the vitality or Qi of the person. Just like tongue diagnosis, it is somewhat general but keep in mind that just like tongue diagnosis, it is not used exclusively as a method of diagnosis. Other examinations will follow and methods of diagno-

sis incorporated that will provide more data for the diagnostic equation. This is really the big picture, however, which outlines the roots of the disease.

The second physical examination makes use of a map I have termed the modified abdominal map, which was developed after I had used other more complicated ones (Fig. 4.6). It involves checking six discrete points for pathology. An analysis of the six points of the modified map shows that it is ideal both in terms of the amount of time the treatment should last and the initial palpation that the patient can sustain. More importantly, it captures the essential characteristics of each of the organs such that a firm yet expedient diagnosis can be made. How to use the modified abdominal map is described in Chapters 6 and 8.

NEW WORDS AND CONCEPTS

Healthy Hara examination – the first palpatory examination in which the fundamental entities of Yin, Yang, Qi and Blood, Excess and Deficiency are determined.

Modified abdominal map – a modern modification of classical abdominal maps in which further diagnoses of Yin, Yang, Qi and Blood are assessed as they pertain to organs.

Organ–meridian complex – the classical Chinese notion of the Zang-Fu organs; that is, the organ in all its physical and energetic manifestations.

QUESTIONS

1. Explain why it is that the various organ maps from the classics don't correspond to the precise Western anatomical organ location.

2. Pick an illness, the common cold for example, and outline the possible seasonal progression it could take.

3. Name the directions that according to the *Five Element classic* correspond to each of the areas depicted in Figure 4.7.

A =

B =

C =

D =

E =

4. Name the organs that according to the *Nanjing* correspond to each of the areas in Figure 4.8.

A =

B =

C =

D =

E =

F =

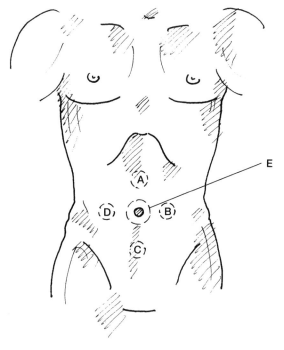

Figure 4.7

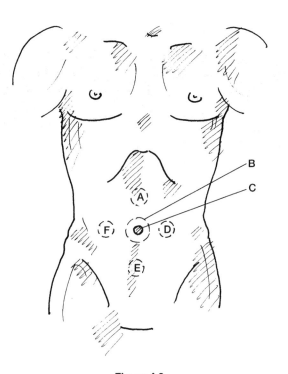

Figure 4.8

5. Name the elements that according to the *Classic of difficult questions* correspond to each of the areas in Figure 4.9.

A =

B =

C =

D =

E =

6. Name the seasons that correspond to each of the areas in Figure 4.10.

A =

B =

C =

D =

E =

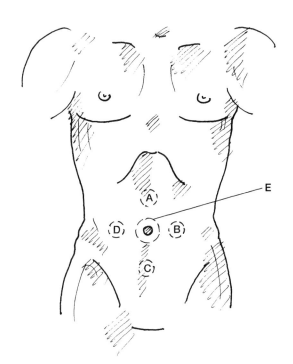

Figure 4.9

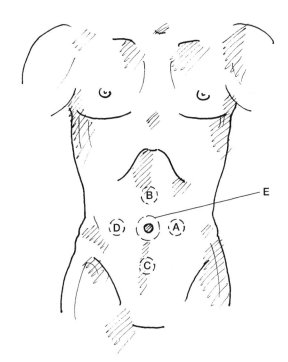

Figure 4.10

5

Theoretical clarifications

Before specifically outlining how to perform the various palpatory examinations, some important theoretical discussions must be covered since the interpretations of many of the palpatory findings are based within this theory. They are inter-related topics, somewhat complex but helpful to take fullest advantage of the palpatory process. These topics are so energetic that I am sure I only possess a glimpse of their meanings. The practitioner is urged to read as many books and articles on them as possible for, by doing so, one's appreciation of these subjects does indeed deepen.

In order to understand the most complex of these theories, the Triple Warmer, we need to start with the building blocks leading up to it, the topics of Mingmen and immunity.

WHAT IS MINGMEN?

As we will see in Chapter 6, in the first palpatory examination, the condition of Mingmen is evaluated. It is assessed by feeling the temperature of a specific area of the lower right quadrant of the abdomen. In health, it should feel warm, indicating that this important energy in the body is functionally sound.

In the few theory books published in English that discuss this topic, Mingmen has been translated as the 'Gate of Life' or the 'Gate of Vitality'. The significance of that concept has had various theoretical interpretations. In ancient times, Mingmen was believed to be a vehicle through which the vitality of life arises. It referred to a philosophical rather than an anatomical concept.

In remote times and reflected in Wang Shu Hc's *Classic of the pulse* (280 CE), the right Kidney was viewed as the gate of life and the left Kidney as the Kidney proper, meaning the anatomical organ of the kidney. Later, Mingmen was viewed more as an area where the energy of the two kidneys converged and performed specific functions and duties. It is a pilot light, so to speak, for metabolic activities, hence its warming aspect.

Classical literature suggests that Mingmen is more than Kidney Yang but in the minds of most modern practitioners there seems to be an equation that Mingmen is exclusively equivalent to the Yang aspect of the Kidney. Let us look a little further at this perhaps incorrect perception.

Jeremy Ross (1984), in his book *Zang Fu, the organ systems of traditional Chinese medicine*, summarizes these opinions.

Some authorities consider Mingmen, the Gate of Life, to be insubstantial, to be located between the Kidneys and to be associated with the fire of the Body. Other authorities associate Mingmen with the Right Kidney, but in either case, Mingmen, or the Gate of Life Fire, is considered to be responsible for warming and activating processes of the body. In clinical practice, the Manifestation of Kidney Fire, Kidney Yang, Mingmen Fire and Yuan Qi are often regarded as more or less identical. (p. 68)

Claude Larree (1995, p. 156) concurs when he cites, 'In a Being the kidneys are double; they are the symbolic receptacles of the origin of life (this will be specified in later works of the Chinese tradition by the name Mingmen, Water and Fire, the authentic and original Yin and Yang)'. But perhaps the renowned Chinese scholar, Zhang Jie Bing, said it best when he so eloquently wrote:

Mingmen totally controls the Kidneys and both Kidneys belong to Mingmen. It is the home of Yin and Yang. It is the passageway of life and death. If Mingmen is depleted, then the five Yin and six Yang organs are diseased and changed. [Therefore] there is no place unaffected [by the depletion]. (Matsumoto & Birch 1988, p. 113)

It is in this passage that he informs us that Mingmen is more than just Kidney Yang; it includes Kidney Yin as well.

Leon Hammer (1988), MD and acupuncturist, continues this thought process. He states:

Kidney Yang also known as Kidney Fire or the Fire of Ming Men is therefore the functional energy that provides 'drive' to all of the Organ systems and circulation. The heat energy, required for the physical and mental digestive function of the Earth element, comes from the Ming Men. Kidney Fire provides the metabolic heat to transform what would otherwise be a relatively inert organism into a dynamic, goal oriented aggressive being. From the beginning it provides the 'force', to the 'life force' and the 'will' to the 'will to live'. (p. 109)

Those who only see Mingmen as Kidney Yang fail to recognize that a flame needs something to burn. This fuel, a Yin, structive material, is necessary in order to provide the flame that can dominate those basal metabolic activities. Hence, those who understand the Law of the Unity of Opposites, or the Law of Yin and Yang, and who have studied the classics recognize that Mingmen has both Yin and Yang components.

The misperception that Mingmen is exclusively equivalent to Kidney Yang is primarily derived from a knowledge of Eight Principle pulse categorization in which the left Kidney is considered as Kidney Yin and the right Kidney is regarded as Kidney Yang (Gardner-Abbate 1996, p. 143). However, classically trained Chinese physicians point out that the assumption that the right Kidney is Kidney Yang rather than Mingmen in its entirety is incorrect.

In my studies with modern classically trained physicians in Beijing, they concluded that no classical literature differentiates Mingmen as equivalent to Kidney Yang or that Kidney Yin and Yang are separate. Consequently, they believe that Mingmen encompasses primary Yin and Yang.* It is the original Kidney Yin and Yang inextricably bound together, just as all Yin and Yang are so connected.† They support this by referencing the pulse diagnosis systems seen in Table 5.1.

In the *Neijing*, the *Yellow Emperor's classic*, the oldest Chinese medical classic and possibly the oldest medical text in the world, Mingmen was

---

* Derived from discussions with classically trained doctors at the International Training Center of the Academy of Traditional Chinese Medicine, Beijing, PRC, 1988.

† My definition

Table 5.1 An historical comparison of various pulse diagnosis systems

Pulse systems	Position	RIGHT HAND			LEFT HAND		
		Distal	Middle	Proximal	Distal	Middle	Proximal
Yellow Emperor's classic (Neijing) ca. 200 BC	Superficial	Chest	SP	Abdomen	Sternum	Diaphragm	Abdomen
	Deep	LU	ST	KI	HT	LR	KI
Five Element classic (Nanjing) ca. 200 BC	Superficial	LI	ST	TE	SI	GB	BL
	Deep	LU	SP	PC	HT	LR	KI
Wang Shu-He: *Pulse classic* ca. 280 BC	Superficial	LI	ST	TE	SI	GB	BL
	Deep	LU	SP	MM	HT	LR	KI
Li Shi-Zhen: *Pulse diagnosis* AD 1564	Middle	LU	SP	MM and LI TE	HT	LR	MM, SI, BL
Zhang Jie-Bing: *Complete book* AD 1624	Superficial	Sternum	ST	TE, MM, SI, KI	PC	GB	BL, LI, KI
	Deep	LU	SP		HT	LR	
Eight Principle pulse system	Superficial	LU	ST	–	HT	GB	–
	Deep	–	SP	KI Yang	–	LR	KI Yin
Contemporary China based on the classics	Superficial	LI, chest	ST	LI, TE, MM	PC	GB	SI, BL
	Deep	LU	SP		HT	LR	KI

MM: Mingmen (Gate of Life) = Kidney Yin and Yang, immutably bound together

believed to be stored at Bladder 1 (Jingming). Later in the *Nanjing*, the *Five Element classic* or the *Classic of difficult questions*, it was purported that Mingmen was found between the two Kidneys and infused in the acupuncture point GV 4 (Mingmen). The pulse classic of the Ching dynasty, the *Maijing*, maintained that Mingmen could be measured from the right side of the pulse in the chi** position. The left chi position reflected the Kidney organ. Later, in the Ming dynasty, it was the view that Mingmen was stored in the external genitalia.

Weisman & Ellis (1985) state:

Kidney Yin and Yang are regarded as being interdependent and complimentary aspects of kidney essential qi. When vacuity of kidney Yin or Yang reaches a certain degree, it may affect its compliment, since detriment to Yang affects Yin and vice versa. The principle of interdependence of Yin and Yang is also of great importance when treating yin-yang imbalances. Jing Yu's *Complete compendium* states:
Yang when requiring supplementation, should be

sought in yin, since with the help of yin, it can arise infinitely; yin, when requiring supplementation must be sought in yang, since with the help of yang, its source is never ending. (p. 243)

Bob Flaws contends that adult physiology is not an absolute balance of Yin and Yang. As warm-blooded mammals, he maintains that we are relatively speaking more Yang than Yin. He suggests a three-to-two ratio. Hence, Mingmen, as Kidney Yin and Yang inextricably connected, is relatively more Yang in nature than Yin. While the function of Mingmen is similar to Kidney Yang, it is not identical to it. This clarified theory has clinical significance for abdominal diagnosis and treatment, as we shall see.

WHAT IS IMMUNITY?

Now that the concept of Mingmen has been explored, it lays the basis for appreciating its importance in the palpatory examination. The next fundamental topic that needs to be clarified is immunity.

** Foot or proximal position

In Western terms, immunity involves a bio-chemical complex of the defense systems of the body and how it produces antibodies to destroy invading antigens and malignancies. The practitioner is urged to read more about the Western concept of immunity to gain a glimpse of the common threads that are woven between Western and Chinese paradigms.

In Chinese medicine, when the body is lacking Qi and Blood, it is termed Deficient. I believe that, fundamentally, most diseases of the human condition are those of Deficiency. Often the Deficiency is of a long-term or chronic nature and assumes new variations the longer that Deficiency continues. It gets compounded with multiple deficiencies and even excesses such as Stagnant Qi, Blood and Phlegm.

Perhaps less than 5% of illness is truly Excess in nature. A significant portion of those diseases which have an Excess component are due to an underlying Deficiency; for example, Liver Qi Stagnation (Excess) that has developed due to Liver Blood Deficiency.

This opinion is supported in Chinese literature by the statement that the antipathogenic factor (Zheng Qi or True Qi) is the internal cause and the leading cause in the occurrence of a disease. In prophylaxis and treatment of disease, therefore, Traditional Chinese Medicine stresses especially the protection of the antipathogenic factor. The efficacy of acupuncture and moxibustion in prevention and treatment of disease is due mainly to their regulating and strengthening the defensive function of the antipathogenic factor and helping to restore the relative balance within the body as well as that between the human body and its environment (Beijing College 1980).

Years ago, when the first group of Deficiency diseases such as AIDS, chronic fatigue syndrome, multiple sclerosis, fibromyalgia and others began to appear in the medical world in increasing numbers, American acupuncture practitioners tried to understand their etiology and pathophysiology. Increasing numbers of patients were turning to non-orthodox medicine because of their dissatisfaction with the medical establishment's treatment of these diseases. Chinese differentiation of disease books were not helpful to these practitioners because they did not contain the information – the ancient Chinese had not seen these illnesses. Therefore, practitioners needed to look at the basic material that they had learned to see if they could apply it to the new modern-day illnesses.

Articles were written in newsletters and journals on the subject of immunity. There arose a debate as to whether immunity was equivalent to Wei Qi or the True Qi of the body; that is, the Zheng Qi. Immunity is related to Wei Qi, but it is more than that. It is a product of the proper functioning of all of the Zang-Fu organ–meridian complexes such that the basic essential substances of life are produced. It is these substances which keep us healthy. How 'immunity' is created is the subject of our final theoretical clarification in this section – the Triple Warmer.

Wei Qi

Before proceeding with that discussion let us recapitulate the functions of Wei Qi. Wei Qi:

- resides on the surface (exterior – skin, muscle, meridian) and regulates the opening and closing of the pores
- maintains proper body temperature in response to external and internal environments
- protects the body from outside evils
- is regulated by the function of the Lungs
- is a subset of the True Qi of the body.

The integrity of the Wei Qi is a function of the True Qi of the body because the Wei Qi is a component of the True Qi, a direct almost proportional manifestation of its solidity and strength. The Wei Qi of the body can only be as good as the True Qi.

While the Wei Qi resides on the exterior and combats exogenous pathogens at that level, it originates in the Middle Jiao, the place where the essential substances start to be manufactured. The ancient texts maintain that it is the Lower Jiao that confronts the pathogenic factors. There is a connection between immunity and the Wei Qi but its origin is at a deeper level.

Chinese physicians and Qi Gong masters concur. They believe that True Qi plays the most important role in immune problems. Immune deficiency diseases then are primarily seen as diseases related to this Qi. The aforementioned diseases such as chronic fatigue or AIDS are not due to the failure of the Wei Qi in the functional roles described above. The discussion on the role of the Triple Warmer will help to explain this.

The fundamental goal of meridian therapy is to address the root cause of illness. In virtually all cases that root cause is due to weak immunity. The aim of palpation, point selection, needling and the other treatment modalities is to augment the True Qi of the body.

THE TRIPLE WARMER

The subject of the Triple Warmer is one of the most fascinating theoretical concepts in Oriental medicine and it also has tremendous clinical significance. It is not a brief topic, nor has much been written about it in a cohesive way. This is not to say that classical literature does not mention it for in fact, it abounds in references that are simultaneously illustrative and elusive. It was a subject that was synthesized relatively late because of the preeminence of other diagnostic frameworks. It thus has a 200 versus a 2000-year history.

Because the body per se does not have a discrete, visible anatomical organ called the Triple Warmer that is subject to dissection or analysis, the topic of the Triple Warmer is almost completely energetic. In this respect, the Triple Warmer epitomizes Chinese medicine as the energetic system that it is. As we know, one of the operating principles of Chinese medicine is that it focuses on function, process and change. It is not an anatomical system that focuses on independent and what are often perceived as fixed somatic structures.

In classical literature, the Triple Warmer was referred to as a 'name with no form', a statement which expresses the idea of the Triple Warmer as an energetic system. Yet the Triple Warmer was also called a 'form, a cavity, with a name', meaning that it had areas of demarcation.

In its simplest terms, the Triple Warmer was viewed as three *jiaos* – variously translated as regions, areas, warmers or 'burning spaces'. They were seen as places where energy was produced, distributed and consumed. The Upper Jiao is the area above the diaphragm. It includes the chest, neck, face and head as well as the arms and shoulders. The Middle Jiao covers the area from the diaphragm to the navel. It is the epigastric region. The Lower Jiao extends from the navel downward. It includes the lower abdomen, thighs, knees, feet and toes.

The role of the Jiaos is explained in the classics in which it was said that the Upper Jiao is like a mist or a fog. Acting as a spray or all-pervading vapor, the Upper Jiao sends Qi and Blood to every part of the body once they have been manufactured. As the *Lingshu* states, 'The Upper Warmer is a prime mover, it distributes the five food tastes, vaporizes into the skin, fills the body, moistens the hair on the body, is like the irrigation of mist and dew and is called Qi'. It is comparable mainly to the respiratory system.

The *Lingshu* continues, 'The Middle Warmer receives the Qi, extracts the juice, changes it into a substance. This is called blood'. The Middle Jiao is like foam, a froth of bubbles. The Middle Warmer Qi goes up and down like foam in a cauldron. It is where the actual production of Qi and Blood begins. It is like frothy soup reflective of the food and drink as they begin their decomposition in the Stomach and is thus named the Sea of Water and Nourishment. It is comparable to the digestive system.

The Lower Jiao, as a drainage ditch, is like a dam that controls water. It is the place where the unusable dregs of food and drink are expelled. The *Lingshu* adds, 'The Lower Warmer permeates the fluid, unites with the bladder, controls emitting and not entering, divides pure and impure'. It is comparable to the urogenital system.

In classical texts, the Triple Warmer is called 'the Official in Charge of Irrigation' and this function is exhibited in the way the Triple Warmer serves as a water passageway. This is an apt summary of the roles of these areas.

Each Jiao has an activation or controlling point, an acupuncture point where the Qi of each Jiao can be utilized or accessed. The controlling point of the Upper, Middle and Lower Jiaos are CV 17

(Tanzhong), CV 12 (Zhongwan) and CV 7 (Yinjiao) respectively. The Front Mu point of the Triple Warmer is CV 5 (Shimen). Yoshio Manaka claims that ST 25 (Tianshu) is the Front Mu point of the Triple Warmer and so we will see that due to this energetic, Stomach 25 becomes an important diagnostic area of the abdomen and the function of the Triple Warmer. The anatomical boundaries of the Triple Warmer and its controlling points are illustrated in Figure 5.1.

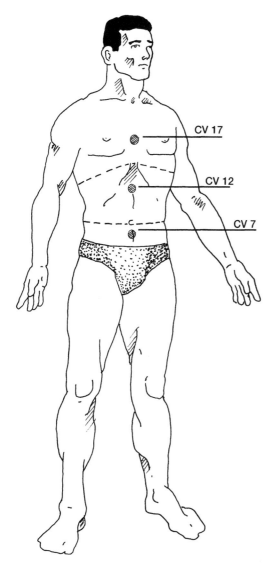

Figure 5.1 The Triple Warmer and its controlling points.

The Triple Warmer also has its meridian component. Like all meridians, the Triple Warmer has a specific meridian symptomatology dependent upon where it traverses and what it is believed to do as a Fu organ in Chinese medicine. As a meridian, it can be used for a number of conditions including febrile disease due to Wind-Heat, Damp diseases, headache, sore throat, scrofula (swelling of lymph nodes due to Phlegm), chest oppression and painful chest. Additionally, it is useful for epilepsy, goiter and motor impairment of the areas it traverses externally. It is a primary meridian for treating any ear pathology.

The Triple Warmer can be used for any syndrome of Spleen and Stomach weakness because of its connection to digestion. The reason should become more apparent after the development of the concept of the Triple Warmer but for now we can see that it activates the Qi of the Middle Jiao. All the points of the San Jiao channel tonify the Yuan Qi, can smooth and regulate the flow of Qi and clear and dredge the Channels. They are foremost in conditions where the flow of Qi and Blood is uneven or where the Qi is in rebellion.

In the Five Element system, the San Jiao is paired with the Pericardium. Just as the Pericardium serves as the 'envelope that protects the Heart from outside evils' so too does the Triple Warmer act as 'the envelope that protects the body from outside evils'. That envelope, like a shield, is made up of the True Qi of the body or our immunity that serves to ward off pernicious influences.

The Triple Warmer is paired to the Gall Bladder in the Six Division energetic framework.* A primary use of the Six Division framework is to explain the invasion of a Cold or Wind-Cold pathogen into the body and how that pathogen's clinical manifestations change if it makes its way deeper into the body. The pairing of these two Yang meridians is called the Shaoyang layer. The Shaoyang is the intermediary energetic level in the body where the Cold

---

* The Six Divisions is a diagnostic framework used to explain the invasion of a Cold or Wind-Cold pathogen into the body and how its clinical manifestations change as it progresses to deeper energetic layers.

pathogen is lodged between the exterior and the deeper Yin levels. It is primarily characterized by alternating chills and fever, a symptom congruent with the hinge-like layer that the pathogen resides in; that is, a half interior/half exterior position.

The Triple Warmer, via one of its points TE 5 (Waiguan), activates the Yangwei channel which controls Yang defensive energy in the body. The Gall Bladder via GB 41 (Zulinqi) activates the Dai channel, the only transverse meridian that encircles the body. The way in which these meridians work together is similar to a spiral that covers every portion of the body in a latitudinal or transverse manner, instead of longitudinally as the other meridians do. This image is captured in Figure 5.2. The Triple Warmer and the Gall Bladder treat diseases on the exterior of the body.

Major lymphatic organs are located along the path of the Triple Warmer, such as the cervical glands of the neck (TE 16, Tianyou area), the thymus (CV 17, Tanzhong area) and the appendix (ST 25 on the right side, Tianshu area). This pathway and its proximity to lymphatic tissue helps to explain the Triple Warmer's more traditional connection to immunity.

The Triple Warmer is also called the 'Commander and Chief of all of the Qi of the Various Organs'. The classics confirm this when they state that the Triple Warmer is 'the road to nutrition, the beginning and end of all Qi'. It manufactures and disseminates the Qi and the Blood throughout the entire body.

We can see, then, that the Triple Warmer has a role in the conversion of food and drink into the essential substances that are the basis of our immunity. In its most complex form, the Triple Warmer is the theoretical construct which explains how all the Zang-Fu organs work together to produce the building blocks of life – Qi, Blood, Jing, Body Fluid, Shen and Marrow – which ultimately constitute our immunity. This is what Kiiko Matsumoto calls 'the Big Envelope' that protects the Shen from outside evil.

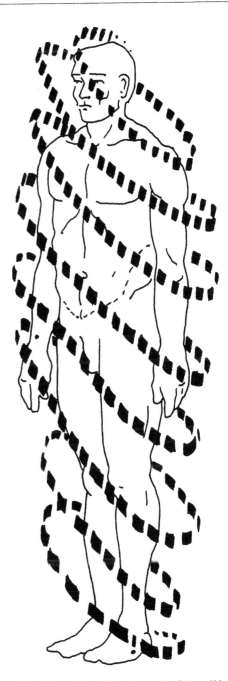

Figure 5.2 The relationship between the Dai and Yangwei channels.

It is through the mechanism of the Triple Warmer that the body is viewed as a whole instead of as discrete parts or even the sum of its parts. It is the secret to seeing the body as a whole

---

TE = standard abbreviation of the World Health Organization (1989) for Triple Warmer.

instead of as individual spheres of organ function or dysfunction. It is an empowering concept that Western medicine lacks and this deficit can limit the quality of patient care it provides.

Kiiko Matsumoto and Stephen Birch (1988) provide an added dimension to the connections between the Triple Warmer, immunity and Source points (we will see that they are major clearance or treatment points on the Hara specifically for Deficiency cases). They write:

The main function of the San Jiao is to govern the various forms of Qi and serves as a passage for the flow of Yuan Qi and body fluids. The Yuan Qi originates in the Kidneys but it is the San Jiao that serves as the pathway for the Yuan Qi to promote the functional activities of the Zang-Fu organs and the tissues of the whole body. The Triple Warmer functions as the messenger of the source qi. The Source points are closely connected to the source of the vital Qi in the body. The Source points of the five organs (yin organs) are the places to which the Triple Warmer comes, the place where the Qi can stay. The hara is the center, the ultimate source of qi. The Triple Warmer is the energetic connection of the hara to all the Source points of all the meridians. Before all other treatment is administered, we need to treat the condition of the Hara. (p. 66)

An understanding of the concepts of Mingmen, immunity and the Triple Warmer can provide us with information to keep people healthy. Their integrity can be felt by abdominal diagnosis and palpation. This is the subject of the next several chapters.

NEW WORDS AND CONCEPTS

Eight Principle pulse categorization – a system of pulse diagnosis which evolved in relation to the Eight Principle diagnosis framework.

Essential substances – the building blocks of life according to Chinese medicine. They are Qi, Blood, Jing, Body Fluids, Shen and Marrow.

Immunity – the True Qi of the body, the Zheng Qi. It is the product of the proper functioning of all the Zang-Fu organ–meridian complexes such that the basic essential substances of life are produced.

Law of the Unity of Opposites – the Law of Yin and Yang.

Mingmen – Kidney Yin and Yang inextricably bound together.

Six Division energetic framework – the diagnostic framework discussed in the *Shang Han Lung* or *Treatise of cold induced disorders* about 220 CE by Zhong Zhong-jing, which explains the invasion of a Cold or Wind-Cold pathogen into the body and how its manifestations may change if it progresses through six distinct energetic zones of the body.

Triple Warmer – the theoretical construct used to explain the production and distribution of the essential substances.

QUESTIONS

1. Why isn't Wei Qi a good definition of immunity in Chinese medicine?

2. How do you think the concepts of Mingmen, immunity and the Triple Warmer are important in relation to abdominal palpation?

3. What aspect of Chinese medical theory helps us to see the body as a whole instead of as individual spheres of organ function?

4. Discuss (list) all the components that determine the quality of our immunity.

How to perform the palpatory examinations

6

General palpation skills and physical examination I

GENERAL PALPATION SKILLS

Palpation is the process of examining the surface of the body to detect the presence of disease and to observe the patient's reaction to pressure (Weisman & Ellis 1985, p. 141). It is also the mechanism by which that disease may be treated.

Disease has myriad manifestations; it may appear in the guise of heat, cold, moisture, distension, pain or in several other forms. In order to detect these clues and to diagnose correctly, the practitioner must be assured that the information gleaned through palpation is accurate. Therefore, the practitioner must bring a certain level of consciousness to the process of palpation, as to all phases of diagnosis and treatment (Gardner-Abbate 1996, pp. 12–13). Box 6.1 summarizes the general palpation skills that constitute that consciousness and they are discussed below.

Box 6.1   General palpation skills

1. Presence, sensitivity, centering
2. Proper draping, professional decorum
3. Clean, warm hands and short nails
4. Timing (such as not keeping the hands on an area too long or pressing the point too long)
5. Practitioner comfort: protection of the shoulder by adjusting the height of the table
6. Observation of the patient by palpating from the side of one's dominant eye
7. Skill: being comfortable with the procedures

Presence, sensitivity, centering

When beginning the palpation process it is important for practitioners to be mindful of the procedure they are about to undertake. In using this method of diagnosis, the practitioner is directly establishing contact with the Qi of the patient. Appropriate therapeutic touch calls for an awareness of the patient's energy, sensitivities and comfort levels, both physically, such as their perception of the ambient temperature, and emotionally, including any possible guardedness.

As a professional, the practitioner needs to be aware of all these things to ensure that the correct information is gleaned from the palpatory examination. The practitioner's mind should be wholly focused on the procedure, a procedure that involves interaction with the patient, and the practitioner should be present, sensitive and centered.

Proper draping, professional decorum

Because practitioners are both palpating and simultaneously observing, it is imperative that they are able to see the corresponding body parts. While this is crucial, it does not imply that the patient should not be properly draped. Draping is that proper professional decorum that provides the appropriate level of modesty between the parties. Additionally, the patient should always be protected from catching cold by being covered. Patients may be instructed to put on a patient gown so that it is easy to palpate various parts of the body or they may remain in their clothing if it can be readily moved for the physical examinations. After palpation of specific areas is completed the practitioner should immediately reposition the clothing or cover the patient with a blanket or drape.

Clean, warm hands and short nails

Hands must be washed prior to palpation to guard against the transmission of any infectious disease, in particular hepatitis B. Minimally, the nails of the palpating fingers must be short in order to perform the palpation steps correctly.

This is not negotiable; proper palpation cannot be done with long nails. Washing the hands with warm water prior to palpating will also make the practitioner's hands more comfortable for the patient, particularly if the practitioner's hands run on the cold side.

Timing

When the palpation process is initiated, hands should not be kept too long on any one area as they may change the perception of temperature the longer they are kept in contact with the patient's skin. In general the whole process of palpation should move along. The practitioner should not linger too long on any one point or area of the body when checking temperature or when pressing points or diagnostic areas.

Practitioner comfort

Because palpation is physical, practitioners will be required to use their own strength. Some of this strength will come from the fingers but the largest part of the practitioner's energy comes from the Dan tian and then is directed through the body, to the shoulder and out through the fingers onto the part of the body being palpated.

The protection of the practitioner's shoulder is therefore important. If the table that the practitioner is using to treat the patient is too low or too high, the practitioner's shoulder will be subject to stress. Proper table height can alleviate this stress and practitioners are encouraged to find this height for themselves. It is generally a few inches below the practitioner's hip level.

Observation

The practitioner needs to observe the patients to see how they respond to palpation, whether it hurts, is too deep or vaguely discomforting. The sensation we elicit if the point is 'dis-eased' can be a deep aching feeling, pain, tenderness, even that the patient likes it, or a combination of pain and enjoyment. The more it hurts, the more significant is the pathology represented by that point. It becomes a significant diagnosis point or, in the case of treatment points, a key point to ease abdominal tenderness.

While patients will report certain findings to the practitioner, so too will their body language. These are not always consistent. In performing palpation there is no need to look at the point once it has been located and inspected. Instead, watch the patient's face as the points are being palpated to get a more accurate assessment of the patient's experience; for instance, do patients grit their teeth yet say that the palpation is fine? Usually you will be able to see the reaction on patients' faces before they report it.

Another factor that can help is always to palpate from one side of the patient, preferably from the side of your dominant eye so that this eye is closer to the patient. How to find the dominant eye is described in Box 6.2. In most people, their dominant eye and their dominant hand are on the same side. If this is not the case, the practitioner can palpate from whatever side is more comfortable. The point is that practitioner comfort and observation of the patient are important.

Skill

The whole palpatory examination provides clinicians with the data they need to treat the patient if they have an adequate skill level. Admittedly, it is difficult to learn palpation from a book so practice and conscientiousness are essential.

These guidelines can be applied to any palpation of the body, be it points, structures or organs within any medical paradigm that utilizes palpation as a method of diagnosis and treatment. They can likewise be used as a prelude to needling or any other treatment modality.

PHYSICAL EXAMINATION I: THE HEALTHY HARA EXAMINATION

When inspecting the abdomen, there are essentially nine characteristics that constitute what could be called the features of the healthy abdomen or Hara. Each of these parameters is discussed in detail below and summarized in Figure 6.1*. Following the discussion of the features of the healthy Hara, Table 6.3 highlights pathological abdominal findings and their diagnostic meanings. Before interpreting the findings of this first abdominal examination, be sure to review the general palpation skills covered in this chapter, for the diagnosis can only be as good as the methods used to gather the information that will go into its construction.

Characteristics of the healthy Hara

Temperature

Feeling the abdomen both in general and in specific locations gives an indication of temperature. First, feel the epigastric and lower abdominal regions by lightly scanning those areas with the palmar surface of the hand. The overall temperature should be fairly uniform, tending towards warmth. The practitioner next simultaneously inspects the epigastric area more closely and the lower right quadrant of the lower abdominal region in the Stomach 25–28 area. (Figure 6.2 demonstrates the areas to be examined in performing temperature evaluation.)

Briefly place the palm of one hand on CV 12 (Zhongwan) and the other on ST 25R (Tianshu)

Box 6.2   How to find your dominant eye (Chaitow 1991)

- Make a circle with your first finger and thumb and, holding the arm out in front of your face, observe an object across the room, through that circle, with both eyes open.
- Close one eye. If the object is still in the circle, you will now have your dominant eye open.
- If, however, the image shifts out of the circle when only one eye is open, open the closed eye and close the open eye and the image should shift back into clear view, inside the circle.
- Thus, the eye which sees the same view as you saw when both eyes were open is the one to use in close observation of the body.

---

* Copies of this as well as all forms that the author developed can be found in Section 4 of this book. Practitioners are encouraged to make copies of them and to use them as diagnostic intake forms as they learn how to integrate the palpatory examination into their diagnostic work-up.

ABDOMINAL DIAGNOSIS: THE HEALTHY HARA EXAMINATION

Patient's name: _____ Date: _____

Major complaint: _____

Check (✓) in the Normal column if the patient has this healthy characteristic, check (✓) in the Abnormal column if the finding is abnormal.

Characteristics (The Healthy Hara)	Significance/Comments Keep hands there a short amount of time	Normal	Abnormal	Diagnosis
1. Temperature: a) fairly uniform	As warm-blooded mammals, the human body is more Yang than Yin.			
b) cooler above umbilicus	Why should there be a cool Stomach and *not* a warm Stomach? Warmth consumes Yin which leads to ST Yin Xu and Heat which leads to KI Yin Xu.			
c) warmer in the lower right quadrant (LRQ), the Mingmen area	LRQ = Yin, Yin, Yin. Needs Mingmen Fire to balance it. Therefore should feel warm.			
2. Moisture: a) slightly moist	Not dried up, withered, scaly or fatty deposits.			
3. Resilient: a perpendicular assessment. Check: CV 12, ST 25L, ST 25R, CV 6, CV 4 a) bouncy, elastic, not hard or mushy (If abnormal note quality found in Abnormal column.)	1. Hard, Excess, replete, aggravated by pressure = tense, unhealthy tissue. 2. Mushy = Deficiency, vacant, soft or full but not aggravated by pressure; pain may be relieved. 3. Hardness on top often has Deficiency below or the reverse. Patient says doesn't feel anything.			
CV 12				
ST 25L				
ST 25R				
CV 6				
CV 4				
4. Strength: a surface assessment done at CV 12 and ST 25L a) looser above umbilicus especially at CV 12	1. Substernal tension is the cause of many problems; seen in TCM as KI Yin Xu (because tight = ST Yin Xu). ST Yin Xu leads to KI Yin Xu. Mental degeneration begins with a tight stomach.			
b) stronger on left side ST 25 (Tianshu) (If abnormal, comment on quality found.)	2. Strong ST 25 (Tianshu) = sufficient Blood.			
5. Shape: a) even, symmetrical, including umbilicus, rib cage and size of the sternocostal angle (SCA). Not sunken, fat, thin, puffy, etc. (see Fig. 6.1B)	1. Sunken, thin = Deficiency 2. Puffy, fat = Yang Deficiency 3. Narrow SCA = ST Yin Xu → KI Yin Xu			
6. Pulsation at CV 6: a) palpable in the middle to deep position	Upon palpation should feel pulse at CV 6 (Qihai) = energy of the Kidneys communicating with each other. More important than radial pulse.			

Figure 6.1A

7. Depression along Ren channel and slight depression at CV 12 and above umbilicus	Ren Channel, primordial channel, formed after the first cell division from 1 to 2 cells. Structural meridian. Controls all the Yin meridians. Good constitution, good genetic inheritance.			

8. Breathing:
  a) noticeable rise and fall of
  abdomen below umbilicus
	To bring LU Qi to KI area. The Kidney grasps the Qi.			

9. Point inspection (for pathology)	See Table 6.2			
10. Other (specify)				

General diagnosis: _____

Treatment plan: _____

Figure 6.1A *continued*

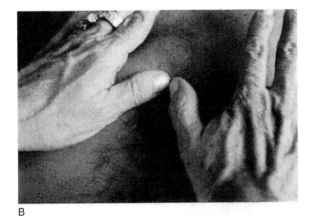

B

Figure 6.1 A: Abdominal diagnosis form: the healthy Hara examination. B: Narrow sternocostal angle, i.e. less than 90°.

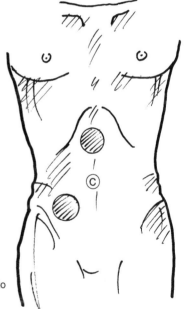

Figure 6.2 Where to perform temperature assessment.

and compare the temperature. Relatively speaking, Zhongwan should be cooler than Tianshu. CV 12 (Zhongwan) is located directly over the center of the Stomach.

It should be cooler because the Stomach is the source of all Yin. If this area is warmer, ask patients if they have just eaten as the digestive process may make the Stomach warmer. If they have not recently eaten, this pattern may be suggestive of Heat or Fire in the Stomach with all their pathological scenarios. The danger of a Hot Stomach is that if Yin is not produced, the Stomach, as the source of all Yin, will not be able to furnish Yin to the other organs.

Stomach Yin Deficiency may furthermore lead to Kidney Yin Deficiency because Earth controls Water according to Five Element theory. Kidney Yin energy is fundamental to all life. All the etiological factors that promote Heat in the Stomach should be considered as leading to this finding. Bear in mind that stress is the leading causative factor of Stomach Yin Deficiency. Table 6.1 offers a fairly comprehensive list of factors contributing to Stomach Heat.

Table 6.1 Factors contributing to Stomach Heat

Etiological factors	Mechanisms
Food	
1. Ingestion of energetically Hot foods into the Stomach either in excess or in excess relative to the patient. The most common offenders are hot, spicy, pungent foods, e.g. chili, curry, red meat, chocolate, sugar, and other acidic foods.	1. Direct entry of Hot foods into the Stomach, causing it to overheat.
2. Over-eating of Damp foods that are difficult for the Spleen and Stomach to break down, e.g. dairy products, greasy, damp, oily or rich foods.	2. When the Spleen fails to transform and transport the digesta, Stagnation may ensue. Stagnation frequently transforms into Heat and/or Fire, which serves to perversely heat up the Middle Jiao.
Alcohol	
One of the greatest offenders, especially wine (Evil Wetness) or other 'hot' alcoholic beverages, e.g. whiskey, tequila.	Causes Heat in the Stomach either directly or because of the failure of the Spleen to transform and transport.
Stress	
Most stress is indicative of the inability of the Liver Qi to flow freely.	When Liver Qi stagnates due to any reason, it overacts on the Earth element, causing Spleen Qi to become deficient and Stomach Qi to ascend and often heat up.

In contrast to this, the Stomach 25 (Tianshu) area on the right is the place on the abdomen where the function of the Mingmen energy can be evaluated. It is the 'yinniest' area of the abdomen because it is on the right side (Yin), below the navel (Yin) and on the front of the body (Yin). To counterbalance its nature to be cool (Yin), it needs to be balanced by the Fire of the Kidney. It is directly on the other side of the right Kidney, classically thought of as Mingmen, the Gate of the Fire of Life, the vitality of life. It is Kidney Yin and Yang inextricably bound together, the pilot light (Yang) as well as the fuel of life (Yin). As Chapter 5 discusses, it is slightly more Yang than Yin. Table 5.1 provides an historical comparison of various pulse diagnosis systems that demonstrate that Mingmen was classically considered to be on the right side of the body and this is reflected in the pulse diagnosis systems.

The warm Mingmen signifies that the Kidney energy is sound and the cool Stomach suggests that the Stomach is fulfilling its job of creating Yin. This configuration of 'cool above and warm below' means that the fundamental structive energies of Yin and Yang are intact. Clinically we frequently see the reverse, that is, 'hot above, cold below'. This is a perverse pattern and represents the counterflow of Qi.

Temperature assessment is the most important factor in the evaluation of the patient's condition because it tells us about the Yin and the Yang. Initially, novices learning palpation commonly report that this is a difficult parameter to determine. Practice in temperature assessment will allow the practitioner to formulate the proper diagnosis.

Remember, don't keep your hands on the areas being checked for too long or your perception of the temperature may change. This aspect of the healthy Hara examination should be done first and quickly, as the temperature of the patient's body may change if it is uncovered for too long, generally in the direction of cooling.

Moisture

The moisture of the skin can be determined by inspecting the skin of the abdomen with the hand and gently stroking it. Sometimes the moisture is more likely to be seen than felt because normal moisture makes the skin subtly glisten. Healthy skin should be slightly moist, not dry, withered, oily, scaly or with fatty deposits (skin tags). Moisture is indicative of sufficient Body Fluids including Yin, Blood and Jin Ye fluids.

Dry skin thus is indicative of Heat, Blood, Yin or Jin Ye fluid deficiency; it usually feels rough or scaly. Oily or sticky skin is abnormal moisture that indicates the presence of Dampness. Cold moisture indicates Yang Deficiency.

Perform this step as the second part of the physical exam because the longer the abdomen is exposed, the more likely it is that the moisture will change, especially in a dry climate or a hot room.

Resilience

The abdomen should be elastic and resilient and not feel painful upon palpation. Resilience refers to the bouncy ability of the tissues to respond with elasticity to the degree that they were pressed. It is a quality of softness that should not be confused with a mushy, vacant feeling. Resilient areas do not feel hard or stretched like a drumskin. Resilience is determined with a perpendicular assessment; that is, the direction of the palpation is to push perpendicularly into the abdomen, release and determine the degree of response.

Resilience is checked in the epigastric area at CV 12 as well as below the navel, specifically along the Conception Vessel channel at CV 4 (Guanyuan) and 6 (Qihai) and at ST 25 on both the right and the left. Figure 6.3 illustrates the areas to palpate for resilience. Proper resilience in the lower abdomen indicates that the Original Qi of the Kidney is good, whereas resilience in the

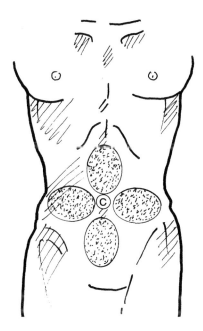

Figure 6.3   Areas to check for resilience.

epigastric region means that the Qi of the Upper Jiao, the Gathering Qi of the Heart and the Lungs, is flowing smoothly. Resilience at ST 25R is indicative of Lung Qi performing its functions and on the left that Liver Qi is flowing smoothly.

The opposite of resilience is tension. When the upper part of the abdomen feels hard and knotted the Qi of the Lung and the Heart is constrained and the patient may have emotional problems. The abdomen should not feel tight, tense or hard. It should not be discomforting to the patient, that is, aggravated by pressure. If so, it indicates an Excess condition. Many Excess conditions are due to the lack of free flow of Qi and Blood. Western interpretations are that the excess is caused by an acidic condition arising from increased meat consumption, stress, insufficient oxygenation, build-up of lactic acid and other reasons.

When CV 12 (Zhongwan) is tight, the pressure and tension produce constraint of Qi flow. This Stagnation can produce Heat. Heat can turn to Fire and consume Yin. When Yin is consumed, Phlegm can be produced. Phlegm, a pathological product, has many physical and psychological presentations. These can be read about in numerous sources (Cheung 1996, Gardner-Abbate 1995a).

The resilience of ST 25L tells us about the condition of the Blood, whether it is sufficient, deficient or stagnant. If this point feels strong when it is rubbed horizontally on the surface of the skin, it means that the structive energy of the Blood is present and that the Blood is sufficient. When it feels hard and tight it suggests Qi and Blood Stagnation.

ST 25 (Tianshu) on the left is a Blood Stagnation reflex point. Serizawa (1988, p. 110) corroborates this when he says, 'When there is strong tension or tenderness on the left side of the lower abdomen, this is traditionally associated with Blood stagnation'.

Mushiness on the other hand is a Deficiency pattern which feels empty and vacant. The area does not feel aggravated by pressure; in fact, the patient may enjoy the palpation, further support of the degree of Deficiency. Thus, if the area feels sunken or weak, it indicates Blood Deficiency. The final pattern is one of feeling mushy on the top of the area palpated but hard below or the reverse; such hardness resembles the hardness of a rock. This pattern suggests a combined Excess/Deficiency pattern. The Excess is generally due to an underlying Deficiency.

Strength

Strength is different from resilience. Whereas resilience reflects buoyancy or elasticity, strength feels solid, not hard or tight. It is a surface versus a perpendicular assessment, meaning it is not determined by pushing perpendicularly into the tissues but by rubbing the surface of the areas being diagnosed.

Strength is checked at two sites: the substernal region, specifically CV 12 (Zhongwan), and Stomach 25 (Tianshu) on the left. This is illustrated in Figure 6.4. In the substernal region, rub the CV 12 (Zhongwan) area and feel for a sensation of solidness on the surface. Strength at this point corroborates the strength of the Qi of the Middle Jiao and lack of strength indicates Qi Deficiency of the Middle Jiao.

Stomach 25L (Tianshu) should feel strong. This signifies that there is good Original Qi. The lack

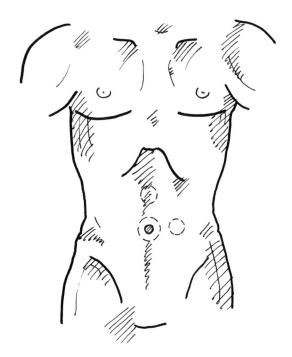

Figure 6.4 Areas to check for strength.

of strength or solidness indicates weakness of Qi and Blood. Comparatively, the strength of ST 25 (Tianshu) on the left should be greater than that felt at CV 12 (Zhongwan) because it reveals the adequacy of the physical substrate of the Blood.

Shape

The shape of the healthy abdomen should be even and symmetrical, full and softly rounded, not thin, gaunt, puffy, overweight or obese. There should be no areas of sunkenness at any spot. Carefully check important points such as CV 6 (Qihai), CV 4 (Guanyuan) and CV 9 (Shuifen) for the pathological characteristics listed above.

Likewise, the navel needs to be inspected for symmetry; there should not be depressions around it nor any puffiness except for a slight depression at CV 9. The navel can be examined either at this point or as one of the subsequent examinations that will be covered in this book. For ease of explaining the characteristics of the healthy Hara, the information on navel inspection and diagnosis is discussed separately in Chapter 10.

Examine the rib cage for symmetry, checking to see that all the ribs are aligned evenly and that one side is not higher than the other. The area under the ribs should not appear swollen or distended. Such findings may be caused by Liver Qi Stagnation if found on the right in the hypochondriac area or Spleen Qi Deficiency if seen on the left. Other diagnoses such as an enlarged Liver or Spleen are also possible although the most common generalized meanings are those first mentioned.

Pulsation

Upon palpation, the practitioner should be able to feel a pulse at the point CV 6 (Qihai). This pulse is felt in the middle to deep position on the abdomen when one pushes into the point, meaning it is not on the surface nor is it located too deeply. It is not a pulse that should be seen but one that should be felt. This point is the place where the energies of the two Kidneys communicate with each other. For this reason it is more important than the radial pulse. A weak pulse at this point means that the energy of the Kidneys is weak, which is a common finding. You may need to search for the pulse. Let the patients know what you are doing. Look at them as you feel for the pulse to avoid causing them too much discomfort. Ease up on the point if it causes too much pain and simply conclude that the Kidney energy is Deficient.

Depressions

A clear depression above the umbilicus should be seen on the front of the body along the Ren channel (Fig. 6.5). This depression along the midline is only found above the umbilicus. The Ren channel is one of the first two channels formed after conception (Matsumoto & Birch 1988, p. 181). As an early, formative, structive meridian, its vitality is reflected in the presence of this depression. The Ren channel also controls all the Yin meridians so when the Ren channel is visible, it is probable that the other meridians are structurally and functionally sound as well.

Breathing

Without telling the patient to breathe, just inspect the patient's abdomen during normal breathing and watch for a noticeable rise and fall of the abdomen below the umbilicus. When the lower

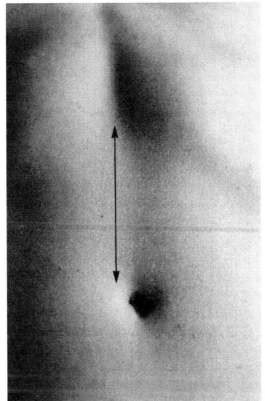

A

B

Figure 6.5 A & B: Depression of the Ren channel.

abdomen rises and falls it means that the Lung is sending its Qi down to the Kidney and the Kidney is grasping it. Failure of the Lungs to send energy to the Kidney means that its Qi cannot be grasped and Kidney Qi Deficiency results. Clinically, most patients fail to breathe deeply and you will not see this bellows-like movement often, except in people who consciously cultivate breathing practices.

Point inspection

Inspect the abdomen for other signs of point pathology such as moles, rashes, petechiae, depressions, lumps and knots. Table 6.2 lists the various pathological characteristics of points and the clinical significance of these findings that I have garnered from clinical experience.

In reviewing the clinical significance of the healthy Hara examination, it should be evident that what this examination determines is the fundamental condition of the Yin, Yang, Qi and Blood, with an emphasis on the Qi of the Kidney, the root of the Qi. For summary purposes, the areas of healthy abdominal assessment are combined into Figure 6.6 while Table 6.3 summarizes the significance of the pathological findings of the healthy Hara examination.

When to use the healthy hara examination

The healthy Hara examination should be the first physical examination conducted on the patient. It is easy to conduct, taking about 5 minutes to complete. Since many patients are not used to atten-

Table 6.2 Signs of point pathology and their clinical significance

Pathology	Clinical significance
Rashes	Heat in the Blood, may be Damp-Heat if oozing, Yin Xu Heat, Heat leading to Blood Stasis
Moles	Excess Heat/Fire or Yin Xu Heat/Fire
Warts	Heat in the Blood
Petechiae	Stagnant Blood
Asymmetries	Need to evaluate in relation to where they are
Boils	Damp-Heat, Toxic-Heat
Lumps	Qi Stagnation, Blood Stagnation, Damp, Phlegm, desiccated feces
Lesions	Damp-Heat, Toxic-Heat
Varicosities	Blood Stagnation and/or extravasation
Scars	Potential organ/meridian disturbances
Bruises	Blood Stagnation and/or extravasation
Swellings, edema, puffiness, bloating	Damp, Water, dilute Phlegm, Phlegm, Yang Xu
Redness	Heat of the excess or deficient type
Bone growths	Phlegm
Dryness/wetness	Blood Xu, Yin Xu/Dampness, Yang Xu
Inversions/eversions	Weak Yin meridians/weak Yang meridians
Knots	Qi Stagnation, Dampness
Abnormal hair presence or absence	Hormonal imbalance or Deficiency of affected area
Fat pad at GV 14	Yang Deficiency
Fat/overweight	Qi and Yang Xu with retention of Damp
Leathery	Blood or Yin Xu
Withered	Blood or Yin or Yang Xu
Prolapses	Spleen Qi Xu
Growths	Phlegm, Stagnant Blood
Size of sternocostal angle (narrow)	Lung Qi Xu/Kidney Qi Xu
Visible pulsations	Heart Qi Xu
Depth of breathing (shallow)	Lung Qi Xu
Shoulder posture (concave/convex)	Lung Qi Xu/Excess in Lungs
Muscle bands	Free ionized calcium (Damp)
Flushing colorations	Excess Heat or Yin Xu
Birth marks	Blood Stagnation
Hairy patches	Hormonal imbalance

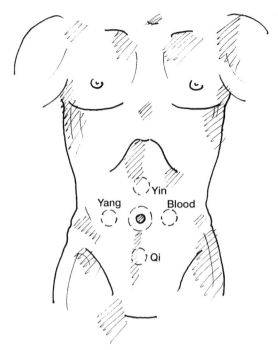

1. Temperature = Yin (CV 12) and Yang (ST 25R); also felt all over
2. Moisture = Yin, Blood and Body Fluids; also Yang Deficiency; felt all over
3. Resilience = Qi (CV 14, CV 12, CV 6, CV 4, ST 25R and L)
4. Strength = Blood (CV 12, ST 25L)
5. Shape = Qi; observe all over
6. Pulsation = Kidney Qi
7. Depression along the Ren Channel = Yin
8. Breathing = Kidney Qi
9. Point Pathology = other pathology; all over

Figure 6.6   The root meaning of the abdominal diagnosis and where to find it.

tion being paid to their abdomen, explain to them both what you are doing and why. Explain that, by feeling their abdomen you can learn many things about their organs and their fundamental energy. If they are interested you can relay your findings to them, such as the temperature of the stomach and the Mingmen area or any other finding. Record your findings on the form in Figure 6.1.

The form is conveniently organized with many useful features, analyzed below.

- In the furthermost left-hand column the characteristics of the healthy Hara are found.
- In the middle column the clinical significance of those characteristics is explained.

- Space is provided for you to record whether the patient has the normal, healthy characteristics or if they are abnormal. We are looking for as many normal characteristics as possible. However, attention will be paid to the abnormal ones for these will require treatment.
- The 'Diagnosis' column is where you will record the meaning of the abnormal finding. The meanings are too numerous to be listed on this form and can be found in Tables 6.2 and 6.3.
- Based upon this form, which assists you in organizing your data, you can then advance a treatment plan.

Even if you did not read the rest of this book, you could use the information gleaned from this examination to prepare a treatment plan if you are theoretically inclined to treat the root or the big picture. Points, herbs or other modalities could be chosen based on the analysis of the patient's pattern of energy. For instance, if the Mingmen area was cool and there was an imperceptible pulse at CV 6, you could choose points from the repertoire of acupuncture points to tonify the Yang of the Kidney, such as ST 36, CV 4 or KI 7. This treatment plan, although broad, could be administered by itself or as the skeletal outline of treatment to other points that might be selected from other diagnostic data.

My approach is to build upon this first exam and to employ all the multiple exams presented in this book. As such I administer this exam on the first patient visit to gain the broad outlines of their disorder. However, I then proceed to the second physical examination that will be covered in Chapter 8.

This exam does not need to be repeated at every patient visit, although it could be because of its ease of administration. But because the broad root energies of a patient do not change that quickly, I tend to conduct this exam about every six visits to check on how these parameters may have changed.

NEW WORDS AND CONCEPTS

Abdominal clearing – the process whereby pathology is removed from the abdomen by

Table 6.3 Pathological significance of the Hara

Finding	Meaning
Temperature	
Cold skin without perspiration	Insufficient Yang
Hot without perspiration	Fever in superficial layers; Excess condition
Warm/hot CV 12 (Zhongwan)	Heat/Fire in Stomach leading to ST Yin Xu and possibly Kidney Yin Xu and systemic Yin Xu
Cool/cold Mingmen	Kidney Qi vacuity
Moisture	
Dry, rough, withered	Yin, Blood, Body Fluid Deficiency
Oily, sticky	Dampness
Cold moisture	Yang Deficiency
Resilience	
Hard abdomen (overall)	Blood Stagnation, Heat in Yangming
Masses at specific locations, hard in nature, resist dispersion under pressure	Accumulation of Blood Stasis or Phlegm, extravasated Blood, Heat Stasis; connect to specific organs
Firm, palpable masses, severe abdominal distension	Full patterns such as Blood Stagnation; connect to specific organs
Soft abdominal masses that move	Qi Stagnation
Tenderness with abdominal rigidity and rebound tenderness	Perforated viscus
Abdominal distension, tenderness, abdominal rigidity	Mesenteric vascular infarction
Muscle guarding, tenderness	Full pattern such as acute diverticulitis
Aggravation by palpation	Full condition (Shi or worms)
Soft lower abdomen	Weakness, Deficiency; connect to specific organs
Tense feeling ST 25 (Tianshu) L	Qi and/or Blood Stagnation
Loose feeling at ST 25R	Weak immunity, Lung Qi Xu
Tight feeling at ST 25R	Exogenous pathogenic invasion, possible concomitant LU Qi Xu
Loose mushy feeling at ST 25L	Liver Blood Deficiency
Combination of hard and soft at ST 25L	Liver Qi Stagnation due to Liver Blood Deficiency
Hard and knotted substernal region (CV 14 area)	Lung and Heart Qi constraint, constriction of the Hun (emotional problems)
Strength	
Weak feeling at ST 25 (Tianshu) L	Blood Deficiency
Weak feeling at CV12 (Zhongwan)	ST Yin Xu, weak ST/SP energy
Shape	
Pitting when pressed	Dampness
Swollen abdomen	Yang Xu
Bloated, distended abdomen	Replete intestinal Qi
Sunken, depressions	Deficiency
Puffiness	Yang Xu
Swollen right ribs	Liver Qi Stagnation
Swollen left ribs	Spleen Qi Xu
Pulsation at CV 6 (Qihai)	
Lack of	Kidney Qi Xu
Depression along Ren channel	
Lack of	Weak Yin organs and Ren channel function
Breathing	
Lack of	Lung and Kidney Qi Xu
Point pathology	See Table 6.2

palpation of points distal to the abdomen, i.e. the clearance points.

Dan tian – the area below the umbilicus, particularly in the CV 4 (Guanyuan)–CV 6 (Qihai) area, where the root of the Qi, the energy of the Kidney, resides.

Healthy Hara – an abdomen exhibiting no pathological characteristics.

Resilience – a soft, bouncy, elastic feeling of the abdomen.

Strength – a feeling of solidness determined by palpation.

QUESTIONS

1. What is ST 25L (Tianshu) a reflex point for?

2. Explain why the CV 12 (Zhongwan) area should be cool and why the ST 25R (Tianshu) area should be warm.

3. Name the nine normal characteristics of the healthy Hara examination.

4. Name five common signs of point pathology and the clinical significance of each.

5. What is the leading causative factor of Stomach Yin Deficiency?

6. What is the difference between strength and resilience?

7. What factors may have contributed to the tight CV 12 of the patient in Case 6.1? That is, describe the relationship between the patient's tight CV 12 and her overall symptomatology.

ABDOMINAL DIAGNOSIS QUIZ

Test your knowledge of the basic information found in Chinese introductory texts. Match the answers found in Column B with the clinical manifestations found in Column A. Some answers may be used more than once.

Column A

1. Urination is normal and the abdomen does not feel hard. With distension or fullness and tympanic note on percussion (like a drum)

2. Feels like a rubber bag, containing water with a splashing sound and a fluctuating sensation upon palpation

3. Immovable hard masses with pain at a definite site

4. Unfixed soft masses without pain

5. A cluster of masses palpated in the left abdomen with constipation

6. Rebounding pain in the lower right abdomen (suggest appendicitis)

Column B

a. Stagnant Qi

b. Stagnant Qi and Blood

c. Accumulation of fluid

d. Retention of dry stools

THE HEALTHY HARA EXAMINATION QUIZ

Match the diagnosis found in Column B with the area of abdominal inspection listed in Column A. Note: Some answers may be used more than once.

Column A
1. Temperature
2. Moisture
3. Resilience
4. Strength
5. Shape
6. Pulsation
7. Depression along the Ren channel
8. Point pathology

Column B
a. Qi
b. Kidney Qi
c. Yin
d. Yin and Yang
e. Blood
f. Other pathology

Match the clinical significance of the palpatory findings listed in Column A with the corresponding diagnostic findings described in Column B.

Column A
1. Tight stomach
2. Substernal tension
3. Palpable pulse at CV 6 (Qihai)
4. Tension at ST 25L (Tianshu)
5. Cool/cold Mingmen
6. Depression along Ren channel
7. Hard, unresilient tissues

Column B
a. Good genetic inheritance
b. Viewed as Kidney Yin Deficiency
c. Blood Stagnation
d. An etiological factor leading to ST Yin and ultimately KI Yin Deficiency
e. Indicative of Qi Xu, excess acid condition
f. Energy of the Kidneys communicating with each other
g. Insufficiency of KI Yin and Yang

Case 6.1 Emotional problems detected and treated at the tight CV 12 (Zhongwan) area

The patient was a female, age 35, with no real major complaint. She made an appointment for a check-up because her friend had been satisfied with the medical care I had given her. If she had to pick a complaint, she said that it was that she was emotionally high-strung and in general was stressed from her work.

Upon conducting the interview, the following subpathologies were identified.

- Tension ran in her family. She relayed that her grandparents suffered from nervous disorders.
- She was not happy as a child. She was a victim of incest and emotionally is still bothered by it.
- She reported feeling tightness in her intestines with a tendency towards constipation. She had constipation as a child.
- Her breasts are tender and she bites her nails.
- She also feels facial, hand and leg tension.
- She overthinks at 3–4 am when she wakes up.
- She has a ravenous appetite, abdominal distension and gas and eats a lot of soy products and raw foods on a daily basis. She is very thirsty, drinks alcohol and 'too much coffee'. She likes water and prefers salty foods followed by spicy.
- Her period is heavy, bright red with clots, with some vaginal discharge from time to time although it is not bothersome.
- She feels hot in the daytime.
- Her grandparents and mother had heart problems. She has pinpoint pain in the heart.
- She has mild allergy symptoms; you can hear phlegm in her voice.
- She had hearing loss as a child; father and grandparents had hearing loss too.
- She has darkness under her eyes and acne on the face.
- She has hip joint pain, nighttime urination, 6–7 times per night, and suffers from exhaustion from time to time.
- Her tongue was reddish-purple and flabby with a red tip. The surface was rough with small Yin Xu cracks throughout. There was no coat except for a greasy one in the Lower Jiao.
- The pulse was thin, weak and superficial in all positions. It was slightly stronger on the right and more slippery.
- The general abdominal exam (healthy Hara) was performed and the most significant finding was a shallow, tight, hard CV 12 (Zhongwan).
- Her primary diagnoses point to Liver Qi Stagnation with Heat, Yin Deficiency of the Stomach, Kidney Qi Xu and some Damp-Heat in the Lower Jiao.

Because of the abdominal findings, the course of treatment emphasized resolving the tightness at CV 12 (Zhongwan). Fifteen treatments were necessary to resolve this. As the tightness abated, so too did every subpathology listed above that was revealed in the interview, with the exception of the hearing loss.

'Abdominal clearing' (see Chapter 8) was used prior to every needle treatment to clarify the root. When the abdomen started clearing, her symptoms started to resolve quickly. When the tightness at CV 12 (Zhongwan) was resolved, the patient reported feeling 'warm, nurtured and taken care of'. Prior to one of the last treatments, the patient had an abnormal uterine bleeding at ovulation after which she felt 'a new freedom in her abdomen' (see Chapter 11). I considered this a functional healing crisis.

The patient was very receptive to deep breathing and awareness of her body and complied well with advice given to her. She felt better after the course of treatment; that is, less highly strung and she reported less stress at work. In fact, now she viewed it as a challenge.

Clinical notes

Mental degeneration: stages of progression, beginning with a tight stomach (from Lee 1992)

Stage 1 – Unhappiness, internal tension, nervousness; the person does not know what to do and is in conflict but seems calm on the outside, saying little if anything about internal troubles. The stool is small – sign of tenseness.

Stage 2 – The mind runs in a loop – the patient mentally repeats what was said over and over.

Urination increases, skin thickens and becomes wrinkled; there will be weight loss and dehydration. Appetite dwindles, as does the ability to laugh and sleep. The patient hates fire and won't cook.

Stage 3 – The patient can't think, hates noise, especially the sound of tapping on wood (Liver vs Kidney); such sounds produce shaking, depression and fearfulness. If the Heart is involved, he talks nonsense and won't listen, singing songs with no meaning at inappropriate times, laughing to himself or yelling. People with such imbalances complain bitterly about the treatment you give them, scold and threaten to sue. This is solid Heart imbalance. Needle HT 7 (Shenmen) for a short time and don't take their insults and outrages personally. When the Heart is deficient, the patient will be unhappy, crying constantly; the pressures of adversity will seem unbearable. Again needle HT 7 (Shenmen), but leave the needle in longer.

Stage 4 – At this stage, patient has no shame; she may run naked through the streets, singing loudly and climbing trees, and may be suicidal or homicidal. This is due to too much Stomach Heat – bleed ST 45 (Lidui), the Jing (well) point.

If the person loses sense or consciousness and the ability to talk, there is too much solid Heat and Phlegm in the Stomach. Sedate ST 40 (Fenglong). If violent and raving, the person should be shut in a room for 2 days and made to drink his own urine. This causes him to vomit up the Phlegm, after which he will return to his senses.

Schizophrenic patients who repeat themselves, whose voices go from a whisper to a shout in the same sentence, may not be getting enough Blood to the brain. Use Barefoot Doctors' needles down the spine and HT 5 (Tongli).

At any stage, ST 36 (Zusanli), SP 6 (Gongsun), LI 11 (Quchi), LI 4 (Hegu) or LU 7 (Lieque) will help to calm the patient and restore balance to the internal organs so that the Heart can again house the spirit.

7

The relationship between the etiological causes of disease and the pathophysiology of tension

As the practitioner of Oriental medicine knows, the etiological causes of illness fall into several categories. However, the feature that they share in common is that they may induce illness in one of two ways. First, if the strength of the pathogen surpasses the individual's ability to cope with it through the mechanism of their True Qi or anti-pathogenic Qi (immunity or Zheng Qi), disease can occur. In this scenario the pathogen is so virulent and persistent that it overcomes the body's defense mechanisms. Second, disease may develop if the immunity or True Qi of the body is weak.

Of these two, the Chinese generally believe that the leading cause of disease is the second reason postulated above, that is, weakness in the anti-pathogenic Qi, the Chinese concept of immunity. Hence, as we have noted, the Japanese system of therapeutics or a meridian-style acupuncture emphasizes treating the root, which generally stems from a weakness in the immunity of the individual. As we saw in Chapter 5, immunity is ultimately the outcome of strong Kidney energy in concert with the proper functioning of all the Zang-Fu organs that produce the Yin, Yang, Qi and Blood of the body. That is why the first physical examination, the healthy Hara, is performed. It provides the big picture, the bottom line, on the condition of the Yin and Yang, the Qi and Blood.

The causes of illness in Chinese medicine fall into five major categories.

1. The exogenous pathogens (the climates and factors which mimic them such as viruses or bacteria)

2. Endogenous pathogens (the emotions or the emotions elicited from Zang-Fu organ disharmony)
3. The miscellaneous causes of illness (such as diet, exercise, radiation, trauma)
4. The secondary pathological products (stagnant Blood and Damp-Phlegm)
5. Weakness in the antipathogenic Qi

All these pathogens affect the body in different ways and yet there are similarities. For instance, exogenous cold causes contraction and Stagnation thereby retarding the flow of Qi and Blood. In the case of endogenous factors, the Vital Qi may become stagnant in an individual who is grieving excessively or is depressed. Phlegm may turn into arthritic bone deformities. Regardless of the precise way in which each pathogen impinges upon the body, ultimately each disturbs its proper functioning, generally making it weak or by creating tension in the tissues of the body. Box 7.1 depicts how these pathogens lead to tension and therefore to illness. While the information is presented in a linear fashion, the lines of causality can be bent into circles, showing us the viciousness of this cycle. This same concept is shown in Figure 7.1.

Tension is a palpable stiffness or tightness of the tissues of the body. In Chinese medicine, this tension is viewed as lack of free flow of Qi and Blood. The classics remind us that the normal human condition is not one of tension: 'When people are born they are supple, and when they die they are stiff. When trees are born they are tender, and when they die they are brittle. Stiffness is thus a cohort of death; flexibility is a cohort of life. That is, the healthy body is supple' (Cleary 1993, p. 21).

Box 7.1 The etiological causes of illness

A→	B→	C→	D→	E→	F→
Etiological factors a. The exogenous pathogens (Wind, Cold, Damp, Dryness, Heat, Summer-Heat) b. The endogenous pathogens (anger, joy, fear, fright, grief, worry, melancholy) c. The miscellaneous pathogens (lifestyle variables including nutrition, exercise, trauma, stress, sex, breathing, vaccinations, operations, drugs, infection, inflammation) d. Secondary pathological products (Dampness, Water, Dilute Phlegm, Phlegm) e. Weakness in the antipathogenic factor	Derangement in flow of Qi a. Decreased (deficient) b. Stagnant c. Rebellious d. Sinking Derangement in the flow of Blood a. Deficient b. Stagnant c. Extravasated d. Hot	Tension, stiffness, detectable pain, may also be vacancy	Muscle tissue, meridian/organ contraction; expansion in another area	Decreased circulation (inadequate cellular nutrition)	Illness, structure, body becomes blocked, lumpy, shrinks, empty, which becomes a further etiological factor

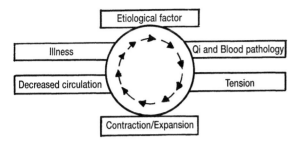

Figure 7.1 The cycle of tension.

Physiologically, when this tension or lack of free flow develops, the surrounding as well as underlying structures can concomitantly become affected and illness can ensue. As the Chinese remind us, without Qi and Blood there is no place in the human body that can be living and healthy (Weisman & Ellis 1985, p. 23). Muscle becomes constricted, lumpy or knotted; Qi and Blood do not flow smoothly through the meridians. This Qi and Blood pattern may affect the organ–meridian complexes. Figure 7.2 illustrates

in energetic terms and diagrammatic form how the pathophysiology of tension affects the body. As the figure demonstrates, Stagnation on all these levels – skin, muscle, meridian, Blood vessel and organ – is interrelated.

The Western paradigm's perception of tension is essentially the same but it is expressed in different language.

- It is maintained that where there is deoxygenation there may be cell, tissue and possibly organ death. This deoxygenation can come about as a result of stress or tension.
- Tension weakens the arterial system leading to decreased oxygenation and cellular nutrition (Qi and Blood problems).
- The venous system is affected, creating a build-up of carbon dioxide and lactic acid and increased pooling of Blood (stagnant Blood).
- Lymph vessels become compressed, thus impairing the lymphatic system. This weakens the immune system also.

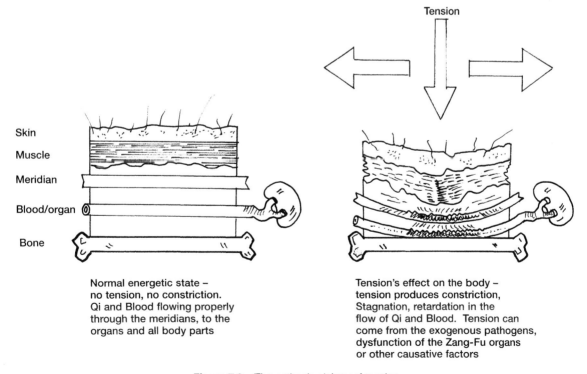

Skin

Muscle

Meridian

Blood/organ

Bone

Normal energetic state –
no tension, no constriction.
Qi and Blood flowing properly
through the meridians, to the
organs and all body parts

Tension's effect on the body –
tension produces constriction,
Stagnation, retardation in the
flow of Qi and Blood. Tension can
come from the exogenous pathogens,
dysfunction of the Zang-Fu organs
or other causative factors

Figure 7.2 The pathophysiology of tension.

● The nervous system is aggravated, creating irritation, pain and firing of nerves (Heat Stasis, Stagnation and Fire syndrome manifestations).

The scientific theory of stress provides an excellent outline as to why specific symptoms develop and why tension is one of its cardinal benchmarks. Until the 19th century, stress referred to external forces on physical objects rather than to internal psychological states. Modern use of the term can be traced to 20th-century physiological psychologist Walter Cannon and Canadian physician Hans Selye. Cannon defined the classic 'fight-or-flight' reaction that occurs when the sympathetic portion of the nervous system is activated to prepare for emergency.

Selye defined a stressor as an event that places inordinate demands upon the body and the natural adaptive bodily defenses that cope with it. This process is called the general adaptation syndrome and includes three stages: the alarm reaction, resistance and exhaustion.

During the alarm stage, hormone levels increase and there is strong physical and emotional arousal. If this reaction is not sufficient to cope, the resistance phase begins. Resistance is either successful or unsuccessful; that is, the stressor is either tamed or takes over. If coping is not successful, hormonal reserves are exhausted and fatigue, exhaustion, depression, anxiety or even death can set in (DeVito 1994).

Stress, then, has the effect of creating tension in the individual. Stress is a state of disequilibrium in a living creature – a complex of injurious defense mechanisms caused by any harmful stimulus.

Stress is an imbalance in the autonomic nervous system which is composed of two divisions: the sympathetic and the parasympathetic. The sympathetic nervous system is responsible for allowing flight and fright reactions. It is the functional mechanism for quick, survival responses. It works best when it is only used for these relatively rare reactions. The parasympathetic nervous system is responsible for the everyday normal physiological functions such as digestion, circulation and excretion. It is important to point out that both of these systems can become affected by stress, not just the sympa-

thetic. There are five basic response patterns to stimuli that make up these two branches of the autonomic nervous system (ANS), detailed in the Clinical notes at the end of the chapter.

Tension or stress is a leading healthcare problem in modern life. About two-thirds of all visits to doctors are stress related. While stress is a fact of life, the way one experiences stress is to a certain degree individualized. There are also many common clinical manifestations of stress that affect the body systemically and their import should not be discounted. Box 7.2 provides a fairly comprehensive list of the physiological effects of stress and Box 7.3 details common illnesses caused by stress.

While tension or stress is ordinarily detected in Chinese medicine through a wiry or taut pulse*, or through specific areas of pain because Stagnation manifests as pain, the Chinese do not emphasize palpating other areas of the body for tension. Yet this tension is detectable in the body if we take the time to feel it.

When tension is palpated, patients are obviously touched. They may not even know that they have this tension until it is uncovered. As was pointed out in Chapter 1, when these areas are felt, the patient often questions why that particular area feels this way. As Mark Seem would say, the patient's body-mind energetic is probed and reminded of its somatized state (Seem 1990, p. 71). Simultaneously, the palpation of these tissues frequently frees up the tension such that palpation is not only diagnostic but also therapeutic.

As Seem notes (p. 71), in releasing constriction, not only are pain and tension in the affected areas alleviated but circulation in the lymph, venous, arterial and nervous systems is boosted, improving overall regulation of the body-mind and enhancing immunity.

French-Vietnamese acupuncturist, the esteemed Nguyen Van Nghi, in discussing treatment strategies states, 'One must ascertain which energetic layer is disrupted – Wei, Ying or Jing – intervening at the appropriate level to bring the

---

* Jin mai = the tight pulse; xian mai = the wiry, bowstring pulse.

Box 7.2   The physiology of stress

Stress causes adrenocorticotropic hormone (ACTH) release from the pituitary gland. ACTH stimulates the adrenal glands to release corticosteroid hormones such as hydrocortisone and epinephrine, resulting in the physiological events described below. Additionally, hydrocortisone has an effect on the hippocampus of the brain. The hippocampus stores memory. Certain severe types of stress such as depression and posttraumatic stress lead to permanent hippocampal shrinkage.*

1. Increased heart rate, the pulse quickens
2. Muscles tense
3. Blood pressure rises
4. The senses sharpen
5. Stored energy in the form of glucose and fat is made available to cells, increasing ketones and fat cells in the Blood such as cholesterol
6. Stress hormones called catecholamines make the Blood thicker and more prone to clotting, likewise increasing the risk of heart attack and stroke
7. The stress hormone cortisol encourages fat to be dumped into the midsection of the body
8. Pupil dilation increases peripheral vision that can result in blurry vision
9. Ear ringing or clicking can develop due to steady contraction in auditory muscles
10. Shallow breathing deprives the body of oxygen
11. Blood vessels constrict in arms and legs
12. Increased sweat results in decreased minerals that carry electrical signals to muscles, causing muscle cramps and decreased body temperature
13. Decreased secretions in the mouth make the mouth dry and cut back on natural bacterial control
14. More air is swallowed, causing belching and flatulence
15. Fungi multiply
16. The immune response to viruses is dampened
17. The number of infection-fighting white Blood cells decreases and there are changes in their function plus the activity of other immune system cells is impaired
18. Warts and skin reactions such as hives or psoriasis can occur due to chemicals released by the nervous system
19. Forgetfulness, indecisiveness and difficulty concentrating can result
20. Severe stress, as in the case of posttraumatic stress disorder, clinical depression or Cushing's syndrome, can cause hippocampal shrinkage of the brain. The hippocampus stores memory.
21. The habitual overreaction of one side of our nervous system causes wear and tear on our nervous system – another good description for the aging process.

---

* It is interesting to note that with age, adrenal output increases, also leading to hippocampal shrinkage and a common symptom of old age, memory loss.

Box 7.3 Common illnesses caused by stress

Aging, short-term memory loss, indecisiveness
Anxiety, depression, mood swings
Asthma, shortness of breath, allergies
Backache, neck, shoulder and jaw pain
Cancer, cold sores, common cold
Constipation
Fatigue
Headaches, migraines
Heart disease, cardiac arrest, stroke, heart arrhythmias, chest pain and atherosclerosis
Insomnia
Irregular periods, low sexual interest, genital herpes
Seizures, hypertension
Stomachache, flatulence, colitis, irritable bowel syndrome, diarrhea, ulcers, diabetes, overeating, heartburn
Premature delivery, low birth weight, infertility
Psoriasis, rashes, hives, acne
Psychological problems, anger, resentment
Weight gain or loss

entire organism back into harmony'. Mark Seem builds upon this concept.

...the Wei level is the surface. It is yang. It is composed of the main meridians and the secondary meridians (tendinomuscular, divergent, longitudinal luos). As Yang it tends towards excess and reacts constantly to outside stressors producing holding patterns and somatic defense mechanisms. Palpation frees this area up so that the jing or core level can be accessed. The Ying level is the internal, functional layer. It consists of the organs and is energetic. These Zang-Fu organs can be accessed through acupuncture, particularly through the Mu and Shu points. The Jing level is the core level. It is yin. It is prenatal, encoded material that directs growth and development. It is found in the kidney and the Eight Extraordinary Meridians – encoded energetic vectors that lay out the pathways that will later become the regular meridians, organs, and functions. It is the root to treatment and treatment at this level reminds the body of how it should perform. (Seem 1992)

This Jing or root level can be palpated directly when the Wei level is freed up. Also, as we will see, the Confluent points are primary treatment points that play a major role in allowing us to reach the Jing level and thus remind the body of how it should perform.

Acupuncturist and herbalist Jake Fratkin mentions that according to Oriental medical theory, specifically according to Shudo Denmei:

The wei leads the ying qi. What this means is that when we affect the wei through surface needling, this in turn guides and leads the ying Qi that is in the meridian and ultimately the organ. Thus when we do superficial contact needling we actually have greater effect on the interior than deeper needling. (Fratkin 1996a)

This is a further reason why freeing up the surface is so effective in treatment and why the Japanese predilection is to needle shallowly.

As Seem concludes, in short, acupuncture (and palpation) is at once a local, myofascial release (of the surface) and a systemic probe to set the organism back on track (treating the Jing or the root) but not an internal organ functional therapy per se. And lastly, if needed, relevant treatment of disease points to treat the Zang-Fu energetics can be judiciously incorporated (Seem 1992). Table 7.1 summarizes the relationship between the energetic levels of the body and treatment.

From a physiological point of view the role of palpation is to free up the surface of tension and to stimulate the Jing by treating the root. This strategy will become more obvious in Chapter 8 on the energetics of the diagnosis and clearance points and Chapter 11 on the overview of the integrative process.

Any area in the body can become tense. However, certain areas are more energetically predisposed to tension than others because of the physiological roles that they play in the body. These areas include but are not limited to the stomach, navel, scars, thighs, sinuses, neck and back. Consequently, an added dimension to the Japanese physical examination processes will include a detailed examination of each of these areas. Figure 7.3 depicts an integrated view of the important areas of the body prone to tension and how they may affect the health of the Zang-Fu organs. The reasons for the development of congestion in each of these areas and their corresponding treatment are outlined in Section 3.

NEW WORDS AND CONCEPTS

Autonomic nervous system – a part of the nervous system concerned with control of invol-

Table 7.1 The relationship between the energetic levels of the body and treatment

Levels	Nature	Treatment
Wei – surface	Yang – tends toward Excess, reacts to stress; creates bodily armor in the meridians	Local (branch) – remove the Excess, i.e. with palpation or superficial needling
Ying – functional	Interface – the Zang-Fu organs	With treatment of disease points *after* the branch has been freed up and the root treated through palpation
Jing – core	Yin – tends toward Deficiency. Found in Kidney and Eight Extra Meridians	Root – needs tonification with select, limited points, i.e. needles and/or moxa

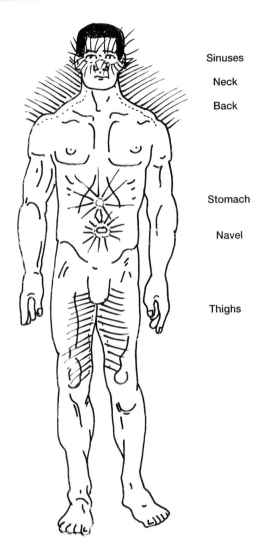

Sinuses

Neck

Back

Stomach

Navel

Thighs

Figure 7.3 An integrated view of bodily energetics via the areas prone to tension.

untary bodily functions such as the heart, the glands and smooth muscle tissue. It is commonly defined as including the sympathetic or thoracolumbar division and the parasympathetic or craniosacral division.

General adaptation syndrome – the natural adaptive bodily defenses that deal with stress.

Hippocampal shrinkage – a phenomenon that can occur due to age or hydrocortisone affinity to the hippocampus. The effect of this occurrence is memory loss.

Jing level – the combined prenatal and postnatal Qi that is stored in the Kidneys. It is a deep core energetic level consisting of stored Essence and genetic potential.

Parasympathetic nervous system – that part of the autonomic nervous system which produces vasodilation of the part of the body supplied, fall of Blood pressure, copious secretion of saliva, increased gastrointestinal activity, slowing of the heart and contraction of the pupil.

Stress – a state of disequilibrium in a living creature; a complex of injurious defense mechanisms caused by any harmful stimulus.

Sympathetic nervous system – that part of the autonomic nervous system which stimulates sympathetic fibers to raise Blood pressure, dilate eyes, depress gastrointestinal activity, accelerate the heart, raise arm hair and secrete small amounts of thick saliva.

Tension – a palpable stiffness or tightness of the tissues of the body; in Chinese medicine a lack of free flow of Qi and Blood.

Wei level – the first and most exterior of the Four Stages that can be invaded by exogenous Heat. It corresponds essentially to the skin and the muscles.

Ying level – the second of the Four Stages, corresponding to the nutritive Qi that is associated with the Blood.

QUESTIONS

1. Describe the mechanism by which tension is created in the body's tissues, resulting in illness.

2. How is palpation diagnostic as well as therapeutic with regards to tension? Compare it to pulse reading in relation to its ability to detect tension.

3. What are the major areas of the body that are prone to tension and why?

4. Name eight etiological factors that can contribute to the development of tense, unresilient tissue. Which do you think is the leading causative factor?

5. What group of points allows palpation to treat the Jing level and thereby treat the root?

6. What must be done in order to access the Jing level?

7. Pick three physiological manifestations of stress mentioned in this chapter. Then, using Chinese medical theory, give a mechanism for the occurrence of each. Try to use the theory of the endogenous pathogens (Seven Emotions) in at least one of your answers.

8. Using both a Chinese medical and a Western medical perspective, explain how the Kidneys are affected by stress.

9. Using Chinese medical theory, explain how stress might lead to hippocampal shrinkage.

Clinical notes

Learn the patterns of stress (O'Brien 1994)

There are five primary stress response patterns. Which is your most common reaction to stressful situations? The most dangerous ones are the mild ones, the constant annoyances that we've grown accustomed to and do little or nothing about. Over time these little episodes of inappropriate behavior can become something serious.

1. The mild sympathetic response. These are life's little annoyances and habitual behaviors that keep us wound up and can be anything that stimulates us regularly or for a prolonged period.
2. The severe sympathetic response. These are the situations or events that cause major mind/ body stimulation, such as being involved in a car accident or being held at gunpoint or assaulted.
3. The mild parasympathetic response. Repetitious, monotonous activities cause our bodies

to begin to shut down. Boring lectures, sitting for long periods and conditioned, dulling responses fit here.
4. The severe parasympathetic response. Depression, seasonal affective disorder (SAD) and responses of extreme withdrawal are a dominant reaction by the parasympathetic half of the ANS.
5. The manic response. This is an emotional and psychological roller-coaster ride. One moment the person is flying high, the next moment he is down or feeling blue. This condition alternately touches both ends of the ANS response spectrum. Some causes are organic and can be treated with drugs and natural light. Other causes have a psychological base and respond well to therapy. This is the hardest response pattern to self-treat. If you feel you have a problem with mood swings, seek professional help. There are treatments that can help most people.

Protect your heart (Doner 1996)

Stress and anger can sneak up on you. You may think you're not angry if you don't scream and fight with people but as far as the nervous system is concerned, anger is a far more subtle emotion. A wide range of attitudes – suspicion, frustration, impatience, aggression, hostility, a lack of concern for others – can all cause a damaging stress response. Suppressing anger doesn't seem to help either. People at both ends of the spectrum who either habitually hold anger in or always express it get into risky territory. To check your hostility levels ask yourself the following questions.

1. Are you generally mistrustful and cynical?
2. Do you secretly think people whom you consider to be 'stupid' or 'pathetic' deserve whatever happens to them?
3. Do you get very angry if someone disrupts your daily routine?
4. Do you often accuse family members of misplacing things only to find that you've done it?
5. If someone at work offers to help you with a task, do you assume they're doing it exclusively to help themselves?

Box 7.4 Adaptive ways to cope with stress

Learn to recognize what causes your stress or your patient's stress, how you react to it and how to deal with it. Construct a stress management program for yourself or your patients. It works! Include some of the following.

- Communication to resolve conflicts with other people, social support and close relationships
- Exercise
- Fun. Take breaks, get away from stressors, get enough sleep and rest
- Good nutrition with foods such as zinc, vitamin C, vegetables and fruits, and foods with serotonin (lack of serotonin affects stress levels)
- Guided imagery, quiet reflection, warm baths, flowers, massage
- Learn new ways to deal with stress
- Listen to music
- Look at change as a challenge, not a threat
- Try progressive muscle relaxation, aromatherapy, reflexology
- Recognize how stress affects you
- Reduce mental irritation, replace bothersome thoughts with constructive ones
- Relaxation techniques such as deep abdominal breathing, yoga, meditation
- Seek information about any problem you have and create strategies for achieving your goals
- Simplify your daily routine, regulate time and tasks realistically
- Take responsibility for your life, set realistic goals, cultivate an inner sense of control, control the things that you can, don't worry about the things you can't

---

6. Do you honk your horn repeatedly when the car in front of you doesn't move quickly after the light turns green?

If you answered 'yes' to any of these questions you might want to try some of the adaptive strategies listed in Box 7.4.

In patients with heart disease, feelings of sadness or tension may double the odds that coronary arteries will narrow, causing a temporary but potentially dangerous drop in the Blood supply to the heart (*Time* 1997).

8

Physical examination II and the palpation process

PART 1: PHYSICAL EXAMINATION II – THE MODIFIED ABDOMINAL MAP AND THE PALPATION SCHEMA

As was mentioned in Chapter 1, abdominal diagnosis is one aspect of meridian therapy that has seen a variety of approaches over the years since slightly different methods were utilized amongst its originators. Therefore we encounter considerable variation when we look at how it is practiced. Be that as it may, since they share a common origin, all the approaches have many more similarities than differences.

One of these areas concerns abdominal maps. As was discussed in Chapter 4, there are various historical abdominal maps but a careful perusal of them illustrates that there is much agreement among them on diagnostic areas.

The particular abdominal map that this book concentrates on is what I have termed the modified abdominal map. One feature of this map is that it is easy to use. It employs only six points that elegantly and accurately serve as a sound and relatively complete basis of diagnosis. Having used it on thousands of patients, I have found that it diagnoses all their presentations and tells us about their condition in general terms.

This chapter is the heart of the book and hence several major items are addressed herein. In Part 1, emphasis is placed on the diagnosis points of the modified abdominal map. First, the clinical significance of each diagnosis point on the abdomen is discussed. Second, the method of palpating each point is covered. Third, the differential diagnosis of the palpatory findings is interpreted. Part 2 covers the palpation process. The clearance or treatment points are explored, specifically how to palpate them and why they work. The differential diagnosis of the clearance findings is then outlined. The development of the treatment plan based upon abdominal palpation, as well as the integration of other diagnostic data is discussed later in Chapter 11.

Because this topic is probably new to the practitioner and additionally consists of several steps, all the material discussed within this chapter is also summarized in convenient tables for rapid clinical consultation. As always, the practitioner is encouraged to use these tables as an aid. The understanding, the thinking process behind what is being done, is most important. If practitioners understand the method, they will be able to move from step to step and will not require the tables that can hinder the course of palpation and diagnosis if they are overly relied upon. Practice with abdominal clearing will facilitate the internalization of the material.

PATIENT POSITIONING, INSTRUCTIONS AND A WORD ABOUT JAPANESE POINT LOCATION

The modified abdominal map consists of six points that are used individually and cumulatively to diagnose the patient. These points are CV 14 (Juque), CV 12 (Zhongwan), ST 25 bilateral (Tianshu), CV 6 (Qihai) and CV 4 (Guanyuan). Each of these points has multiple energetics, which make them valuable for diagnosis. All are palpated perpendicularly, with the exception of the CV 14 area that is palpated obliquely upward. The modified abdominal map is presented here again for clinical convenience (Fig. 8.1).

When undergoing abdominal diagnosis, patients should be as relaxed as possible, lying in a supine position with the face up and arms by their side. While bending the knees is useful for relaxing the abdominal wall, this also makes it more difficult to locate abdominal reactions. Therefore, the abdomen should be diagnosed without the patient's knees bent or supported by a pillow.

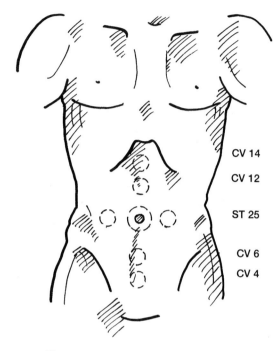

Figure 8.1 The modified abdominal map.

Patients should be instructed to breathe in and then out. As the patient breathes out, look at them and then press to the appropriate depth of palpation, also using the correct angle. Specific instructions will be covered under the discussion of each point that follows.

The proper palpation method of the abdominal points involves using the hand on the same side as your dominant eye or your dominant hand. Nails must be short to palpate the points correctly. The fingers should be positioned next to each other in a gentle curve. The three middle fingers are the palpating fingers. Figure 8.2 illustrates the proper positioning of the palpating fingers. Note that they form a vector that palpates the point as an area and gently establishes contact with the Qi in the point in a less invasive manner than would occur if one were to use one finger to palpate.

Practitioners should slowly touch the patient's skin and press down as if they were going through six discrete layers of tissue. These tissues would include the skin, the muscle, the meridian, the Blood, the organ and the bone. Palpation is

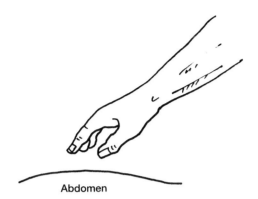

Figure 8.2 The proper finger positioning for palpating the abdomen.

done at the junction of the meridian and the organ. In terms of depth this junction is identical to the depths of insertion one would use if employing a needle. Hence, practitioners should

have both an intellectual knowledge of this depth as well as sensitizing themselves to this depth by feel.

This three-dimensional view of what you are trying to touch is crucial. Knowledge of anatomy and meridian depths of insertion is invaluable. The whole purpose of this process is to establish contact with the energy of the point that is usually just above the organ layer. This image is depicted in Figure 8.3

The palpation technique is not abrupt or harsh. The practitioner slowly presses down to where the Qi of the point resides, which is what you are attempting to establish contact with at the meridian/organ junction. Palpate only to the level that you can, then quickly release the point once you have reached the desired level of palpation. There is no reason to stay on the point once the Qi has been contacted. Sometimes practitioners

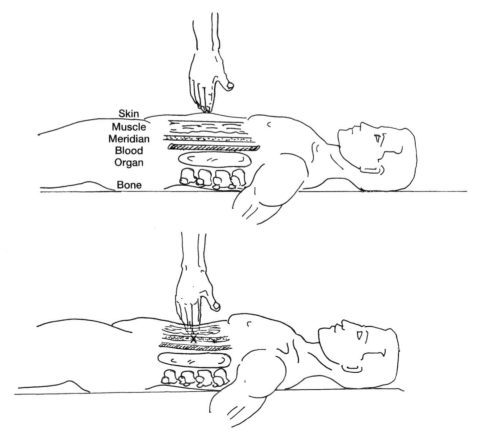

Figure 8.3 The energetic layers of the body in relation to palpation.

linger on the point and stimulate it by rubbing. This is not correct. At this point, the acupuncture point is being contacted, felt, only to diagnose and requires no further stimulation. The palpation of the point is only done once.

As a teacher, the major clinical faux pas that I find with those starting to learn this material is that they tend to palpate the abdomen too deeply, too fast and they stay on the diagnosis point too long. I have found the best way to attempt to correct this is by having the practitioner press the point on a patient followed by me pressing it. The patient can then offer feedback to the novice so that they can readjust their palpation depth, speed and retention time. However, when learning palpation from a text I would recommend pressing on points as deeply as you would press on other points you may be more familiar with, such as Front Mu points. Also reread this material, practice and sensitize yourself to the presence of the patient and the goals of palpation and the depths of insertion you would use with needling.

The depth of palpation and the interpretation of that palpation are the most critical steps when one uses palpation as a method of diagnosis. It is important to point out that a diagnosis per se is not necessarily being established but rather a pattern of energy. Pressing too deeply or not pressing deep enough will yield incorrect results. All the remaining steps in this system through to treatment are contingent upon this emerging pattern. The treatment is directly linked to the interpretations derived from the sensations elicited from palpation so the proper depth is critical.

Prior to the start of the palpation process, patients should be informed about the procedure. You should explain that you will be pressing on certain points on the abdomen that will aid your interpretation of their bodily energy. Explain that you want them to report any sensations that they experience. The most common sensations are pain, discomfort or aversion to being touched. These are all signs of Excess. However, it is not uncommon for patients to report that although there is some discomfort, they like the touch. This is an indication of Deficiency. Patients may report other sensations

such as feelings of warmth or feelings radiating to other areas and it is up to the practitioner to determine their meanings.

It is extremely important that the practitioner look at the patient at all times during the palpation process, just as one should when needling a patient. Patients may say that the palpation is all right because it has not reached a threshold of pain or that they can 'take it', but this process is not about evoking pain or having the patient stoically bear the procedure. It is about interpreting the patient's and your reaction to the palpation.

Initially, patients may say that the palpation is fine and yet be sweating, breathing shallowly or grimacing, again because they are not familiar with the proceedings. Once they become used to this process they are better at giving practitioners the feedback they are looking for.

Usually what the clinician feels corresponds to what the patient feels. For instance, the patient says the point feels tight and the practitioner agrees. Always give the patient the first opportunity to comment on the experience. Then, practitioners should share their perceptions with patients so that they learn how to be aware of the findings. For instance, if the patient says that the point feels tight, you agree and confirm this after the patient has had the opportunity to speak.

There are times when there is a difference between what the patient and the practitioner feel. When this occurs, practitioners should rely upon their perception of the areas palpated. Again, point this out to the patient. For instance, often I will press CV 14 (Juque) and the patient will say that it feels fine but I tell them that I feel it is tense and that I am going to loosen it up by pressing on one of the clearance points. I then go back and repalpate the CV 14 area and they say that it feels looser even though they thought that it was fine to begin with. Patients require a reference point for their perceptions, which is what occurs when you show them how it can feel better and explain things to them. Their body-mind energetic needs to be probed and this is what the palpation process is activating.

Just as there are differences within Chinese medicine, and sometimes even from practitioner to practitioner, Japanese point locations may

Patient's name:_____ Date:_____

Major complaint and accompanying symptoms: _____

_____

Palpate these points	Palpation sensation, degree of tenderness or vacancy	Signs of point pathology	Clinical significance of point pathology or palpation sensation	Clearance points used and degree of clearance obtained
CV 15/14 (Jiuwei/Juque)				
CV 12 (Zhongwan)				
ST 25 (Tianshu) Left and Right				
CV 6 (Qihai)				
CV 4 (Guanyuan)				

General abdominal map: circle points which were tender:

Results of clearance:_____

_____

_____

_____

_____

_____

_____

Figure 8.4 The modified abdominal examination form.

vary from Chinese point locations. When those points are employed in the palpation schema, those differences will be pointed out.

The diagnosis points of the Hara will now be discussed, including their clinical energetics, how to palpate the point, how the point feels and the meaning of that palpatory finding. If you are performing this exam, record the data requested on Figure 8.4. This exam takes less than 10 minutes to perform. Each point is palpated only once.

SIGNIFICANT DIAGNOSTIC POINTS OF THE HARA AND THE DIFFERENTIAL DIAGNOSIS OF ABDOMINAL FINDINGS

CV 14 (Juque)

Clinical energetics

The condition of the Heart is palpated in the epigastric area. The CV 15–14 area is the diagnostic area of the Heart. CV 14 (Juque) proper is the Front Mu point of the Heart and CV 15 (Jiuwei), in the same local area only 1 cun away, has functions similar to the Front Mu of the Heart.

As a Front Mu point, this area indicates the condition of the Yin and Yang of the Heart. It pacifies the spirit, adjusts the Qi, harmonizes the Stomach and benefits the diaphragm. Physical heart problems can be detected from palpation of this point as well as energetic problems such as deficient Heart Blood. This point also signifies Stagnation in the Upper Jiao and lack of free flow of Liver Qi.

Palpation method, sensation and differential diagnosis

First locate CV 14 by measuring 6 cun above the umbilicus. Then by feel, slide down to the first available space you feel you can press into. Then palpate lightly downward about 0.5 cun and obliquely upward simultaneously in a gentle upward swoop a distance of about 1–2 inches. Have the patient breathe out as you press in. The oblique palpation angle is used because the patient may have an elongated xiphoid process or a narrow sternocostal angle that prevents

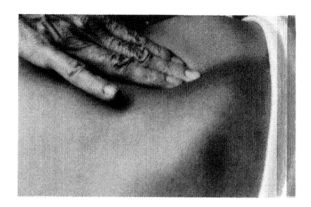

Figure 8.5 How to palpate the CV 14–15 area.

access to the point. The place of entry for the palpating fingers is usually around CV 13 or even close to CV 12 but you will be palpating the CV 14–15 area because of the angle of palpation. Put the three middle fingers together to form a gentle palpating arch. Figure 8.5 illustrates how to palpate this area.

This point is frequently tender and guarded but some patients say that this point feels fine. The practitioner needs to be assured that there is no tightness here. Painkillers may reduce sensitivity at this point.

The skin should not feel as if it were a stretched drumskin. The perception of tightness is very subtle and is perceived through practice. This point presents as uncomfortable or tense for any patient with a diagnosed Heart condition and/or considerable Liver Qi Stagnation. The healthy area should feel soft and resilient and have no pulsation. If the area is hard or there is a strong pulsation, the Qi of the Heart is deficient. An electrical sensation is also indicative of weakness of the Qi of the Heart.

Serizawa (1988) offers additional differential diagnoses. He claims:

Palpable pulsation on gentle pressure is usually a sign of mental excitability – if felt only on deep pressure it is indicative of a weakness in the heart. If there is resistance without pulsation then there is hypersecretion in the stomach, and if the resistance extends to the right hypochondrium then the digestion is impaired and the emptying of the stomach is too slow. (p. 26)

CV 12 (Zhongwan)

Clinical energetics

CV 12 (Zhongwan) is the Front Mu of the Stomach, the Influential point that dominates the Fu organs and the controlling point of the Middle Jiao. CV 12 (Zhongwan) adjusts the Stomach, tonifies the Spleen and Stomach, regulates the Qi and, as the activating point of the Middle Jiao, transforms Damp.

According to Stomach physiology, CV 12 is the source of all Yin, hence its ability to diagnose the Yin of the body. Stress is the most common cause of Stomach Yin Deficiency. When a person experiences stress in this area it becomes tight. This is diagnostic of ST Yin Xu and potentially Kidney Yin Deficiency whereby Earth fails to control Water. Additionally, it can signify the beginning of mental deterioration because when Yin is consumed Phlegm and Heat are produced and these factors can affect the mind.

By virtue of internal pathways, this point is diagnostic of other organ disharmonies. For example, the Stomach main meridian begins at CV 12 (Zhongwan) as does the Lung meridian. The Liver meridian ends there (another reason why it is a reflection of stress), the Spleen internal trajectory starts there and the Triple Warmer, Large Intestine, Ren channel, Heart and Small Intestine meridians all pass through this point.

Palpation method, sensation and differential diagnosis

This point is palpated perpendicularly to a depth of about 0.5–1.0 inches when the patient breathes out. When the point is felt it should have strength (feel solid) and resilience (possess elasticity or springiness like a rubber ball) and not feel hard or vacant. A sensation of tightness generally indicates Yin Deficiency and/or Phlegm or food Stagnation. Vacancy indicates Qi Deficiency in the Middle Jiao. Chapter 6 also pointed out that CV 12 should energetically feel relatively cooler than the lower abdomen.

Serizawa (1988) adds further diagnostics. He says in reference to CV 12 (Zhongwan):

It should be firmer than CV 14–15 area but less tight than CV 6. If it feels like dough, soft and weak, and there is a noticeable pulsation then there is atony of the stomach. If there is deep-seated root-like resistance, there is likely pyloric stenosis and hypertrophic gastritis. If the pulsation is very small like a grain of rice or hard and stick-like, situated between CV 12 and the navel, this would indicate emptiness of the stomach and spleen. A strong aortic pulsation extending up to the sternum can indicate a psycho- and stomach neurosis, whilst a wide resistance on either side indicates mental depression and insomnia. A stick-like induration extending from CV 12 (Zhongwan) down to CV 9 (Shuifen) can also indicate a pancreatic disturbance and too slow emptying of the stomach. Ticklishness in this area, or the area feeling like a balloon or bag of water indicates Spleen Qi xu. (p. 26)

ST 25 (Tianshu) bilateral

Clinical energetics

In Japanese acupuncture, Stomach 25 (Tianshu), like many points, is considered to be an area rather than a finite spot. It is sometimes regarded as the area extending from ST 25 through 28 (Shuidao). I palpate it closer to the traditional point. However, if the patient has signs of point pathology or pain between ST 25 and 28, view it as if it were ST 25.

Stomach 25 has multiple energetics which make it one of the most powerful points in the body. According to the *Neijing*, ST 25 is, as most of us have learned, the Front Mu point of the Large Intestine. As such, it can add Yin to the organ. Another of its most powerful energetics is that it can adjust the Large Intestine, be it deficient in any aspect (Yin/Yang) or excessive, such as having stagnant Qi or Blood.

ST 25 is the meeting of the Yangming energetic layers of the Stomach and the Large Intestine and can be used to regulate them both. It can be used for chronic Deficiency of the Spleen and Kidney. It regulates menstrual flow and reinforces the Qi of the Stomach and the Spleen. It can also be viewed as the reflex point of the appendix, indicating that the lymphatic glands are weak or exhausted.

According to the *Nanjing*, ST 25 (Tianshu) on the right side is the Front Mu of the Lungs, the Master of the Qi. Because of this relationship to energy, it has ability to move stagnant Qi and Blood in the intestines and elsewhere. This connection to the Lungs makes it a reflex point for problems of the nose and throat.

According to Yoshio Manaka, ST 25 (Tianshu) on the right is the Front Mu point of the Triple Warmer. This important energetic makes ST 25 a diagnostic point for immunity. We saw in Chapter 5 that the Triple Warmer can be viewed as the theoretical construct that explains the production of the essential substances that constitute our immunity and certainly the Large Intestine plays a role in retrieving water and nutrients which contribute to our immunity.

Dr Nagano calls this same point the reflex of lymphatic glandular exhaustion. In a nutshell, the concept of lymphatic glandular exhaustion refers to an impaired immune system. In this case the immunity has been impaired not through a failure to produce essential substances via the Triple Warmer but rather as a result of secondary infections developing due to a failure of the body's lymphatic tissue to destroy pathogens at the time of the initial invasion. Thus the lymphatic glands are weak or exhausted. In any case, immunity is compromised.

Western medicine lends further support for the relationship between the intestines and immunity. The fight against infection is one of its key roles. Research has shown that the intestinal tract has an important function in the immune system (Kagoshima 1996). Valuable intestinal bacteria make up the natural and critical ecosystem of the intestines and play an important role in the development of the immune system because they fight exogenous pathogens. These bacteria, called probiotics, consist of approximately 500 species that inhabit the human intestine. They include *Lactobacillus acidophilus*, *Lactobacillus bulgaricus* and *Streptococcus thermophilus*. In sufficient numbers they keep disease-causing bacteria from overpopulating the intestines. They also improve digestion, manufacture B vitamins and boost immune system activity (Challem 1996). This delicate ecosystem can become disrupted due to antibiotic use, diet, stress or even excessive hygienic habits. Hence, the role of ST 25 as an indicator of intestinal function is of prime significance and it is included as a primary point in the modified abdominal map.

ST 25 on the left is located over the area where the portal vein, the only vein that carries nutrients, goes to the Liver. Hence there is an intimate connection between the Liver and ST 25 on the left. As such, this point can be used to diagnose Liver problems, be they Liver Qi or Liver Blood Stagnation and/or Liver Blood Deficiency.

Palpation method, sensation and differential diagnosis

Palpate ST 25 on the left first, then on the right. The reason for this is that ST 25L will be easier to clear because it is on the course of the descending colon. If you cleared ST 25 on the right first, energy could be moved to ST 25L, thus making that point more difficult to clear.

Press into the point when the patient exhales. As described in Chapter 6, the Stomach 25 area should feel resilient on both sides, have strength on the left and be warm on the right. ST 25 is palpated with several fingers, as for all points on the modified abdominal map; that is, the point is felt more as an area than as a discrete fixed point.

Lack of strength on the left means Liver Blood Deficiency. Tightness indicates Liver Qi and Blood Stagnation. A combination of tightness and emptiness means Liver Qi Stagnation with Liver Blood Deficiency. On the right, lack of resilience signifies Lung Qi Xu and/or weak immunity.

CV 6 (Qihai) and CV 4 (Guanyuan)

The CV 6 (Qihai) through CV 4 (Guanyuan) area in the hypogastric region, referred to in Chinese medicine as the Dan tian, is considered to be the Kidney reflex area. It tells us about the condition of the foundation Yin and Yang, otherwise known as the Yuan Qi. These points essentially tell us about the condition of the Kidney.

CV 6 (Qihai)

Clinical energetics

CV 6 (Qihai) is the center of energy in the body. It adjusts and tonifies Kidney Qi, activates the Yuan Qi because it connects to the concentration of Yuan Qi in the body, tonifies the Yin and the Yang and connects to the Chong channel.

CV 4 (Guanyuan)

Clinical energetics

Specifically, this point is the Front Mu point of the Small Intestine. Small Intestine function in Chinese medicine falls under the domain of the Spleen, its principal organ of digestion and assimilation. Due to this function, CV 4 firms up the body, builds Blood, adjusts the Qi, makes the Yang return and builds Kidney Yang, because Earth (Spleen) controls Water (Kidney).

Palpation method, sensation and differential diagnosis

As we saw in Chapter 6, the lower abdomen should feel warm and resilient, indicating the presence of the Yang and the ampleness of the Kidney Qi respectively. Ample Kidney Qi makes this area resilient in feel and slightly protruding in shape.

Kidney Qi is deficient if there are depressions or the area feels cold or if a tight band or tension is palpated deeply. This area should not feel vacant or mushy. All vacancy signifies Deficiency and in this case it is indicative of Kidney Qi Xu. If it feels tight or hard superficially but emptier below the differential diagnosis is Kidney Yin Deficiency. We hope to feel a pulsation upon moderate to deep pressure at CV 6 (Qihai). This signifies that the energies of the two Kidneys are communicating with each other. Checking for a pulse is done at the time of the healthy Hara examination.

For a summary of the clinical energetics of the diagnosis points of the modified abdominal map, the palpation method of each point and the differential diagnosis of the palpatory findings, see Table 8.1.

PART 2: THE PALPATION PROCESS

WHAT ARE THE CLEARANCE POINTS AND HOW DO YOU PALPATE THEM?

Now that the clinical significance, palpation schema, sensation and differential diagnosis of the abdominal points have been explored, we now turn our discussion to the treatment points or what have been conventionally referred to as the *clearance points*. The clearance points are those points located distally from the diagnosis points that remediate the pathology perceived at the diagnosis points, whether that pathology be tightness, tension, tenderness, vacancy, lack of resilience or any other pathological finding discussed above and summarized in Table 8.1. Most of the clearance points are located on the extremities but some are in other areas such as the chest.

As we have proposed, the fundamental premise of abdominal diagnosis is that the abdomen is the reflection of the Zang-Fu organs, the Qi and the Blood, the Yin and the Yang. All pathology will be reflected on the abdomen albeit in general terms as perhaps only the shadow of the disorder. If an individual has any overt or even preclinical disease it can be ascertained from the abdomen and its clearance points. If the patient is healthy and ample in Qi and Blood and the Yin and Yang are harmonized, the abdomen may have no pathology but this is rare.

The abdomen can provide a tremendous amount of information about the state of the Qi if the practitioner has the ability to perceive it. Sometimes when I give students an assignment to diagnose and clear the abdomen, they report that they could not find anything abnormal. If the patient has any sort of a complaint, this cannot be. There are several reasons why they reach this conclusion but usually it is because the abdomen is not being palpated correctly.

The clearance points represent an even earlier, preclinical condition; that is, one before the organs, as reflected on the abdomen, are affected. For instance, let's say you palpate CV 14 and both you and the patient agree that there is no

Table 8.1 The clinical energetics of the diagnosis points of the modified abdominal map, palpation method and differential diagnosis

Point	Clinical energetics	Palpation method	Differential diagnosis
CV 14–15 area (Juque/Jiuwei)	1. Front Mu of the Heart – indicates condition of Yin and Yang 2. Pacifies spirit, adjusts the Qi, harmonizes the Stomach, benefits the diaphragm	Palpate lightly, pressing in slowly in an obliquely upward manner. Should feel soft, resilient, no pulsation. See text for how to locate this point	Physical and energetic Heart problems Tightness = Liver Qi Stagnation If area is hard or there is a strong pulsation = Heart Qi Xu
CV 12 (Zhongwan)	1. Front Mu of the Stomach – indicates the condition of Yin and Yang. Adjusts the Stomach, tonifies the Spleen and Stomach, regulates Qi. The source of all Yin. Reflection of stress 2. The Influential point that dominates the Fu organs 3. Activating point of the Middle Warmer – transforms Damp	Palpate perpendicularly downward. Should feel strong (solid) and resilient (soft), not hard or vacant	Hard = Yin Xu and/or Phlegm or food Stagnation Vacancy = Qi Deficiency of Middle Jiao Tight = Stomach Yin Deficiency
ST 25–28 area (Tianshu/Shuidao)	1. Front Mu of the Large Intestine – indicates the condition of the Yin and the Yang 2. Meeting point of Yangming – ST/LI 3. For chronic Deficiency of SP/KI 4. Reflex point of the appendix	Palpate perpendicularly downward. Do left side first, then right. Should feel resilient on both sides	
	a. On the left side – Blood Stagnation reflex	Palpate perpendicularly downward. Should feel strong on the left side	Tightness = Liver Qi and/or Blood Stagnation Lack of strength = Liver Blood Xu Tight and empty = Liver Qi Stagnation due to Liver Blood Xu
	b. On the right side – Front Mu of the Lungs indicates condition of the Yin and Yang of the Lungs. Front Mu of the Triple Warmer Lymphatic glandular exhaustion reflex	Palpate perpendicularly downward. Should feel resilient	Lack of resilience = Lung Qi Xu or weak immunity
CV6–4 areas (Qihai/Guanyuan)	1. Kidney reflex area – indicative of foundation Yin and Yang (Yuan Qi)	Should be resilient	Vacant, mushy, tight, hard = Kidney Qi Xu

tenderness, no discomfort and no tightness. The implication is that there is no Heart or Upper Jiao problem. Instead of moving on to the next point in line, CV 12 (Zhongwan), go to the first and major treatment point for CV 14 (Juque) which is PC 6 (Neiguan) and palpate it to see if there is any tenderness here. If so, it suggests that while there is no abdominal reflection, the earlier manifestation may be developing as signified by the tenderness at the clearance point. The patients should be taught how to treat and monitor themselves in this manner, with pressure. The clearance points are excellent points for the prevention of any undiagnosed pathology.

In another instance, let's say that you palpate ST 25 on the left and there is no tenderness, meaning no Liver Qi or Blood Stagnation or Liver Blood Deficiency. Instead of going to the next diagnosis point, ST 25 on the right, check the primary clearance point for ST 25L which is SP 10 (Xuehai). If there is no tenderness at that clearance point there is no early diagnosis of any potential Liver Qi Stagnation, Blood Stagnation or Blood Deficiency and ST 25L does not require further attention.

There are some cases in which the patient clearly has a major complaint and other pathologies and yet the patient does not react. Drugs such as steroids and painkillers, stress, emotional and psychological problems or advanced Deficiency can cause this insensitivity. Postsurgical patients who have had organs removed may also be somewhat unresponsive to abdominal palpation. Elderly patients whose vital Qi may be weak are often unresponsive to palpation, as they are when you needle them and seek to contact the Qi. For the extremely weakened patient who tends to have multiple deficiencies, abdominal clearing may have less relevance than the healthy Hara examination. Remember the root picture is revealed in that examination. Herbs may be more valuable therapeutically or another mode of treatment, for instance auricular acupuncture.

Other patients who are excessive in nature use their musculature as external bodily armor and this prevents the abdominal points from being contacted. Athletic patients sometimes fall into this excessive category. Note that not all athletic musculature is healthy. Healthy tissue, while toned, needs to be resilient. For these two types of patient, palpation may have limited value. I have found that often these patients do not even like acupuncture. They are restless on the table and aggravated by discreet needles and prodding fingers. But the Tiger Thermie warmer, with its combination of mechanical pressure and light soothing heat, has the effect of relaxing them without the aforementioned aggravations. If you can establish rapport with these patients, administer short treatments, which act like peeling off the layers of an onion to reach the center. Results can be obtained with these patients and indeed, through treatment, they can become softer and more open on many levels if they engage in this therapy. Figure 8.6 illustrates abdominal palpation of the normal patient, the deficient patient and the excessive patient.

The multiple factors that affect the interpretation of abdominal clearing are discussed below and summarized in Box 8.1.

Depth, pressure and angle

Palpating the diagnosis points or clearance points too deeply or too shallowly, or with too much or not enough pressure, will give a false reading. The patient's feedback may sway you towards this. This is due to several factors. One is that the abdominal points, which are the diagnosis points, usually do not hurt when palpated unless there is a severe pathology. Remember, they are only touched or contacted, not stimulated. The typical sensation patients report on these points is that they feel tight. Additionally, deficient patients tend to like deep touch and often they will tell you to go deeper on the abdominal points.

Other patients may say that the clearance points hurt. However, they must be pressed correctly which is generally with a deep dispersive rub to activate the point so that it can perform its treatment function. Insufficient pressure on the clearance points will fail to produce an appreciable clearance value.

Interestingly, while beginners tend to push too deeply on the diagnosis points, they correspondingly tend to press too lightly on the clearance

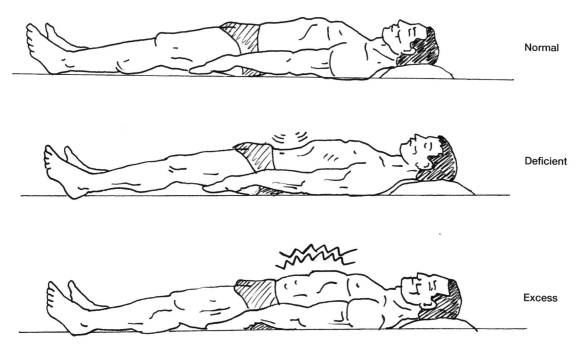

Figure 8.6 Abdominal palpation for three distinct types of patient.

Box 8.1 Factors that affect abdominal clearing

- The leading factor that affects abdominal clearing is pressing too deeply on the diagnosis point.
- Incorrect location of the diagnosis and clearance points. Usually, it is the clearance points, due to the use of Japanese locations.
- Improper angle and/or depth of palpation of the diagnosis and clearance points.
- Insufficient pressure on the clearance points, perhaps due to reluctance to cause discomfort.
- Lag time between palpation of the diagnosis point and the clearance point and then rechecking the diagnosis point. Move along. Know the protocol.
- Staying at the same level of palpation when rechecking the diagnosis point. If 'cleared', you may have greater access to the point. Or the patient may suggest that you can go deeper or that you are not on the same point.
- Ability to clear previous points.
- Interpretation of the findings.
- Patient positioning. Patients should be reclining on their back with the legs and arms comfortably extended to allow the practitioner to adjust the Qi and Blood through clearing. Do not put a pillow under their legs; that is, do not elevate them. Do put a pillow under their head.
- The patient may be taking certain medications such as steroids or painkillers which affect their ability to report discomfort to you. Other factors that may affect their response are that they may be under stress, have emotional or psychological problems or neurological disorders or the vital Qi may be very weak.
- Body type of the patient.
- Organ removal or severe emotional problems may make the patient unable to report accurately on palpation sensations.

points. This may be because of the known sensations of tenderness at the clearance points and the practitioner's hesitation to cause discomfort. These points must be pressed firmly with a deep invigorating pressure because we are trying to clear as much as possible by hand. In effect, we are removing excesses or bringing energy to the area so that the root deficiencies can be narrowed down prior to treatment with needles, moxa or herbs. It takes energy or stimulus to do this, hence the need for the clearance sensations.

In any event the practitioner must learn the proper depth for palpation and not succumb to the patient's instructions. The angle of palpation is also critical so that the correct area is palpated and the practitioner needs to know the proper angle of palpation.

Point location

Incorrect point location, of either the diagnosis point or the clearance point, will affect abdominal clearing. Most commonly, the clearance point is located incorrectly, particularly because many have Japanese locations. The locations of the clearance points that are different in the Japanese method are found in Figures 8.8–8.17.

Timing

Lag time, that is, too much time between pressing the diagnosis point and the clearance point and then rechecking the diagnosis point, can inhibit abdominal clearing. One only needs to stay on the clearance point for 2–3 seconds, no longer. The practitioner needs to reduce this delay by knowing the clearance procedure and not looking things up. Lag time can accumulate if the practitioner engages too much in conversation with the patient or is unfamiliar with the clearance protocol.

The clearance protocol is so effective that when you are rechecking a point patients may claim that you are not pressing with the same force or to the same depth or even in the same place. Once points are cleared, greater accessibility to the tissues can be gained. Therefore the practitioner needs to be mindful of where to repalpate the point, how deep to go and only go to that level. You can assure the patient that you were on the same spot by having them hold it or marking it but usually the disbelief only occurs at the beginning of treatment. When patients see how well it works, they no longer question your accuracy.

Clearance of subsequent points

Difficulties in clearing previous diagnosis points will interfere with the clearance of each subsequent diagnosis point and the overall abdominal map. Hence, clear each abdominal point by hand as much as you can. That is one reason why several clearance points are provided for each diagnosis point. They are sequenced in order of their clinical efficacy to be efficient and to reduce unnecessary palpation.

Interpretation

The interpretation of patient response and what you as a practitioner are feeling is critical in order to proceed to the treatment phase. For instance, if the area palpated is tight but you don't interpret it as tight, you probably won't treat it as tight. This in turn will contribute to the incorrect development of the treatment plan which does not include treating tightness. Do not discount patient feedback, especially as you first learn how to feel the body. Ultimately, however, the skilled practitioner's perception is more important.

THE PALPATION SCHEMA

The clearance points are palpated with firm, deep, dispersive pressure immediately after each diagnosis point is evaluated. Each diagnosis point is pressed only once, as are the clearance points. The operating principle behind the clearance points is that they reflect the preclinical state even more than the diagnosis points. They are usually exquisitely tender and this puts them into the category of what would be called a passive point. A passive point is an acupuncture point that elicits pain or tenderness upon some type of mechanical stimulation or pressure. The fact that it is tender signifies that the physiological role which that point plays in the body has gone awry. Just like the diagnosis points, the clearance points are not necessarily needled. They do, however, enter into the evolving diagnosis and are excellent points for the patients to work on at home.

The goal of the palpation process is to clear (i.e. remove pathology and return to normalcy) each diagnosis point as much as possible by hand so that a minimum number of needles will be needed to consolidate the treatment plan. The clearance points should clear 50–100% of each point's pathology, which effectively also clears the abdomen 50–100%.

The palpation schema is an artistic process and so users can modify it as they start to garner their own clinical experience. The process described below is the one that I prefer. However, there are some modifications that one can make based upon supporting signs and symptoms. A common modification will be discussed after the usual clearance process is presented.

The abdominal clearance procedure

1. Starting with CV 14–15 and working downward, palpate each diagnostic point once in the order of their presentation and clear it at least 50% with each set of clearance points. Moving from top to bottom helps to bring the patient's energy down. This is a fundamental treatment strategy whereby the Qi is directed towards the Dan tian in the lower part of the body so that it can be rooted.

2. Apply the appropriate pressure to each clearance point for about 2–3 seconds, no longer. Each point is palpated only once. I have observed that beginners tend not to press this point deeply enough but also stay on the clearance points too long. There is no need to stay on the point longer than a few seconds; however, it is necessary to palpate deeply enough. Once you have contacted the Qi and evoked a reaction from the patient, the energetics of the point have been initiated and time is not needed.

Clearance points have known sensations; for example, SP 4 (Gongsun) is consistently very painful on virtually everyone. Prepare the patient to experience this feeling before palpating the point by telling them what to expect so they will be mentally prepared for the point sensation if it is pathological. Such sensations are summarized later in Table 8.3.

3. Before moving on to the subsequent clearance points for the same diagnosis point, assess the significance of the palpatory finding; that is, wait for the patient to give you feedback about how the point felt upon palpation. Provide feedback to the patient about what you are feeling. For instance, confirm that you too feel the point is tight if both of you think so or tell them you feel tension in the point even if they don't, so that they can become attuned to this awareness.

4. Immediately, with little lag time in between, repalpate the diagnosis point and see how things have changed. The aim is to clear by hand somewhere between 50% and 100% of each abdominal point's tenderness. Note that there are several clearance points for each diagnosis point. The order in which I have arranged them for palpating reflects their degree of clinical clearance. For instance, PC 6 clears CV 14–15 on average at least 50%. It makes more sense to first palpate a point that has greater clearance value than several points that only contribute minutely to the process.

5. Move to the next clearance point in line for a diagnosis point until you get 50–100% clearance of the abdominal point. There is no need to go to a subsequent point if you have already managed to get 80–100% clearance on the diagnosis point. For example, if you obtain 100% clearance on CV 14 with PC 6, you can move to the next diagnosis point, CV 12, instead of going on to the other clearance points for PC 6 that are LU 7 (Lieque), KI 6 (Zhaohai), KI 25 (Shencang) and CV 12 (Zhongwan).

6. The aim of clearing the abdomen is also to get 50–100% clearance of the general abdominal map. Ultimately, we are trying to get the highest clearance value on each point. It is important to stress to patients that the clearing is actually part of the treatment process and a rather powerful one at that. Certain patients and certain conditions can be treated exclusively through this procedure. The *Neijing* reminds us that the aim of treatment is to effect a change and as the practitioner will see, clearing the abdomen produces dramatic results. Patients generally report that they like palpation; they feel better after this process, most notably if they have been suffering from an acute problem. They say they feel 'grounded, energetic and cen-

tered' and they do experience an improvement in symptoms. Repeatedly they compare the clearance to magic, perhaps further support for the power of palpation as the 'magic hand'. Cases 8.1 and 8.2 found at the end of this chapter are illustrative of the singular power of abdominal palpation.

7. Some clearance points will actually make the diagnosis points worse, in which case, go back to the previous clearance point and reclear the abdominal point. For instance, let's say that you cleared CV 12 with ST 34 (Liangqiu) and achieved 50% clearance. You want to clear this point more so you move on to ST 44 (Neiting) and get another 20%. But you want to get 80–100% so you move on to SP 4 (Gongsun). However, SP 4 makes the abdominal point feel worse, not better. In this case go back to the previously successful clearance point and repalpate ST 44 and bring the abdominal point back to its 70% clearance.

8. Many of the clearance points are only palpated on one side due to the fact that certain meridians' energetics are more right or left sided. (See Table 5.1 on the affinity of particular meridians to be more left or right sided as reflected in the historical pulse diagnosis systems.) Some points are palpated bilaterally. In such cases, palpate each point, one at a time, not simultaneously. Most of the Kidney points are palpated bilaterally and this is reflected in most pulse systems. The Kidney is the root of the Qi.

The abdominal palpation schema is so effective that to get 80–100% clearance of the abdominal map is not hard. However, there are factors that can interfere with this end result and they are mistakes that the novice practitioner tends to make. They are discussed here so that practitioners can keep these problems in mind as they learn how to clear the abdominal map. These factors are summarized in Box 8.1.

Another clearance approach is a successful modification of the abdominal clearance protocol. In this case, the first step is to open the Dai channel and its couple, the Yangwei mai, because of the intimate way that they work together.

Sometimes the Dai channel, the only transverse meridian, may be blocked. Blockage of the Dai channel can influence the functioning of all the other meridians that pass through it in a longitudinal manner as well as their internal channels. Hence, it can be judicious to open the Dai channel before adjusting energy anywhere else in the body so that this blockage does not hamper your efforts. When the Dai channel is no longer blocked the energy in the meridians is more likely to be amenable to being adjusted.

Dai channel obstructions can come about due to excessive weight in the lower abdomen, scars in that area, gravity, tight clothing, childbirth or wearing high heels. The Dai and its couple, the Yangwei, work synergistically together to open up any horizontal blockage in the person.

If specific symptomatology suggests that the Dai channel is involved, I open that first; for instance, if patients say that they feel numbness or heaviness in their legs in the course of the interview. Otherwise, I open the Dai channel when I am at the level of the waist, specifically at the ST 25 left side. In the absence of Dai channel symptomatology, I tend to use the standard abdominal clearance protocol presented above.

THE CLINICAL ENERGETICS OF THE CLEARANCE POINTS

The order of palpation of the clearance points with Chinese or Japanese locations is summarized in Table 8.2. Twenty-six clearance points are listed and these are the main ones. It is rare that all of them are used. Other points may also be clearance points but they are not listed here because potentially any point can be a clearance point. If other points are needed to address the condition but not necessarily affect an abdominal clearing because of the severity of the condition or other factors (i.e. they may need to be needled), they fall into the realm of what I call treatment-of-disease points. Additional disease points will be presented in Section 5.

A perusal of the clearance points in Table 8.2 shows that they tend to fall into several categories in the point classification system, namely

Table 8.2 The clearance points in the order of palpation, point location, side of the body to palpate and type of point

Diagnostic points	Clearance points in order of palpation, location and side to palpate. Chinese (C) or Japanese (J) location	Type of point
CV 14–15 (Juque/Jiuwei)	PC 6 (Neiguan) L (C)	Luo and Confluent
	LU 7 (Lieque) R (C) and alternate	Luo and Confluent
	KI 6 (Zhaohai) B (J)	Confluent
	KI 25 (Shencang) L (C)	–
	CV 12 (Zhongwan) (C)	Front Mu
CV12 (Zhongwan)	ST 34 (Liangqiu) R (J)	Xi (cleft)
	ST 44 (Inner Neiting) B (J)	Water point
	SP 4 (Gongsun) B (J)	Luo and Confluent
ST 25 (Tianshu) L	SP 10 (Xuehai) L (J)	Sea of Blood
	TE 5 (Waiguan) R (C)	Luo and Confluent
	GB 41 (Zulinqi) L (J and C)	Confluent
	LR 5 (Ligou) L (J and C)	Luo
	LR 3 (Taichong) B (C)	Front Mu
	LR 14 (Qimen) R (C)	Luo
ST 25 (Tianshu) R	LU 1–2 (Zhongfu, Yunmen) B (C)	Front Mu
	LI 4 (Hegu) B (C)	Source
	TE 3 (Zhongdu) B (J)	Source
	SI 3 (Houxi) B (C)	Confluent
	TE 5 (Waiguan) B (C)	Luo and Confluent
	GB 41 (Zulinqi) L (J and C)	Confluent
CV 6 (Qihai) and 4 (Guanyuan)	KI 1 (Yongquan) B (C)	Sedation
	KI 6 (Zhaohai) B (J)	Confluent
	KI 3 (Taixi) B (J)	Source
	KI 7 (Fuliu) B (C)	Tonification
	BL 62 (Shenmai) R (J)	Confluent
	KI 16 (Huangshu) (J)	Front Mu (Manaka)

L = Left
R = Right
B = Both

Xi (cleft) points, Luo points, Source points, Confluent points or Front Mu points. Because of the traditional energetics of these categories of points, it is logical that they would be effective clearance points.

Let us review the energetics of these categories of points.

● **Xi (cleft) points** – points of accumulation and blockage. Reflex points of the meridian
● **Luo points** – special vessels of communication between channels. They can be used in several ways: transversely to connect with the coupled organ–meridian complex in cases of both Excess or Deficiency; longitudinally to stimulate the organ–meridian complex itself

● **Source points** – points where the Original Qi of the organ is infused
● **Confluent points** – points that open an Extraordinary Meridian and reinforce the action of the main meridians
● **Front Mu points** – points where the Yin and Yang of the organ collect

Chapter 18 discusses the unique applicability of these points and includes illustrative case histories.

In this next section, the clinical energetics of the clearance points are discussed along with their differential diagnosis, point location, palpation sensation and other notes. Table 8.3 summarizes the palpation method of the clearance points.

Table 8.3 Palpation method of the clearance points, sensation and differential diagnosis

Diagnostic point	Clearance point	Palpation method and sensation	Differential diagnosis
CV 14–15 (Juque/Jiuwei)	PC 6 (Neiguan)	Left side only Perpendicular, with deep pressure Very tender	Tense, stringy = Liver Qi Stagnation Tense on top, mushy below = Liver Qi Stagnation with Liver Blood Deficiency Mushy = Liver Blood Deficiency
	LU 7 (Lieque)	Right side only Rub on the styloid process of the radius or in the alternative location Not much sensation, if any	Lung and Ren channel pathology
	KI 6 (Zhaohai)	Both separately, strong transverse rub Exquisitely tender	Yin Deficiency
	KI 25 (Shencang)	Left side only Transverse rub in the intercostal space Achy	Lung, Heart and Kidney problems
	CV 12 (Zhongwan)	Perpendicular, about half to one inch Tight	Tight = Stomach Yin Xu, Phlegm, food Stagnation Vacant = deficient Qi of Middle Jiao
CV 12 (Zhongwan)	ST 34 (Liangqiu)	Right side only Deep perpendicular rub Very tender, gripping	Stagnation in Stomach of Heat, Damp or Wind
	ST 44 (Inner Neiting)	Both separately Deep dispersive rub up and down (longitudinally) Exquisitely tender	Stomach/Large Intestine Heat
	SP 4 (Gongsun)	Both separately Deep dispersive rub against the bone Excruciatingly tender	Dampness, Spleen/Stomach disharmony
ST 25 (Tianshu) Left	SP 10 (Xuehai)	Left side only Deep transverse rub Very tender, gripping	Liver Qi and Blood Stagnation Liver Blood Deficiency
	TE 5 (Waiguan)	Right side only Perpendicular pressure Can be tender	San Jiao pathology as well as Yangwei disturbance
	GB 41 (Zulinqi)	Left side only for both Chinese and Japanese locations Deep transverse rub Extremely tender	Liver Yang rising due to Liver Yin Deficiency
	LR 5 (Ligou)	Left side only, use three locations Deep rub in the cleft or against the bone Usually very tender	Excess or Deficient in Liver/Gall Bladder energy
	LR 3 (Taichong)	Both separately Deep transverse rub Generally feels achy to tender	Liver Qi Stagnation due to Deficiency
	LR 14 (Qimen)	Right side only Gentle transverse rub in the intercostal space May be achy	Liver Yin/Yang disharmony
ST 25 (Tianshu) Right	LU 1–2 (Zhongfu, Yunmen)	Both sides separately Moderate transverse rub in the intercostal space Achy, usually more at LU 1	Lung pathology

Table 8.3 Palpation method of the clearance points, sensation and differential diagnosis (contd)

Diagnostic point	Clearance point	Palpation method and sensation	Differential diagnosis
	LI 4 (Hegu)	Both sides separately Deep dispersive pressure Very tender	Large Intestine pathology
	TE 3 (Zhongdu)	Both sides separately Rub in between the tendons May be achy	San Jiao pathology, Kidney Yin and/or Yang Xu
	SI 3 (Houxi)	Both sides separately Rub against bone Occasionally slightly tender	Small Intestine pathology as well as Du channel
	TE 5 (Waiguan) GB 41 (Zulinqi)	See above See above	San Jiao pathology Dai channel pathology
CV 4–6 (Guanyuan, Qihai)	KI 1 (Yongquan)	Both sides separately Deep dispersive pressure Generally extremely tender	Blood disturbances
	KI 6 (Zhaohai) KI 3 (Taixi)	See KI 6 (Zhaohai) above Both sides separately Firm pressure against heel May be tender	Yin Deficiency Kidney Qi Xu
	KI 7 (Fuliu)	Both sides separately Moderate pressure Achy	Kidney Yang Xu
	BL 62 (Shenmai)	Right side only Deep transverse rub Usually tender	Yang Excess in head
	KI 16 (Huangshu)	Palpate all around the navel at an angle towards the navel	Kidney Qi Xu

Diagnostic point 1: CV 14 (Juque) – CV 15 (Jiuwei)

The area should feel soft and resilient and have no pulsation.

Clearance points: PC 6L (C), LU 7R (C), KI 6B (J), KI 25L (C), CV 12 (C) (C = Chinese, J = Japanese, B = both)

<u>PC 6 (Neiguan)</u>

1. **Location** – standard location. Two cun above the transverse crease of the wrist, between the tendons of the m. palmaris longus and flexor carpi radialis. Use left side.
2. **Palpation method and sensation** – deep perpendicular pressure. In almost every case this point is very tender. This is due to the multiple roles which PC 6 (Neiguan) plays in the body.
3. **Energetics** – PC 6 is the first and most important point used in the entire palpation schema. Additionally, it is the first clearance point in a series of potential points for the CV 14 (Juque)/CV 15 (Jiuwei) area. Its precise job is to remove Stagnation anywhere in the body with a special effect on the Upper Jiao. As Mark Seem says, it is the most powerful distal point on the hand Jueyin for opening the chest (Seem 1989a). For a comprehensive argument on the importance of PC 6 as a treatment point see my previous book or my journal article on the same topic (Gardner-Abbate 1995b, 1996, pp. 133–147). These energetics are briefly summarized below.
   - As a longitudinal Luo point, PC 6 regulates the Qi and Blood of the Heart, opens the Heart orifice and calms the spirit, mind and Heart. It expands the diaphragm, decongests the chest and diaphragm, broadens the chest and controls the chest above the Stomach. It can drain off excessive stuck energy of the Upper Jiao, the Heart and the chest in particular, including stuck emotional energy that can cause stagnant Qi and Blood.
   - As a transverse Luo point, it connects to the Triple Warmer. Thus, it can calm and harmonize the Stomach, promotes the functional Qi of the Middle Burner and regulates the function of the Triple Warmer, including the harmonization of all three Jiaos.
   - As Master of the Yinwei mai, it opens the Yinwei channel to distribute Qi to the Stomach, chest and Heart. It links all the Yin channels together. Additionally, as Master of the Yinwei mai it is coupled to the Chong meridian that is virtually identical to the Kidney meridian, only more superficial. Thus, it has a connection to the Kidney.
   - By virtue of its internal pathway which passes through the chest and CV 17 (Tanzhong), its own Front Mu point, as well as the fact that it is the Influential point which dominates the Qi, it suppresses rebellious Qi and disperses stagnant Liver Qi. As a result, it suppresses pain, stops vomiting and regulates the Jueyin meeting of the Three Arm Yin (HT, LU, PC).
   - All the extra meridians meet here.
   - It is useful for miscommunication between the Upper and the Lower Jiao, particularly the uterus, because there is a special vessel called the Bao Luo which connects the Pericardium (Xin bao) with the uterus (Bao gong).
   - The Pericardium in ancient times was considered to be so intimately connected to the Heart that it was not viewed as a separate organ. We know that the Heart is linked with the brain, emotions and mental function. Due to this inextricable connection, when PC 6 (Neiguan) is used in treatment it has the added function of benefiting the Heart, the brain, the emotions and the mental state. Consequently it is one of the most important points to use in treatment (Johns 1997). Of all the acupuncture points, it is my favorite.

   A visual representation of the relationships of the Pericardium to various parts of the body is depicted in Figure 8.7.
4. **Differential diagnosis**
   - Commonly this point feels tense and stringy = Liver Qi Stagnation
   - It can feel tense on top but mushy below = Liver Qi Stagnation with Liver Blood Deficiency
   - If it only feels mushy, it indicates Liver Blood Deficiency

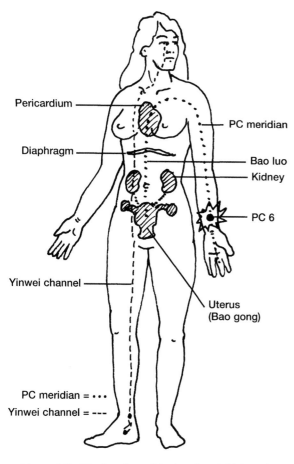

Pericardium

PC meridian

Diaphragm

Bao luo

Kidney

PC 6

Yinwei channel

Uterus
(Bao gong)

PC meridian = •••
Yinwei channel = ---

Figure 8.7 The functions of Pericardium 6 (Neiguan).

5. **Notes** – as in all cases, even if CV 14–15 does not seem abnormal you should check PC 6 (Neiguan) since this, like all the clearance points, is even more preclinical than the diagnosis point. PC 6 usually provides between 50% and 100% clearance of CV 14–15. If 80–100% clearance is obtained you can move on to clearing CV 12. If less than 80% is obtained, palpate LU 7 (Lieque) so that you can attain a higher clearance value.

LU 7 (Lieque)

1. **Location** – standard location. Superior to the styloid process of the radius, 1.5 cun above the transverse crease of the wrist. In the depression on the styloid process of the radius. Right side. There is also an alternative location that is parallel to this description, on the course of the radial artery.

2. **Palpation methods and sensation** – Lung 7 is the second point to palpate to obtain further clearance of CV 14–15. It is a small point but it can be palpated and when it is involved the patient may report that it is tender. Only palpate LU 7 on the right side with a rub in the cleft of the styloid process of the radius. The supplemental location of LU 7 described above may also be used.

3. **Energetics**
   • Lung 7 (Lieque) is the Luo point of the Lung channel. As the longitudinal Luo, it has the ability to tonify the Qi of the Lungs as well as that of the whole body because the Lungs is the Master of the Qi. It stimulates the descending and dispersing function of the Lung, eliminates Wind, circulates defensive Qi, releases to the exterior, increases Wei Qi and is a general body tonic. It opens to the nose and communicates with the Large Intestine as a transverse Luo to assist it in removing the dregs from the body.
   • As a general Luo point, it promotes the free flow of Qi in the body, picks up the energy of the body and is one of the best Controlling points for rebellious Qi in the chest.
   • It is the Master of the Ren channel which makes it an extremely efficient point in opening the Ren channel and allowing its energy to flow upward. The Ren channel has responsibility for all the Yin channels and nourishes the fetus. It passes through the uterus.
   • By virtue of its Luo point function as well as Triple Warmer physiology, it benefits the Bladder, opens water passages and eliminates excess water in the body. It sends the Qi downward to be grasped by the Kidney.
   • In the Extraordinary meridian system it is coupled with KI 6 (Zhaohai) and these two points work together like a wheel to put Stagnation in motion as well as regulate water passageways and water metabolism.

4. **Differential diagnosis** – it is indicative of Lung and Ren channel pathology.

5. **Notes** – Lung 7 may provide additional clearance of the CV14–15 area. If you reach a combined clearance on CV 14–15 of 80–100%, move on to clear CV 12 (Zhongwan). Otherwise go to KI 6 (Zhaohai) for further assistance with clearing CV14–15.

KI 6 (Zhaohai)

1. **Location** – the Chinese recognize two locations of KI 6: one is defined as directly below the medial malleolus and the other as 1 cun directly below the tip of the medial malleolus at the junction of the red and the white skin. The Japanese prefer the latter.

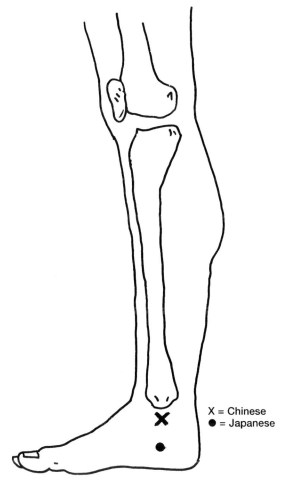

X = Chinese
● = Japanese

Figure 8.8 Two locations of KI 6 (Zhaohai).

Henceforth when I refer to KI 6, I mean this one. Palpate both sides.

2. **Palpation method and sensation** – KI 6 tends to be another of the exquisitely tender points. Palpate KI 6 bilaterally, one at a time, not simultaneously, with a strong transverse rub.

3. **Energetics**
   - As the Master of the Yinqiao mai, it is the best point to nourish KI Yin and clear Deficiency Fire. It is useful for any inflammation (any illness ending in 'itis'), certainly a broad list of diseases.
   - It invigorates the Yinqiao mai, promotes the function of the uterus, opens the chest, brightens the eyes and strengthens the lower back. It distributes Yin to the upper part of the body, thereby benefiting the throat.
   - It benefits deficient and cold Kidneys.
   - It nourishes the Yin, calms the mind and the spirit.
   - It cools the Blood and eliminates Damp.
   - As the adrenal reflex, it strengthens the adrenals, balances hormones and reflects shock, trauma, stress, drug use and chronic illness.

4. **Differential diagnosis** – Yin Deficiency.

5. **Notes** – if KI 6 (Zhaohai) has contributed to the 80–100% clearance, move on to clear CV 12 (Zhongwan). If cumulatively you have not reached this total, continue to clear CV 14–15 with KI 25 (Shencang).

KI 25 (Shencang)

1. **Location** – standard Kidney 25. In the depression on the lower border of the clavicle, 2 cun lateral to the CV channel. Left side.

2. **Palpation method and sensation** – KI 25 is palpated on the left side only. Rub transversely in the intercostal space. When diagnostic, the patient claims that it tends to feel very achy or sore.

3. **Energetics**
   - KI 25 is considered the reflex point of Heart disease. It is good for chest pain and invigorates local Qi Stagnation.
   - It can calm the mind and is useful for anxiety due to Kidney Deficiency.

- It aids Lung Qi to descend and disperse and brings down rebellious Qi. It is used for cough and asthma due to Kidney Deficiency and strengthens the Kidney's ability to grasp the Qi.

4. **Differential diagnosis** – Lung, Heart and Kidney problems.

5. **Notes** – if 80–100% clearance has not been achieved now that four clearance points have been used, several things may be occurring.
   - Consult Box 8.1 on factors that affect abdominal clearing. It will probably be one of these.
   - PC 6 should provide the greatest clearance value. If this did not occur press again on PC 6 to the proper depth.
   - It is possible that the CV 12 area is blocked and not allowing CV 14–15 to be sufficiently cleared, in which case you may need to clear CV 12. This is rare but it can happen.
   - The pathology of the abdominal points may be so advanced that they may need to be needled. Needling of the diagnosis and clearance points will be covered in Chapter 12.

CV 12 (Zhongwan)

1. **Location** – standard location, on the Ren channel, 4 cun above the center of the umbilicus.

2. **Palpation method and sensation** – perpendicularly about a half an inch to an inch. When pathological, it tends to feel tight; sometimes it is empty.

3. **Energetics** – all these energetics contribute to its ability to clear CV 14–15 in the Upper Jiao.
   - Front Mu point of the Stomach; source of all Yin
   - Influential point that dominates the Fu organs
   - Controlling point of the Middle Jiao
   - The Lung meridian begins there, the Liver meridian ends there and the Heart and the Triple Warmer pass through there

4. **Differential diagnosis**
   - If it feels tight, it indicates Yin Deficiency, Phlegm or food Stagnation.
   - If empty, it indicates Qi Deficiency in the Middle Jiao.

Diagnostic point 2: CV 12 (Zhongwan)

The healthy sensation that you are looking for when feeling CV 12 is one of softness and yet strength. It should feel resilient and solid but not tense or mushy.

Clearance points: ST 34R (J), ST 44B (J), SP 4B (J)

CV 12 is generally cleared with all three of the clearance points for maximum effect since they indicate the three major pathologies of the Stomach – Stagnation, Heat and Dampness – because clinically these three pathologies are frequently interrelated. However, sometimes one of these points will make CV 12 worse in which case the pattern as expressed in the energetics of the clearance points is incorrect. If this occurs go back to the previous clearance point and use it again to clear CV 12 as well as any other point this happens on through the modified abdominal evaluation.

ST 34 (Liangqiu)

1. **Location** – slightly more lateral and superior to the standard Chinese location which is 2 cun above the laterosuperior border of the patella. It is directly above ST 35 (Dubi) but is more lateral. Palpate on right side only.

2. **Palpation method and sensation** – palpate on the right side only with a deep perpendicular rub. This point is very tender most of the time. Generally the patient experiences a gripping type pain. Prepare patients for this sensation by telling them what to expect. ST 34 will clear CV 12 well if there is Stagnation in the Stomach. However, if there is Heat or Dampness or a combination of Damp-Heat, the subsequent points may need to be used as well.

3. **Energetics**
   - It is the Xi (cleft) point of the Stomach and as such it clears Heat from the Stomach, harmonizes the Stomach, pacifies the Stomach and rebellious Qi and opens the flow to the meridian. This makes it a reflex point of the meridian.
   - It dispels Stagnation and accumulation of the Yangming, clears the channels, removes

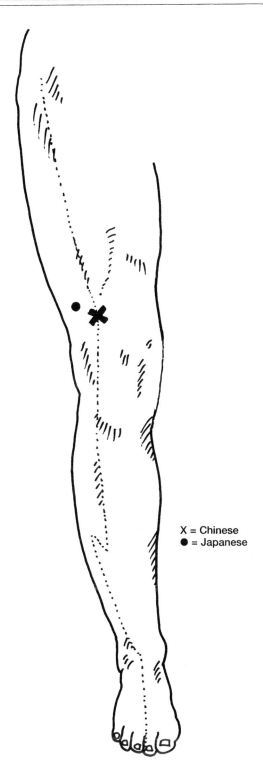

obstructions and quickens collaterals. It is a primary point for acute stomachache and food poisoning. Also locally benefits the knees.
- Expels Dampness and Wind.
- Relieves spasm and stops pain.
4. **Differential diagnosis** – Stagnation of Heat, Damp, food or Wind.

ST 44 (Neiting)

1. **Location** – use the alternative location, the Japanese location Inner Neiting on the sole of the foot at the junction of the margin of the web between the second and third toes. Palpate both sides.
2. **Palpation method and sensation** – press both points bilaterally but not simultaneously, with firm pressure rubbing up and down. Generally they are exquisitely tender.

X = Chinese
● = Japanese

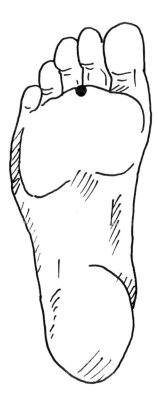

Figure 8.9   Two locations of ST 34 (Liangqiu).

Figure 8.10   Japanese location of ST 44 (Inner Neiting).

3. Energetics

• As the Water point, Ying (spring) point and secondary tonification point, ST 44 cools and drains Heat from the Stomach. It is the most common point for Stomach Fire as manifested in allergic reactions, hydrochloric acid excess, food poisoning, migraines, periodontal gum disease and acute stomachache.

• Regulates the Qi and suppresses the pain of the Stomach channel in relation to Stomach Fire in the face such as toothaches, gum pain, bleeding gums, allergy symptoms, eczema and migraine.

• Cools Heat in the Yangming.

• Promotes bowel movements.

• Regulates rebellious Qi.

• Stops abdominal pain with fever, eliminates Wind from the face.

4. Differential diagnosis – Stomach and Large Intestine Heat.

SP 4 (Gongsun)

1. Location – the Chinese location is in the depression distal and inferior to the base of the first metatarsal bone, at the junction of the red and the white skin. The Japanese location is more directly beneath the base of the first metatarsal bone on both sides.

2. Palpation method and sensation – palpate on both sides separately with deep, dispersive pressure against the bone. Undoubtedly one of the most painful clearance points, if not the most painful.

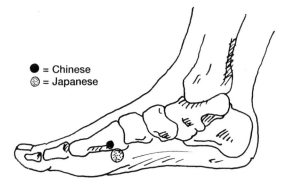

● = Chinese
◉ = Japanese

Figure 8.11 Two locations of SP 4 (Gongsun).

3. Energetics

• Luo point; regulates circulation of the Middle Burner, tonifies Spleen and Stomach Deficiency, removes Damp, regulates Spleen/Stomach disharmonies, pacifies the Stomach, dispels fullness and obstruction, circulates Blood and energy, brings down rebellious Qi and turbidity.

• Master of the Chong mai, dispels Cold from the Heart and abdomen. Regulates the Chong mai, affects adrenals, stops bleeding, regulates menstruation.

4. Differential diagnosis – Dampness, Spleen and Stomach disharmony.

Diagnostic points 3 and 4: ST 25L&R (Tianshu)

Should feel resilient on both sides and have strength on the left.

Clearance points for ST 25L: SP 10L (J), TE 5R (C), GB 41L (J & C), LR 5L (J & C), LR 3B (C), LR 14R (C)

Clear ST 25L first. Remember that ST 25L may be related to Liver Qi and Liver Blood Stagnation, one of the reasons why we want to clear this point first. Its location at the junction of the descending colon also necessitates that it is cleared first.

SP 10 (Xuehai)

1. Location – cup your right palm to the patient's left knee, with the thumb on its medial side and the other four fingers directed proximally. The point is where the tip of your thumb rests. This is the Japanese location of the point. Note that it is more medial to the Chinese. Use the left side.

2. Palpation method and sensation – palpate on the left side only with a deep dispersive rub. SP 10 is another extremely painful point and tends to produce a gripping feeling. Prepare the patient for this sensation.

3. Energetics

• SP 10 (Xuehai) is a Sea of Blood point. It is the Spleen that controls the blood. It moves

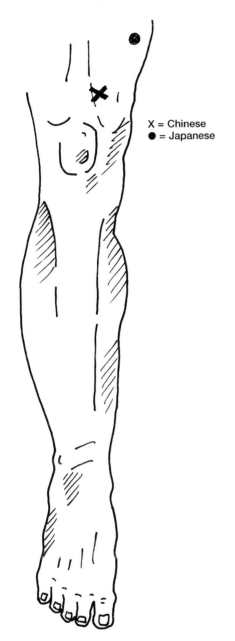

X = Chinese
● = Japanese

Figure 8.12   Two locations of SP 10 (Xuehai).

- Intersects with the Chong mai, hence helps to regulate the Blood, especially the menses.
4. **Differential diagnosis** – Liver Qi and Blood Stagnation, Liver Blood Deficiency.

TE 5 (Waiguan)

1. **Location** – standard location 2 cun above TE 4 between the radius and the ulna, right side.
2. **Palpation method and sensation** – deep perpendicular pressure on the right side only. The point can be tender.
3. **Energetics**
   - Luo point – expels Wind-Heat, releases the exterior, removes obstructions from the channel, benefits the ear, subdues Liver Yang, opens the orifices to influence hearing, transforms mucus, disperses goiter, relaxes sinews and tendons, clears vessels, strengthens arms, sends a vessel to all three heaters, affects Yang organs and digestive energy, a primary point for food poisoning.
   - As Master of the Yangwei mai, it circulates Yang defensive energy to the entire body.
4. **Differential diagnosis** – any San Jiao pathology as well as Yangwei disturbance.

GB 41 (Zulinqi)

1. **Location** – use both Chinese and Japanese locations. Chinese location is in the depression distal to the junction of the fourth and fifth metatarsal bones, on the lateral side of the tendon of the extensor digiti minimi of the foot. The Japanese location is anterior to the cuboid bone. Both are on the left side.
2. **Palpation method and sensation** – check both; each tends to be extremely tender although usually the Japanese location is more so. Press only on the left with a deep transverse rub.
3. **Energetics**
   - Shu (stream) point, Wood point, horary point – resolves Damp-Heat, promotes the smooth flow of Liver Qi, resolves Damp-Heat in the genital region, spreads and drains the Liver and the Gall Bladder, clears Fire and

stagnant Blood especially in the lower abdomen. It regulates the circulation of Blood, especially of the menses. It harmonizes the Blood, cools Heat in the blood, eliminates Damp, perfuses the lower abdomen, tonifies and strengthens the Blood.

TE = standard abbreviation of the World Health Organization (1989) for Triple Warmer.

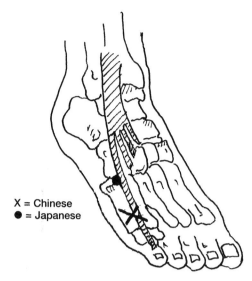

Figure 8.13 Two locations of GB 41 (Zulinqi).

extinguishes Wind, brightens eyes and sharpens hearing, transforms obstructing Phlegm-Heat, removes coagulation and Stagnation of Blood and Phlegm from the Jueyin, for women's problems due to Liver imbalance.
  • Master of the Dai mai – regulates the girdle vessel and, with the Yangwei channel, distributes Yang defensive energy throughout the body.
4. **Differential diagnosis** – Liver Yang rising due to Liver Yin Deficiency.

Supplemental points

Almost 90% of the time, SP 10L, TE 5R and GB 41L will clear ST 25L. However, if they do not provide sufficient clearance, the following supplemental points may be used.

LR 5 (Ligou)

1. **Location** – palpate the three locations of LR 5 to see which is most effective. This point is very tender, left side.
   • Chinese location 1 – 5 cun above the tip of the medial malleolus on the medial aspect and near the medial border of the tibia.

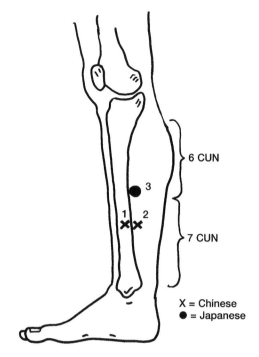

Figure 8.14 Three locations of LR 5 (Ligou).

   • Chinese location 2 – 5 cun above the tip of the medial malleolus posterior to the medial border of the tibia.
   • Japanese location – midway between SP 9 (Yinlingquan) and the tip of the medial malleolus, posterior to the medial border of the tibia.
2. **Palpation method and sensation** – palpate on the left side only. Palpate each point separately, rubbing in the cleft or against the bone, depending upon the location. Usually very tender.
3. **Energetics**
   • LR 5, the Luo point of the Liver channel, like all Luo points, can be used as a longitudinal or transverse Luo. As a longitudinal Luo, it can be used to stimulate its own organ–meridian complex and to drain Excess from the meridian such as Damp-Heat, stagnant Qi and toxicity. Liver Excess manifests on the right. It promotes the free flow of Liver Qi. Can be used for any type of inflammation as designated by the disease name ending in the suffix, 'itis'.

- As a transverse Luo it can be used to connect to the Source point of its coupled meridian, the Gall Bladder, thus harmonizing Wood energy.
4. **Differential diagnosis** – indicative of excess or deficient Liver/Gall Bladder energy.

LR 3 (Taichong)

1. **Location** – standard location, in the depression distal to the junction of the first and second metatarsal bones, both sides.
2. **Palpation method and sensation** – rub each separately with a deep transverse rub in between the tendons. Generally feels achy to tender.
3. **Energetics** – Liver 3 is the Shu (stream) point, Earth point and Source point of the Liver. As such, it can be used to tonify, balance and strengthen the Liver in cases of Deficiency. Liver Qi Stagnation arising from Deficiency manifests more on the right. Liver Excess presents more on the left. Due to this Excess Deficiency syndrome, the points are pressed bilaterally.
4. **Differential diagnosis** – for Liver Qi Stagnation due to Deficiency.

LR 14 (Qimen)

1. **Location** – standard location, on the mamillary line, two ribs below the nipple, in the sixth intercostal space, right side.
2. **Palpation method and sensation** – palpate the right side only, gently rubbing transversely in the intercostal space. An achy feeling can be evoked.
3. **Energetics** – Liver 14, as the Front Mu point of the Liver, can be used to adjust the Yin and Yang of the Liver. When the Liver is deficient, Liver 14 helps to supplement that Deficiency or if the Yang is excessive, it regulates the Yang.
4. **Differential diagnosis** – it works as a clearance point for Liver Yin/Yang disharmony.

Clearance points for ST 25R: LU 1–2B (C), LI 4B (C), TE 3B (J), SI 3B (C)

LU 1 (Zhongfu)–2 (Yumen)

1. **Location** – standard locations, both sides.
   - Lung 1 – 1 cun directly below LU 2.
   - Lung 2 – directly below the acromial extremity of the clavicle, 6 cun lateral to the Ren channel.
2. **Palpation method and sensation** – bilaterally, one at a time with a moderate transverse rub. Lung 1 is usually more achy. Palpate on the right side first.
3. **Energetics**
   - Lung 1 is the Front Mu point of the Lungs. It benefits the Yin of the Lung and tonifies Lung Deficiency. It is the point of entry of energy into the body and so can increase the energy of the entire body. It expands and relaxes the chest, disperses fullness from the chest, stops pain and cough, stimulates the descending of Lung Qi, clears the Upper Burner, as well as Heat from the Lungs. It opens relevant emotional blockages.
   - It is the meeting of Taiyin, Lung/Spleen.
4. **Differential diagnosis** – any Lung disturbance.
5. **Notes** – the Lung 1–2 area should be firm and not sunken. Serizawa, quoted in Denmei (1990, p. 95), states, 'An abundance of Lung Qi is indicated when the upper thoracic area is large, there is ample flesh and the area is firm to the touch. A deficiency of Lung Qi is indicated when the skin in this area is dry and the flesh feels soft or the ribs can be seen easily. If the thoracic wall is sunken over the points LU 1–LU 2 this is also a sign of emptiness in the Lungs'.

LI 4 (Hegu)

1. **Location** – standard location, between the first and second metacarpal bones, approximately in the middle of the second metacarpal bone on the radial side, both sides.
2. **Palpation method and sensation** – a firm, deep dispersive rub against the bone. This

point is generally very sore. Palpate bilaterally one side at a time.

3. **Energetics**
   - LI 4 is the Source point of the Large Intestine meridian. It brings energy down, clears the Large Intestine channel, clears Heat from the orifices of the head and face, expels Wind, relieves the surface, elevates the clear and descends the turbid. It removes obstruction from the channels, disperses Cold, regulates the Qi of the Large Intestine, removes obstruction from the Large Intestine, regulates the bowels, causes sweating, suppresses pain, stimulates its descending and dispersing function.
   - It is calming and antispasmodic, soothes the mind, promotes labor, strengthens Qi Xu and subdues Stomach Qi.
   - It spreads Lung Qi, is the point of entry of the Lungs to the Large Intestine and tonifies Taiyin.
4. **Differential diagnosis** – any Large Intestine pathology.

TE 3 (Zhongdu)

1. **Location** – Japanese location: in the depression distal to the junction of the fourth and fifth metacarpal bones, both sides.
2. **Palpation method and sensation** – bilaterally, one side at a time in between the tendons. Achy when pathological. Palpate the right side first.
3. **Energetics** – Shu (stream) point, Wood point and tonification point. Promotes salivation, releases a tight neck that is a sign of Kidney Yin and/or Yang Deficiency.
4. **Differential diagnosis** – any San Jiao pathology, Kidney Yin and/or Yang Deficiency.

SI 3 (Houxi)

1. **Location** – standard location, when a loose fist is made, the point is proximal to the head of the fifth metacarpal bone on the ulnar side, in the depression at the junction of the red and the white skin, both sides.

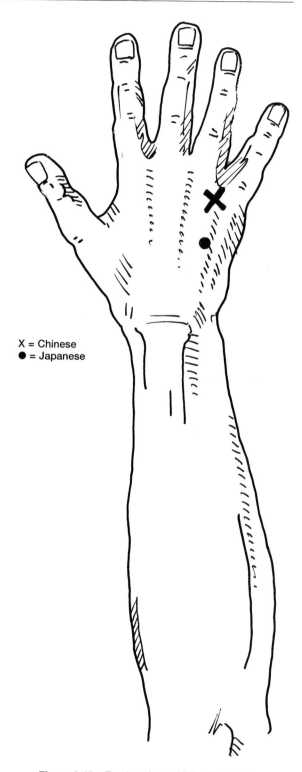

X = Chinese
● = Japanese

Figure 8.15 Two locations of TE 3 (Zhongdu).

2. **Palpation method and sensation** – it is a somewhat awkward point to press but when there is pathology, the point is tender. Press bilaterally, one side at a time against the bone. Palpate on the right side first.
3. **Energetics**
   - Shu (stream) point, Wood point, tonification point. Removes obstructions from the channel, expels Wind-Heat, meridian reflex area, promotes lactation, pituitary gland reflex (master gland of the body regulating hormones), for hormonal abnormalities.
   - Master of the Governing Vessel. Eliminates interior Wind from the GV channel, expels exterior Wind, disperses Heat from the exterior, benefits sinews, comforts tendons and muscles, moves and controls the Governing Vessel, disperses excess Yang of the GV channel, resolves Dampness affecting the chest and Gall Bladder, relaxes the muscle channels, clears the spirit, consolidates the surface, regulates the Yang energy of the head, because the channel passes through the head, the brain and the pituitary gland and has an effect on hormones.
4. **Differential diagnosis** – any Small Intestine or Governing Vessel channel pathology.

TE 5 (Waiguan) – see above under ST 25L

GB 41 (Zulinqi) – see above under ST 25L

Diagnostic points 5 and 6: CV 6 (Qihai) and CV 4 (Guanyuan)

These points should feel resilient.

Clearance points: KI 1B (C), KI 6B (J), KI 3B (J), KI 7B (C), BL 62R (J), KI 16 (J)

KI 1 (Yongquan)

1. **Location** – standard location, in the depression appearing on the sole of the foot when the foot is in plantar flexion, approximately at the junction of the anterior and middle third of the sole, both sides.

2. **Palpation method and sensation** – palpate both points separately with deep dispersive pressure. I call this the 'raise the dead' point which gives you an image of how strong the stimulus of this point can be. Simultaneously, when feeling KI 1, assess the temperature of the feet. Temperature assessment is the most important aspect of palpation of the limbs. A lack of warmth in the extremities is a sign of Yang vacuity.
3. **Energetics** – Jing (well) point, Wood point, sedation point. Adjusts Blood pressure, promotes circulation of Blood due to vascular disturbance of the lower limbs, tonifies Yin, clears Heat, subdues Wind, quiets the spirit, subdues empty Heat, calms the mind, restores consciousness, clears the brain, tonifies Kidneys, benefits Essence, nourishes Yin, suppresses Liver Fire, opens orifices. It is the most important point for regulating the Blood pressure and Blood circulation to the upper part of the body.
4. **Differential diagnosis** – Blood disturbances.

KI 6 (Zhaohai) – see above under CV 14–15

KI 3 (Taixi)

1. **Location** – Japanese Kidney 3 is the point we want to press. This has the same location as Chinese Kidney 5 (Shuiquan) which is in the depression anterior and superior to the medial side of the tuberosity of the calcaneum, both sides.
2. **Palpation method and sensation** – palpate both points separately, rubbing firmly against the heel. It may be tender.
3. **Energetics**
   - Source point, Shu (stream) point, Earth point. Regulates the uterus, nourishes the fetus, thyroid gland reflex (thyroid hormones stimulate the metabolism of every cell just as the Kidney is the basis of all functions in the body).
   - Tonifies Kidney Yin and Yang (KI Qi), replenishes Yin, tonifies Essence, increases

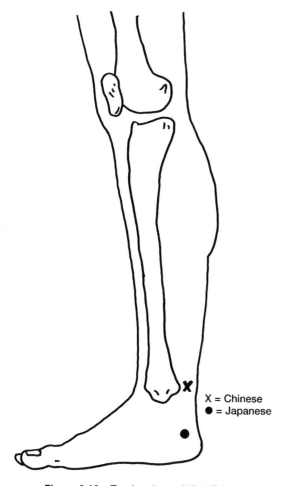

X = Chinese
● = Japanese

Figure 8.16 Two locations of KI 3 (Taixi).

3. **Energetics** – Metal point, tonification point, Jing (river) point. Benefits the Yang, regulates the Qi of the Kidney, clears Heat, eliminates Damp, strengthens Wei Qi, regulates pores, dispels dryness, disperses Stagnation, moves water, organ reflex point of Kidney, regulates Bladder, menses, water pathways, stimulates or restrains sweating, strengthens back, unblocks pulses, restores collapsed Yin.
4. **Differential diagnosis** – Kidney Yang Xu.

BL 62 (Shenmai)

1. **Location** – Japanese Bladder 62 is the point we want to palpate. This has the same location as Chinese Bladder 61 (Pucan) which is posterior and inferior to the external malleolus, directly below BL 60, in the depression at the junction of the red and the white skin, right side.
2. **Palpation method and sensation** – palpate on the right side only with a deep transverse rub. Usually it is tender.
3. **Energetics** – Master of the Yangqiao mai, which originates from the Kidneys. Regulates the Yang energy of the head.
4. **Differential diagnosis** – imbalance of Yang energy of the head.

water of the whole body, moistens the Heart, subdues Fire, benefits Essence, bones, marrow, strengthens lower back and knees, clears Deficiency Heat by nourishing Yin, reflects the condition of the thyroid gland.
4. **Differential diagnosis** – Kidney Qi Xu.

KI 7 (Fuliu)

1. **Location** – standard location, 2 cun above KI 3 on the anterior border of tendocalcaneus, both sides.
2. **Palpation method and sensation** – palpate each separately with moderate pressure. Tends to be achy.

KI 16 (Huangshu)

1. **Location** – a radius of 0.5 of a cun around the entire navel.
2. **Palpation method and sensation** – go around the navel in about 6–8 places. Palpate each point separately on an angle towards the navel.
3. **Energetics** – Kidney 16 is the Front Mu point of the Kidney according to Yoshio Manaka. It supports the Kidney and can tap into the prenatal Qi. It is a Spleen reflex according to the *Nanjing* abdominal map, a point of the Chong mai, an associated point of the intestines and connects with the Heart.
4. **Differential diagnosis** – Kidney Deficiency.

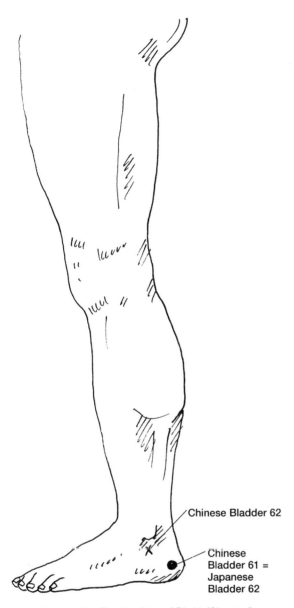

Figure 8.17   Two locations of BL 62 (Shenmai).

Chinese Bladder 62

Chinese Bladder 61 = Japanese Bladder 62

WHEN TO PERFORM THE SECOND PHYSICAL EXAM

This second physical examination is performed every time the patient is seen – it is the heart of the treatment plan. Utilizing only six diagnosis points and usually about 8–10 clearance points, it can quickly and accurately summarize the organ and meridian pathologies of the patient.

The first few times you clear the abdomen there may be a lot of pathology to deal with. However, as you systematically treat the patient every week based upon the pattern of presentation, the number of problematic points on the abdomen quickly reduces to just a few. This is especially true if the patient participates in the healthcare process by stimulating these points between treatments. This core pattern reflects the root pathology which is often a Kidney pathology. However, to ascertain the correct diagnosis, this physical exam is conducted at every visit to assess the full condition of the patient.

At this juncture the patient can be treated with needles to reinforce the clearance achieved by hand. Because a significant amount of quite powerful treatment has already been done by hand, we want to minimize the amount of further treatment yet simultaneously reinforce what has been accomplished. Acupuncture plans to a certain extent are artistry and thus practitioners have the freedom to construct any treatment plan they choose. However, a treatment plan consonant with the data collected from the modified abdominal exam makes the most sense if one is using this system. More will be said about point selection and treatment plans in Chapter 11. Since the navel is part of the abdomen, it can be examined and its treatment integrated with the abdominal treatment.

The case studies that follow provide an appreciation of the immediacy and power of abdominal clearing.

NEW WORDS AND CONCEPTS

Clearance points – treatment points which remove pathology from the abdominal diagnosis points.

Latent points – healthy acupuncture points of the body that do not exhibit any signs of point pathology. They do not spontaneously fire and are not tender when palpated or mechanically accessed.

Longitudinal luo – a vessel that stimulates the organ–meridian complex that it is on. For instance,

---

Case 8.1 Food poisoning treated with abdominal clearing and the clearance points ST 34 (Liangqiu) and ST 44 (Inner Neiting)

The patient was a student who had just eaten a quick spicy meal at a fast food restaurant. Immediately after eating she had an intense pounding headache in the frontal area of the head along with spasmodic and colicky stomach cramps which were extremely painful. She was doubled over in pain and felt nauseous to the point of vomiting. It appeared she had eaten contaminated food. She didn't think she could attend class nor for that matter even get home so I offered to clear her abdomen. She was skeptical of this whole procedure but agreed to it only because she felt so sick.

Throughout the clearing process, as I pressed the clearance points on her feet and wrists, she twisted and turned and yelled that the problem was in her stomach and intestines and her head, not anywhere else. However, I proceeded. The two clearance points which were the most painful were ST 34 (Liangqiu), Xi (cleft) point of the Stomach channel, and Japanese ST 44 (Inner Neiting), the water point. Both are clearance points to move obstruction and clear Fire in the organ.

With the patient in a reclining position I applied a strong dispersion technique by hand to ST 34R. Within a few minutes the stomach pain stopped. However, she still had the headache so I continued to work on CV 12 by proceeding to the next clearance point, the alternative location to ST 44. Shortly thereafter the headache and the nausea stopped.

After I had cleared the six points of the modified abdominal map, the student was amazed that the headache, nausea and stomach cramps had disappeared. In only a few minutes she was able to walk to class feeling fine but admittedly baffled by what had just occurred.

Case 8.2 Acute dysmenorrhea treated with abdominal clearing and the clearance point SP 10 (Xuehai)

The patient was a 25-year-old student suffering from intense menstrual cramps before class. Due to the extreme discomfort, she didn't think that she would be able to sit through the long class that afternoon. Since we had a few minutes before class began, I suggested clearing her abdomen.

Her abdomen was very sensitive, especially at ST 25 (Tianshu) on the left. This Blood Stagnation reflex point correlated with the menstrual cramps. The primary clearance point for this area is SP 10 (Xuehai) on the left. Without the use of needles, I applied a strong dispersive palpation technique to this point for about 5 seconds. It successfully cleared ST 25 on the left because SP 10 invigorates Blood circulation and the Spleen controls the Blood. Within a few seconds the student no longer had the menstrual cramps and she was able to attend class in comfort.

---

when needling LU 7 (Lieque), the Luo point of the Lung meridian, with a certain technique, it connects to the organ of the Lung as well as stimulating the meridian.

Lymphatic glandular exhaustion – the name given by Dr Nagano to the theory of how the body becomes weakened by pathogenic factors and the fight between them and the antipathogenic Qi of the body.

Meridian therapy – a system of therapeutics involving palpation of the meridian systems, including the secondary vessels (Extraordinary meridians).

Passive points – points which are tender upon mechanical stimulation such as palpation, because they are unhealthy.

Reflex areas (kidney, thyroid, adrenal gland, appendix, etc.) – areas that reflect the condition of the relevant organ or where a particular disease manifests.

Secondary tonification point – the Grandmother point or the Controlling point. For instance, LU 9 (Taiyuan) is the tonification point of the Lungs because it is the Earth point of the Lungs and Earth is the mother of Metal. The secondary tonification point is the Controlling point. In this case, that is Heart 7 (Shenmen). Heart 7 is the Earth point on the Fire meridian. Fire controls Metal and Earth is the mother of Metal. Thus, it is referred to as a secondary tonification point.

Transverse luo – a vessel which connects to the Source point of its coupled meridian. For instance, when needling LU 7 (Lieque), the Luo point of the Lung meridian, with a certain technique, it connects to the Source point of its coupled meridian, LI 4 (Hegu). Transverse Luos are used to establish equilibrium between a husband–wife pair.

QUESTIONS

1. Explain how clearance points can represent an even earlier preclinical condition (earlier than the abdominal diagnostic points).

2. Why are some clearance points palpated bilaterally and others unilaterally?

3. What connection does ST 25 (Tianshu) on the left have with the Liver? What connection does ST 25 on the right have with immunity?

4. What are the minimum number of clearance points which can be used to clear the abdomen? What is the maximum number?

5. What are the two most critical steps in using abdominal palpation as a method of diagnosis?

6. Name the points of the modified abdominal map on Figure 8.18.

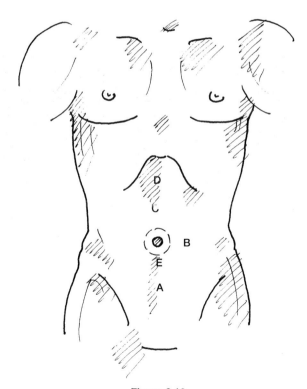

Figure 8.18

7. List all the clearance points in the correct order for each diagnostic point. Designate left, right or both for each point. For each clearance point, give the energetic(s) which enables it to clear the diagnostic point.

8. Explain why a patient with a major complaint and other pathologies might not react to abdominal palpation. (Give at least three reasons.)

9. Which diagnostic point is reflective of stress and why would this be a prime area for reflecting the body's stress?

10. Give the expected healthy characteristics for each of the six abdominal diagnosis points and their expected pathological findings.

11. The fundamental premise of abdominal diagnosis is that the abdomen is a reflection of the body's _____.

12. Clearance points for a given diagnostic point are palpated in a specific order. Explain why.

13. What are the three major pathologies of the Stomach that the CV 12 clearance points treat?

14. What category of points do the clearance points generally fall into? Choose one answer.

- Latent points
- Passive points
- Active points

Clinical notes

Four ways to eliminate Blood Stasis

Blood Stasis is a fascinating concept in Oriental medicine. Although the system has methods for treating this entity, treatment is not easy even though one can formulate a diagnosis of Blood Stasis and a corresponding treatment plan to activate it.

Marcus (1991, p. 46) and others maintain that there are four ways to eliminate Blood Stasis and these are described below. My interpretation of each of these strategies is commented on, particularly the use of certain points in the abdominal clearance protocol to achieve this result.

1. Activating the Blood and transforming Stasis. This is a treatment strategy in which the practitioner aims to promote Blood circulation and thereby wash or sweep away the Stasis. This is the least aggressive of the Blood Stasis methods. In the Japanese system, SP 10 (Xuehai) and KI 1 (Yongquan) are the primary points which can achieve this result.

2. Dispel the Stasis and activate the Blood. In this method, the Stasis is first dispelled and this results in the activation of the Blood circulation. This method is obviously relatively direct. The aim of the treatment is literally to break up the local Stagnation. The application of liniments such as Zheng Gu Shui to the affected area or needling or moxa can accomplish this end.

3. Cracking the Stasis and dispersing the mass. This method is reserved for cases of substantial stagnant Blood such as tumors and cancer. In this case, there are usually palpable masses. This is the most drastic method of eliminating Blood Stasis and is usually accomplished with herbs over acupuncture points. Caution should be used with this method to ensure that the Blood is being dissolved and not just moved so as to cause a metastasis or an embolus. The practitioner should consult a primary care Western physician on common pathways of metastasis and emboli routes and the advisability of treating the patient.

4. Dispelling the Stasis and generating the new Blood. This is a case of Blood Stasis impeding the generation of fresh Blood or the growth of new healthy tissue. This method utilizes a combined Excess/Deficiency approach that is often needed in the case of prolonged Blood Stasis. Again, SP 10 is an efficient point for dispelling the Stasis and nourishing the Blood. There are other points that can nourish the Blood as well and these will be discussed in subsequent chapters.

Figure 8.19 illustrates in graphic form the images that practitioners can keep in mind when encountering these various Blood Stasis presentations.

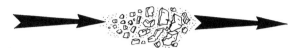

1. Activating the Blood and transforming Stasis – use SP 10

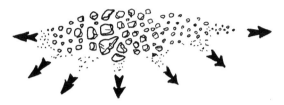

2. Dispel the Stasis and activate the Blood – use liniments, needles, moxa

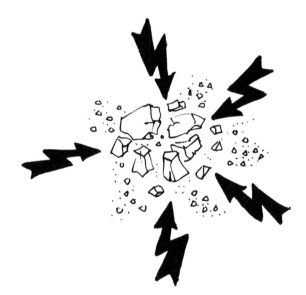

3. Cracking the Stasis and dispersing the mass – use herbs

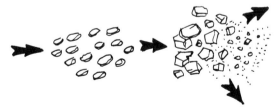

4. Dispelling the Stasis and generating the new or fresh Blood – use SP 10

Figure 8.19   Four ways to eliminate Blood Stasis.

Note: In patients with cancer, I do not recommend abdominal clearance because of the risk of spread or metastasis of the cancer. The healthy Hara examination can be conducted on these patients and they can certainly be needled in select places. With cancer patients, I prefer the use of herbs as implied in the third way to deal with Blood Stasis described above.

Supplemental points for clearance of certain diagnosis points

Additional points to clear right-sided tenderness in the ST 25 (Tianshu) area

BL 2	Zhanzhu
ST 30	Qichong
SP 4	Gongsun

LR 8	Ququan
LR 5	Ligou – for any 'itis'
SP 6	Sanyinjiao
LU 6	Kongzhui – if Lungs are weak
ST 2	Sibai – with weak immune system
TE 16	Tianyou – same as above
SI 18	Quanliao – same as above
ST 12	Quepen – same as above
BL 25	Dachangshu – if ileocecal valve is involved
BL 23	Shenshu – same as above
ST 13	Qihu – 'to reverse a condition'

Additional points for ST 25 on the left

BL 15	Xinshu
BL 18	Ganshu

9

The role of the Eight Extraordinary Meridians in palpatory diagnosis and treatment

To provide a discourse on the topic of the Eight Extraordinary Meridians is not an easy task due to the complex nature of the subject and the fact that there is not universal agreement on their functions. However, the use of the Eight Extraordinary Meridians is an integral part of both the Japanese and Chinese medical systems. Thus, it needs to be explored so we can understand why the clearance points in particular are so effective in treating root pathology.

As we have seen, Japanese acupuncture primarily differs from the way in which Chinese medicine has been practiced in the sense that in the former, meridian palpation and evaluation takes precedence over a Zang-Fu intellectual diagnosis consisting of signs and symptoms pertaining to organs. One of the reasons why the Japanese approach is so efficacious is that it is based upon the natural laws of life that the *Nanjing* expounded. It appreciates internal organ pathways, their points of intersection and the palpatory findings of those points. The Eight Extraordinary Meridians are obviously part of the meridian system and an important one.

Classically trained Chinese physicians would agree that one's acupuncture education is incomplete, if not severely deficient, without an exploration of the functions of the Extraordinary Meridians, their internal pathways, external intersections, the portions of the body they govern, their channel symptomatology and essential functions in the body. As Maciocia (1993) points out, *The study of the Eight Extraordinary Vessels* says, 'If the doctor understands the Extraordinary Vessels, he or she can master the 12 channels and the 15 connecting vessels'.

If practitioners do not understand the clinical usage of the Extraordinary Meridians, they are missing a very large portion of the picture of bodily energetics or physiology. This is not to say that clinicians will not get results in treatment – they will, for such is the nature of a medicine based upon energy, results can be obtained as energy is manipulated. It is common knowledge that herbalists get results without employing the Eight Extraordinary Meridian framework because they work on supporting internal organs by affecting them with biological substances. However, appreciation of the Extraordinary Meridian system, as well as Luo channel physiology and pathology, can elevate practitioners' diagnosis to the most astute and their treatment to the most sublime in the sense of an energetic treatment that matches the energetic configuration of the patient.

The purpose of this chapter is to provide readers with an outline of the Eight Extraordinary Meridians so they:

- can see their valuable clinical roles
- will understand why these points are of such importance in the Japanese system
- will know how to use them appropriately and effectively with palpation, needle selection and their corresponding needle techniques.

THE EIGHT EXTRAORDINARY MERIDIANS AND THEIR RELATIONSHIP TO JAPANESE ACUPUNCTURE

The Eight Extraordinary Meridians, known also as the Eight Curious Vessels, the Secondary Vessels, the Eight Extra Meridians, the Eight Miscellaneous Meridians, the Irregular Vessels, the Miraculous Meridians, the Homeostatic Meridians, the Odd Meridians, the Eight Vessels and the Eight Psychic Channels, are an integral part of the acupuncture meridian system. They are the first meridians created after conception and the resulting early cell divisions (Matsumoto & Birch 1988, p. 181) forming the dynamic

genetic outline that dictates our structural and physical characteristics.

In Chinese terms they are infused with Jing because they came from Jing. This Jing, our Yuan Qi, is a product of our mother's egg (Jing) and our father's sperm (Jing), that combined to form our own Qi or Jing (Yuan Qi, Source Qi, congenital Qi) in the presence of the Shen* of the universe. This rarefied essence contains the instructions for growth, maturation and development. It is the internal dynamic of development, an energetic vector, so to speak.

As acupuncturists know, with the exception of the Conception and the Governing Vessel channels, the Eight Extraordinary Meridians do not have their own set of points by which the energy of their respective channel is reached. However, they intersect with points of the 12 main meridians and these are the points through which the particular physiological energy incarnated in each of the Eight Extraordinary Meridians is contacted. This point of intersection of a main meridian with an Extra channel is called a Coalescent point.

There are eight points from the 12 main meridians which activate the Extra channels and they are called Master or Confluent points. A point on a main meridian connecting to an Extraordinary Meridian is clinically useful because of its ability to tap into the Extraordinary Meridian and activate its function.

Just as each of the 12 main meridians plays a particular role in the body, so too do the Extraordinary Meridians have their own functional characteristics and clinical utility independent of the channels. The 12 main meridians maintain a certain sphere of function for each organ and regulate the superficial flow of energy in the body, sending Qi and Blood to every part of the organism. Most of the Eight Extraordinary Meridians branch out from the 12 primary channels and share functions of circulating Qi throughout the body. They have general roles that they play in the body by virtue of belonging to a primordial group of meridians. Although

---

* Shen in this sense refers to the conditions under which life becomes possible.

they are different from each other, they share some common characteristics.

GENERAL FUNCTIONS OF THE EXTRAORDINARY MERIDIANS

The Extraordinary Meridians are not connected to any organ except for the Kidney because they originate from the Kidney. They do not penetrate the organs. These vessels are not subject to the laws of Yin or Yang; that is, while they work intimately with a coupled meridian and other meridians, they are not bound in a coupled Yin/Yang relationship. The Extraordinary Meridians which deal with Yin are coupled together and the meridians which deal with Yang are coupled together; for instance, the Chong and the Yinwei channels are Extraordinary Meridians which both pertain to Yin.

Homeostatic and supplementing function

Perhaps one of the most important functions that the Extraordinary Meridians possess is a homeostatic quality. Homeostatic meridians have the ability to balance energy in the body. This balancing function has a dual mechanism: first, to absorb excess perverse energy in the body and in effect to annihilate it, and second, to supplement the body with Wei Qi and ancestral energy when it is deficient. As Dr Tran Viet Dzung, Dr Nguyen Van Nghi's protégé, asserts, they have supraphysiologic properties (Dzung 1989). Chapter 27 of *The classic of difficulties*, the *Nanjing*, points out, 'When there are heavy rains, canals and ditches are full to the brim'.

Similarly the Extraordinary Meridians are left out of the channel system so that they can take the overflow from the main channels. Like the gates of a reservoir, they can be used to adjust the Qi flow in the rivers (the 12 organ-related Qi channels) and the level of Qi in the reservoir. They can absorb excess Qi from the main channels and then return it when they are deficient. As we have seen, the purpose of abdominal clearing and treatment is to fulfil both of these roles as well – to remove Excess and to support Deficiency.

Circulatory and enriching function

Part of this supplementation of energy involves circulating Wei Qi and supplementing the body with ancestral Qi. As we have seen in Chapter 5, deficiency of these two types of Qi is the leading cause of illness. The Extraordinary Meridians are adept at providing the body with usable ancestral energy because of their intimate connection with the Kidney. Remember the origin of the Extraordinary Meridians is the Kidney itself. In a sense they are vessels of the Kidney and conductors of Jing. As a result, they are superb for Essence Deficiency illnesses or when the patient experiences a multiplicity of deficiencies. They also harmonize the zones between the 12 main meridians and so they are useful for those areas not traversed by the longitudinal meridians such as the Bladder, Stomach and Kidney that travel upward and downward.

Controlling function

Being so closely associated with the Kidney, they are able to regulate or control lifecycle changes such as reproduction, menstruation and menopause that characterize our human development. Again, lifecycle illnesses are ideally suited to treatment with the Extraordinary Meridians.

Nourishing function

The Extraordinary Meridians have a special relationship with the ancestral organs of the brain, uterus, bones, marrow and Gall Bladder. They circulate Jing and nourish them. Because illnesses of any of these ancestral organs are typically deep seated or areas which may require special attention or access, they are uniquely suited to treatment via the Extraordinary Meridians.

Supervisory function

Each Extraordinary Meridian commands certain portions of the body, certain organs and meridians. For instance, the GV channel governs the neck, shoulders, back and inner canthus and the specific meridian symptomatology associated with each of these areas.

Balancing function

When other techniques such as balancing the pulses or using the 12 main meridians have failed, these channels can be used to treat the complaint and achieve certain therapeutic effect.

Adjusting function

We must remember that while the Extraordinary Meridians are pathways for the flow of Qi and Blood, Wei Qi, Yang and Jing to the surface and the ancestral organs and to particular portions of the body over which they have a supervisory role, they have a structure as well as the structural codes for development. It is this important function that makes the Extraordinary Meridians one of the most useful vehicles for the treatment of musculoskeletal disorders. Because of this feature they can reduce muscle tension, postural or structural stress, be it inherited or acquired. As Mark Seem (1990) says, the Eight Extraordinary

Meridians represent the realm of potential for all energetic function. They encompass our bodily armor and our reaction patterns. Emotional history can have a somatic organization. They are the shock absorbers of the organs.

Tables 9.1–9.3 extracted from my previous book (Gardner-Abbate 1996), provide valuable information in chart form that highlights major uses of the Extraordinary Meridians. Table 9.1 specifically summarizes the general clinical usage of the Extraordinary Meridians as a group. A perusal of these functions should show that their use very much corresponds with the reasons for using abdominal diagnosis. The reader should be able to see the relationship between these functions and why they can address difficult-to-treat conditions, Essence Deficiency syndromes, Heat/Fire Stasis syndromes, Blood Stasis syndromes and the balancing of fundamental energies in the body, one of the greatest strengths of a meridian-style acupuncture which is what the Extraordinary Meridians are a part of.

Table 9.2 specifically delineates particular roles for each of the vessels by showing the portion of the body each governs, their specific physiological function and meridian symptomatology.

Table 9.1 The general function of the Extraordinary Meridians

	Function	Use
1. Homeostatic	Absorb excess perverse energy from the 12 main meridians	To treat fever caused by invasion of an exogenous pathogen
2. Circulatory	Warm and defend the surface by circulating Wei Qi	To increase Yang in body
3. Enriching	Enrich the body with Qi, Blood, and ancestral Qi	To treat deficiencies in those areas
4. Controlling	Serve as reservoirs and conductors of Jing	To treat Essence Deficiency illness and the developmental lifecycle problems
5. Nourishing	Harmonize and nourish the Gall Bladder, uterus, brain, Blood vessels, bone marrow and bone	To treat diseases of the Liver/Gall Bladder, uterus, brain, Blood vessels, bone marrow, bone
6. Supervisory	Exert a commanding role over areas of the body, essential substances and Zang-Fu organs	To treat zones of the body, essential substances and Zang-Fu organs
7. Balancing	Regulate energy	When the pulses are balanced but the patient still complains of symptoms When the 12 main meridians have failed To treat the root causes of a disease
8. Supplementing	Supplement multiple deficiencies	To treat chronic disease, metabolic and hormonal disorders and psychic strain
9. Adjusting	Reduce inherited or acquired structural stress	To treat muscle tension, postural or structural stress

Table 9.2 The specific use of the Eight Extraordinary Meridians

Meridian	Portion of the body governed	Physiological function	Meridian symptomatology
Du	Neck, shoulders, back, inner canthus	Regulates and stimulates Yang energy, increases Wei Qi, and circulates the Yang of the whole body; for attack by pathogens, particularly Wind-Cold at the Taiyang stage. Supervises the Qi of the Yang channels. Has a strong influence on the Liver. Nourishes the brain, Kidneys, spinal cord. Tends to absorb excess energy from the Yang meridians above GV 14 (Dazhui) and supply energy to them when they are deficient below GV 14	Stiffness and pain in spinal column, headache, epilepsy, opisthotonos, diseases of the central nervous system, intermittent fever, Yang mental illness (hallucinations), cold, numb extremities, insufficiency of Wei Qi
Ren	Throat, chest, lungs, epigastric region	Concentration of Yin energy, controls all the Yin meridians. Nourishes the uterus. Absorbs excess energy from Yin meridians below CV 8 and supplies energy if they are deficient above CV 8. For Yin and Blood problems. Commands diseases related to Blood and gynecology, fluid metabolism disorders. Lung/Kidney disharmonies	Leukorrhea, irregular menses, hernia, retention of urine, pain in the epigastric and lower abdomen, infertility in both men and women, nocturnal emission, enuresis, pain in the genitals, rebellious Qi in the chest, hormonal problems during menopause and puberty due to Stagnation of Qi and Blood, dysmenorrhea, fibroids, cysts, hot Blood problems, chronic itching, pharyngitis, Heart disease, stagnation of whole genital system, genital problems due to Stagnation of Qi and Blood
Chong	Heart, chest, lungs	Arouses three Yin of leg (SP, KI, LR). Constrained Liver invading Spleen with underlying Spleen and Kidney Yang Xu	Spasm and pain in the abdomen, irregular menstruation, infertility in men and women, asthmatic breathing, removes obstructions and masses, circulates blood, regulates lifecycle changes, hormonal sensitivity of uterus, weak digestion from poor constitution with Phlegm-Damp accumulation, menstrual problems related to Spleen, Stagnation and obstruction, psychosomatic gastrointestinal disorders
Dai	Retroauricular region, cheek, outer canthus, mastoid region, Shaoyang zones	Promotes pelvic/leg circulation, nourishes hepatobiliary system, supplies deficiencies, influences downward flow of energy. Its disturbances always affect meridians that it encircles at the level of the waist, i.e. SP, ST, KI, Chong, GV, CV. Its energy depends upon the Yangming and GB being sufficient, otherwise the Dai is not nourished leading to pain, paralysis, etc. Controls circulation at the waist and downward. Regulates the warmers above and below	Abdominal pain, weakness and pain of the lumbar area, leukorrhea, hip problems, irregular menses, distension and fullness in the abdomen, prolapse of uterus, muscular atrophy, motor impairment of lower extremities, migraines
Yinqiao	Lower abdomen, lumbar and hip area, pubis	Brings fluid to the eyes and Jing; secondary vessel of the Kidney	Hypersomnia, Yin Xu (Deficiency) especially at night, spasm of lower limbs, inversion of foot, epilepsy, lethargy, pain in the lower abdomen, pain in the lumbar region and hip referring to the pubis, problems of eyes, genitals, bone marrow, genital Stagnation, used mainly for women
Yangqiao	Inner canthus, back, lumbar region, lower limbs	Secondary vessel to Bladder, absorbs excess energy of head (brain, eyes)	Epilepsy, insomnia, redness and pain of inner canthus, pain in back, lumbar region, eversion of foot, spasms of lower limbs, stiff spine, neck, authoritarian personality
Yinwei	Interior syndromes	Preserver of the Yin, principal vessel of the Kidney; binds the Yin	Cardialgia, chest pain, all Yin Xu (Deficiency) especially of the Heart, impaired Pericardium function
Yangwei	Exterior syndromes	Preserver of the Yang, binds all Yang meridians	Chills and fever, imbalance in defensive energy, jaw tension, digestive disturbances, perspiration problems

Table 9.3 Points of the Extraordinary Meridians

Meridian	Meaning of name	Master points	Coupled points	Xi (cleft)/ Luo points*	Coalescent points
Du mai (GV)	Governor vessel. Governs all Yang channels	SI 3	BL 62	GV 1*	X
Ren mai (CV)	Conception vessel. Responsible to all Yin channels and nourishes the fetus	LU 7	KI 6	CV 15*	X
Chong mai (TV)	Sea of Blood, Sea of Arteries and Meridians, Thoroughfare Vessel, Thrusting channel, Penetrating Vessel. Vital channel communicating with all the channels; regulates the Qi and Blood of the 12 regular meridians	SP 4	PC 6	X	CV 1, KI 11–21
Dai mai (DV)	Belt Vessel, Girdle channel. Binds all the channels	GB 41	TE 5	X	GB 26, 27, 28
Yinqiao mai (YINHV)	Yin Heel Vessel, Heel agility, Accelerator of the Yin	KI 6	LU 7	KI 8	KI 6, 8
Yangqiao mai (YANGHV)	Yang Heel Vessel, Accelerator of the Yang	BL 62	SI 3	BL 59	BL 1, 59, 61, 62, GB 20, 29, SI 10, ST 4, 3, 1, LI 15, 16
Yinwei mai (YINLV)	Yin Link Vessel, connects with all Yin channels	PC 6	SP 4	KI 9	KI 9, SP 13, 15, 16, LR 14, CV 22, 23
Yangwei mai (YANGLV)	Yang Link Vessel, connects with all Yang channels	TE 5	GB 41	GB 35	BL 63, GB 35, 13–21, GV 15, 16, ST 8, SI 10, TE 15

All nomenclature = standard abbreviations of the World Health Organization (1989)

Table 9.3 outlines the significant points that play a role with the Extraordinary Meridians. These are their Master and Coupled points, Xi (cleft) points, Luo points and Coalescent points. Note that the Coalescent points in particular represent eight out of the 26 possible clearance points in a system where 6–10 are the norm for treatment.

Appendix 3 offers a comprehensive list of clinical manifestations derived from research of several texts and lectures. Readers may use them to refresh their memory on specific clinical conditions that may lend themselves to treatment with the Extraordinary Meridians.

Extraordinary Meridian points

Note that in the 26 major clearance points, all the eight Master and Coupled points of the Extraordinary Meridians are represented. Clinically they are also the points that have the highest clearance value and therefore constitute the skeletal outline of the treatment. In a hierarchy of points for abdominal clearing, each has a

specific function. Without the employment of these eight points, the body-mind probe could not be as deep or dramatic and abdominal clearing could not be achieved.

Let us briefly highlight what each Extraordinary Meridian point does in the schema in the order in which they are palpated. All these point energetics were discussed in depth in Chapter 8 in terms of how they related to clearing of the abdomen. They are alluded to now in the context of the Extraordinary Meridians so that we can see their use in meridian-style acupuncture.

PC 6 (Neiguan)

As was mentioned in Chapter 8, it is my belief and that of many clinicians, such as Seem, Van Nghi and others, that in order to reach the root and access core energetic disharmonies, the surface (or the Wei level or the musculature) must be freed up. Another way of saying this is that local Excess and Stagnation must be set in motion before we can get to the underlying deficiencies that need to be tonified. This is the role of the very first point in the clearance procedure, PC 6 (Neiguan).

PC 6 (Neiguan), in my opinion, is the primary treatment point for Stagnation anywhere in the body but particularly in the upper part of the body. As a result, it has a special relationship with the Liver, the organ responsible for the free flow of Qi in the body. It is connected to the Heart, the Liver, the diaphragm and the uterus. All the Eight Extraordinary Meridians meet there. It also stimulates the production of the essential substances.

SP 4 (Gongsun)

Essentially, Spleen 4 (Gongsun) has the cumulative effect of strengthening the critical function of the Spleen and Stomach, the source of postnatal Qi. This function includes supporting SP Qi and Yang, creating Blood and transforming Dampness and harmonizing the Stomach.

TE 5 (Waiguan)

Waiguan, as Master of the Yangwei channel, increases and circulates Yang defensive energy in the body. It works closely with its couple, the Dai channel, to circulate vital defensive energy throughout the entire organism.

GB 41 (Zulinqi)

GB 41 (Zulinqi) opens the Dai channel, the Girdle vessel, the only horizontal support system of the body. If this meridian is not opened then any subsequent redirection of energy could be impaired if it cannot bypass this blockage. Again, as an energetic medicine, results can be obtained in treatment without opening the Dai channel but they may be even more effective when this pathway is not blocked and energy can efficiently move from top to bottom and vice versa via the meridians which traverse the Dai channel.

LU 7 (Lieque)

Lung 7 (Lieque) stimulates the Lung in its capacity as the Master of the Qi. It moves Qi and the Blood that follows the Qi. It works closely with

the Kidney, like a wheel, to circulate energy and distribute Yin and Body Fluids to every part of the body.

KI 6 (Zhaohai)

Kidney 6 (Zhaohai), the source of all Yin, provides Yin to the entire body.

SI 3 (Houxi)

By opening the Governing channel, this point allows Yang energy to circulate properly.

BL 62 (Shenmai)

This point regulates the Yang.

In summary, these points show us that the cumulative effect of the Extraordinary Meridians is:

- to move Stagnation anywhere in the body (PC 6)
- to strengthen the source of postnatal Qi (SP 4)
- to circulate Wei Qi (TE 5)
- to open the Dai channel (GB 41)
- to promote the circulation of Qi and Blood (LU 7)
- to nourish the Yin (KI 6)
- to allow the proper circulation of Yang (SI 3)
- to regulate the Yang (BL 62).

Because of their ability to diagnose as well as treat these basic substances and energies, the points of the Eight Extraordinary Meridians are clinically significant. They fundamentally monitor the state of the immune response. As early, formative, structive energies they are uniquely susceptible to stressors such as poor diet, overwork, drugs and excessive emotions that are part and parcel of modern-day life and that can compromise the True Qi of the body.

HOW TO USE THE EIGHT CONFLUENT POINTS WITHIN THE JAPANESE SYSTEM

In regard to an actual treatment plan, the Extraordinary Meridians can be used in five major ways.

1. As the broad outline to treatment
2. As a Master/Coupled set
3. As Extraordinary Meridians with other relationships to each other
4. As part of the Jing treatment
5. As part of the navel treatment (see Chapter 10).

As the broad outline to treatment

When Chinese doctors are asked how they use the Eight Extraordinary Meridians they typically reply that they are aware of what are called Extraordinary Meridian treatments or Jing treatments. However, they say that they do not employ these strategies per se but rather use the points for their unique energetics that assist in achieving the objectives of the general treatment plan. This is a strategy many practitioners employ.

As a Master/Coupled set

The Extraordinary Meridians can also be used as a Master/Coupled set and this is a common usage. In this case, the Confluent point of each pair is needled. Using this system, the point on the upper part of the body is needled first followed by the point on the lower extremity. Unilateral needling is universally employed. Historically there are varied opinions on which side of the body to needle. My personal preference is to choose points based upon whether their energetics are more left or right sided.

This treatment strategy seems to employ a minimum of two and more commonly four points as part of the treatment plan. My tendency in this case is to needle these points first and then to add other points if needed. Other directives can be to insert the Master point of one channel first to open it, followed by any supplemental points and then finally to close the circuit with the Master point of the associated channel. For instance, the Dai channel could be opened by using GB 41 (Zulinqi), followed by needling some other points that would make sense in the treatment, followed by the Coupled point, the Master of the Yangwei channel, TE 5 (Waiguan).

As Extraordinary Meridians with other relationships to each other

In this strategy, Extraordinary Meridians which are not associated in a coupled relationship but have a connection to each other are needled. For instance, in the treatment of menopause, hot flashes are effectively treated by regulating the Yinqiao and Yangqiao channels which are not Coupled channels but have an energetic connection of regulating the Yin and the Yang. Here, KI 6 (Zhaohai), Master of the Yinqiao channel, and BL 62 (Shenmai), Master of the Yangqiao channel, are needled in a tonification direction to bring Yin energy up and Yang energy down to regulate the Yin and Yang energies that are not in harmony. Thus the manifestations of hot flashes are quelled.

The Jing treatment

The Jing treatment is a Chinese-style treatment in which all the Confluent points supplemented with CV 6 (Qihai) are needled to access the Extraordinary Meridians as supraphysiologic vessels. This is a very potent and profound treatment, which contacts the Qi, specifically the Jing Qi that is located at a very deep level. After this treatment patients usually feel rested and balanced. They are usually not superficially energized and should be encouraged to rest and not to disperse or use their Qi after treatment.

There are various ways to administer this treatment. I tend to use it under the following conditions that exactly correspond to the functions of the Extraordinary Meridians outlined in Table 9.1.

- When the patient has a multiplicity of deficiencies
- When diagnosis is complex but Deficiency is the predominant presentation
- When there are clear signs of Jing Deficiency
- When there are excesses such as Blood Stagnation or Fire syndromes
- As a balancing treatment
- When the ancestral organs may be involved
- When the pulses are balanced but the patient still complains of symptoms
- When exogenous pathogens are not being dealt with by the 12 main meridians

- When the patient experiences chronic disease, emotional, hormonal or psychic strain
- When the 12 main meridians have failed
- When the patient's complaints match the symptomatology of the Extraordinary Meridians.

As usual, the eight needles are inserted unilaterally. Various sources (French, English and others) have their own philosophical predilection as to which side of the body to needle according to one's gender, the order of insertion and withdrawal of the needles and other ideas. Practitioners are encouraged to gain their own clinical experience and to use those methods that make the most sense to them. My particular methodology is summarized in Table 9.4.

NEW WORDS AND CONCEPTS

Ancestral organs – also known as the Extraordinary organs: the brain, uterus, bone, marrow, Gall Bladder and Blood vessels. With the exception of the Gall Bladder, they do not have a meridian counterpart.

Ancestral Qi – the Qi one is born with. Also referred to as congenital Qi, Yuan Qi or Source Qi.

Coalescent point – a point of intersection of a main meridian with an Extraordinary Meridian.

Coupled point – a Master point of an Extraordinary Meridian that is paired to another Extraordinary Meridian.

Jing Deficiency – a weakness of the essential substance of rarefied energy stored in the Kidneys and the Extraordinary Meridians.

Master point – also known as a Confluent point. It activates an Extraordinary Meridian.

QUESTIONS

1. How do the Eight Extraordinary Meridians perform a homeostatic function in the body?

2. What types of disorder are the Eight Extraordinary Meridians most useful for and why? Include specific illnesses.

3. Based on the knowledge of the Eight Extraordinary Meridians given in this chapter, explain again how abdominal palpation functions to treat the root.

4. When were the Eight Extraordinary Meridians created?

5. How are the Eight Extraordinary Meridians different from the 12 regular meridians?

6. What types of clearance point have the highest clearance value?

7. How could the theories of the Eight Extraordinary Meridians be compared with Western theories of genetics (DNA specifically)?

8. List some signs and symptoms of Jing Deficiency.

9. List the 11 conditions for which the Jing treatment is indicated. Using your knowledge of the functions and energetics of the Eight Extraordinary Meridians, explain why the Jing treatment would be effective for each of these 11 conditions.

10. In the Jing treatment, TE 5 (Waiguan) and GB 41 (Zulinqi) are the first pair of Confluent points to be needled. How would you explain this?

11. In the Jing treatment, most of the Confluent points are needled in the direction of the meridian, with little or no manipulation. Why is this? Compare it to Chinese needle techniques. From the charts given in this chapter, make a general comparison between Japanese and Chinese needling techniques.

Table 9.4 How to use the eight Confluent points in treatment – the Jing treatment

Point order	Master point	Coupled point	Side of body to palpate	Palpation method	Sensation	Point location	Needle technique (Japanese needles best = 1G)
TE 5 (Waiguan)	Yangwei mai	GB 41 (Zulinqi)	Right	Deep palpation to PC 6, perpendicular pressure. Relatively speaking, palpation on this side will be more shallow because Yang side is more muscular and Yin more mushy	Not as strong as subsequent points but when relevant, patient perceives sensation at the point	Standard TE 5 location	Perpendicular insertion 0.5–0.8 in. No or small manipulation depending upon patient's constitution
GB 41 (Zulinqi)	Dai mai	TE 5 (Waiguan)	Left	Vigorous rubbing	Point is shallow and extremely painful in general	Compare two locations: standard GB 41 location and Japanese location in the depression anterior to the cuboid bone	For either location, obliquely 0.3 in. In the direction of the meridian (toward toe)
PC 6 (Neiguan)	Yinwei mai	SP 4 (Gongsun)	Left	Deep perpendicular palpation to TE 5	Very tender when pathological	Standard PC 6 location	Insertion 0.5–0.8 in. No or light manipulation depending upon patient's constitution
SP 4 (Gongsun)	Chong mai	PC 6 (Neiguan)	Right	Solid rub against bone	Extremely painful in most cases	Standard SP 4 location	Perpendicular or oblique insertion 0.3–0.5 in. If oblique, needle in direction of meridian (toward heel)
LU 7 (Lieque)	Ren mai	KI 6 (Zhaohai)	Right	Massage in cleft of the styloid process of the radius	Not much comes up on palpation because of the size of the point but it can. Other signs and symptoms will support the use of the point	Standard LU 7 location	Obliquely 0.3 in. In direction of the meridian (toward thumb). Sometimes I go up the arm for dispersion using the point as a longitudinal Luo
KI 6 (Zhaohai)	Yinqiao mai	LU 7 (Lieque)	Both	With thumb push into the point	Characteristically tender, usually more on one side than another. Choose the more tender	One of the alternative Chinese locations defined as 1 cun below medial malleolus, but slightly superior to the junction of the red and white skin in a depression generally marked with a (X) fold in the skin	Posteriorly horizontally 0.1–0.2 in. in direction of meridian (toward heel)

SI 3 (Houxi)	Du mai	Left	Obliquely upward against bone	In terms of frequency, does not come up that often, except when indicated and then there is some sensation that the patient reports	Standard SI 3 location	Perpendicular or obliquely upward (toward fingers) 0.3 in.
BL 62 (Shenmai)	Yangqiao mai	BL 62 (Shenmai) Right	This is a shallow point; rub it firmly	Generally very sore	Japanese BL 62 location which is closer to the Chinese BL 61 location	Obliquely 0.2–0.3 in. In the direction of the meridian (toward toes)
CV 6 (Qihai)	X	SI 3 (Houxi) Center	Press perpendicularly 1–1.5 in.	Dislike if in pathology, sometimes invasive and guarded. In pathology, either a sensation of mushiness indicative of Deficiency or hardness which is Excess due to underlying Deficiency. Resilient and good tone in health	On the midline of the abdomen 1.5 cun below the center of the umbilicus	Perpendicularly 1–1.5 in. Summon Qi to the area and tonify

10

Physical examination III: the navel as a microsystem for diagnosis and root treatment

While the diagnostic significance of the navel has historical roots in the *Nanjing*, this part of the anatomy also has useful clinical applicability for illnesses in the modern world. The navel reflects various organ-related phenomena useful in the diagnosis and treatment of specific clinical conditions such as asthma, allergies and skin disorders and more. In this chapter an introduction to the navel as viewed in Western medicine is followed by an exploration from the perspectives of Chinese and Japanese traditions which are supplemented with treatment strategies, cases and photos. Included herein is a method for strengthening Spleen, Lungs and Kidney – the root Qi of the body – via the navel region that is clinically effective and can be applied immediately in practice.

Early in Oriental medical training, the student learns that the umbilicus or navel, which corresponds to the acupoint CV 8 (Shenque: Spirit Gate), is regarded as a 'forbidden point' for needling. They then discover that the application of moxibustion to this area of the abdomen is permissible for specific conditions, such as loose stools or increasing the will to live. However, they rarely see it used clinically and they may not use it often, if at all, when they become practitioners. Nevertheless, in Oriental medicine there are important uses of the navel as a microsystem with its own diagnostic parameters and treatment strategies that extend well beyond the conditions for treatment in Oriental medicine, including the diseases cited above.

CLASSICAL FOUNDATION FOR ABDOMINAL DIAGNOSIS AND MICROSYSTEMS

We have seen that the abdomen, or the Hara as the Japanese term this region, is the cavity where the living Qi, the life force of the Zang-Fu organs, resides. As such abdominal diagnosis and palpation, including the microsystem of the navel, are capable of revealing occult disturbances, thus enabling insight into appropriate root treatment.

Located centrally on the abdomen, the umbilicus holds special significance. According to Matsumoto & Birch (1988), commenting on Chapters 16 and 56 of the *Nanjing*:

...the Chinese imaged the universe in the abdomen centered around the north pole star, CV 3, ST 25, ST 23 and the umbilicus. The area around the north pole star, which is the center of heaven, was termed the middle palace, ruled by earth. The *Nanjing*, in partial emulation of the macrocosmic view, placed the earth phase in the center of the abdomen around the umbilicus, mirroring the central location of the middle palace. The other four phases (elements) lie around the center. (p. 333)

Figure 10.1 presents the *Nanjing* abdominal map of the navel.

The *Nanjing* views the navel region as the center of heaven, ruled by Earth, and by virtue of Five Element correspondences, its pertaining organs are the Spleen and the Stomach. Based on this association, practitioners of classical Chinese medicine have used the navel as a means of treating the Spleen, the Lungs (because Spleen is the 'figurative' mother of Lungs) and the Kidney (because Earth 'figuratively' controls Water). Practitioners continue to treat the navel with various modalities for addressing disharmonies of these three major organs; these will be discussed following an introduction to the navel as viewed from the perspectives of Western and Oriental medicine.

THE NAVEL FROM WESTERN AND ORIENTAL PERSPECTIVES

As we know, the navel is the scar on the abdomen marking the location where the umbilical cord joined the body in embryonic life. In most adults it

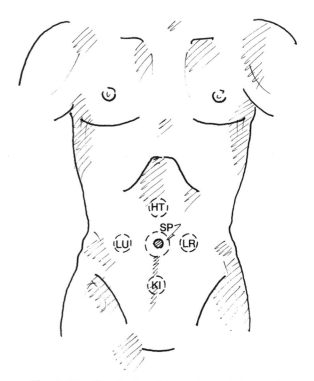

Figure 10.1 The *Nanjing* abdominal map of the navel.

is marked by a depression; in others it is marked by a small protrusion of skin. It is located at the level of the interspace of the third and fourth lumbar vertebrae and interrupts the linea alba about halfway between the infrasternal notch and the pubic symphysis.

The flexible umbilical cord, consisting of two arteries and one vein, is the critical part of the placenta, a highly specialized organ that connects the fetus to the mother. Its function is that of carrying nutrients, proteins, vitamins, salts and oxygen to, and removing deoxygenated Blood and waste products from, the unborn fetus. One of the final roles of the umbilical cord is to deliver antibodies to the child through the Blood at the time of birth. At the time of delivery, after umbilical pulsation has ceased, these antibodies are released, a process which takes about one minute. These antibodies are critical to the establishment of immune function in the newborn child.

While the cord is still connected there are many things leaving the body for the final time. If the time for this is cut short and foreign substances are not allowed to escape, but are trapped by the knotting of the umbilical cord, then there remains in the body foreign substances which the T-cells must recognize and attack. This leads the T-cells to misread the information and also to consider some of the body's own tissue as being foreign. It begins to attack this tissue and continues to do so through life. This may precipitate allergic reactions and if the immune system is weakened as well, autoimmune disease may develop. (Matsumoto 1987)

Severing the umbilical cord before the pulsation has ceased or before the spontaneous ejection of the placenta (usually 15–30 minutes after birth) has the net effect of limiting transfer of these antibodies, as well as a significant amount of placental Blood. Therefore, within seconds, the immunity of a new human life may already be impaired.

Studies conducted more than 30 years ago demonstrated that delayed clamping of the umbilical cord enables newborns to receive far more Blood than with immediate clamping, a common obstetrical practice (Raloff 1996). Clamping delayed by even 5 minutes has been shown to give the infant an additional 80–90 ml of Blood based on an average fetal capacity of +310 mL. Researchers have found that the onset of iron deficiency anemia among infants in developing countries can be delayed by waiting for one minute before severing so that the umbilical cord can deliver placental Blood and cease pulsing (Raloff 1996). According to one source, 'A perennial argument with the cord is when to cut it. Humans used to let it be, at least until the placenta was ejected (usually within 20 minutes), until the 17th century. The practice then began of cutting it and tying it off, leaving a short stump' (Smith 1968, pp 121–124).

The cord is usually clamped and cut off, forming a stub about one inch in length approximately one minute following delivery. The stub dries and usually falls off within 1–2 weeks and then scar tissue forms. Tying or clamping the cord incorrectly or cutting it too close to the abdominal wall can lead to serious digestive disorders, small bowel obstruction, excess bleeding or even possible death.

Voluminous worldwide research on retrieval of cord Blood has shown it to have numerous applications. For example, it is an ideal source of Blood

for the newborn in the event of transfusion, either at the time of birth or in the future – a form of biological insurance. Containing a great quantity of stem cells, which play a role in the body's immune and Blood systems, fetal Blood is being harvested and banked to treat, for example, leukemia and severe anemia and used as an alternative to bone marrow transplantation. Interestingly, since cord Blood has more immunological tolerance than bone marrow in the donor, the recipient does not need to be closely matched (Stephenson 1995).

Japanese medicine appreciates that the navel is our first scar. They refer to it as the Birth Trauma Mu and the area around the navel, that is the KI 16 (Huangshu) area, as the Missing Organ Shu (point) (Matsumoto 1987), in which 'organ' refers to the placenta.

The term 'scar' is applied to a healed wound, ulcer or breach of tissue; it consists of essentially fibrous tissue. In Oriental medical theory, a scar may restrict Qi and Blood flow to various places, organs and meridians; thus, scars have the potential to cause an organ–meridian disturbance.

However, not all scars produce this effect. The level of disturbance that a scar can create depends upon many factors: location, shape, depth, the duration of its existence and how well it has healed. Due to the navel's relatively large size and depth, it is more likely to present the characteristics of a pathological scar; that is, acting to inhibit meridian and organ function. It can be the agent of many organ and meridian pathologies locally and at a distance. This is one major reason why we want to diagnose and treat it in the abdominal examination.

Like all scars, the navel must be palpated to determine the level of involvement. Palpable tension can interfere with the circulation of Qi and Blood. Methods for palpating the navel will be discussed later in this chapter.

The navel is located in an area structurally prone to tension. Basically it is a 'knot' or physical formation in the center of the body where critical physiological functions occur, especially from an Oriental perspective.

When we inspect a patient's navel, it is important to note that its current shape is probably not the same as at the time of birth. It may change in response to system energetics, weight patterns, pregnancy, abdominal surgery and other factors. The average person and the average practitioner may not be aware of this simply because they do not closely observe the navel. However, the underlying energetics can impact the presentation of the navel and the treatment of the navel can impact the underlying energetics.

THE HEALTHY NAVEL

According to Oriental medicine, the navel is regarded as the entry point for the life force. The *Nanjing* characterizes the healthy navel as deep and well shaped with strong surrounding tissue and full pulsation, signs of strong resistance and a long life. The healthy navel is not too shallow, not too deep, not too wide, not too thin and not too tiny. It should be in the center and 'tucked in'. It should have no visible pulsation above it or off center and no depressions around it, except for a very slight one above it. It should look like the 'sun with emanating rays' within the navel ring.

DIFFERENTIAL DIAGNOSIS OF THE PATHOLOGICAL NAVEL

Navel diagnosis involves a microsystem that is easy to learn; few criteria are involved in its assessment.

1. Begin by looking at the borders of the navel. There should be no interruptions, indentations or collapsed borders or depressions except for a very slight one superior to (above) it.

Depressions are indicative of Deficiency (Xu). Using an abdominal map based on the *Nanjing*, looking closely at the corresponding area surrounding the navel can provide a diagnosis of Deficiency of a pertaining organ. You may need to gently feel for subtle depressions. The larger the depressions, the greater the Deficiency in the corresponding organ–meridian complex.

Spleen/Stomach Deficiency is diagnosed at the upper border of the navel, Liver Blood Deficiency to the left of the navel, Lung Qi Deficiency to the right and Kidney Qi Deficiency below (see Figs 10.2–10.5).

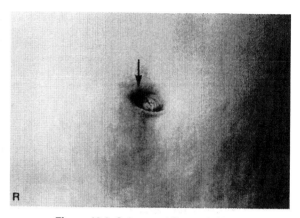

Figure 10.2 Spleen and Stomach Qi Xu.

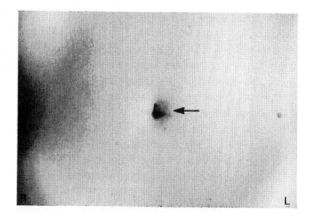

Figure 10.3 Liver Blood Deficiency.

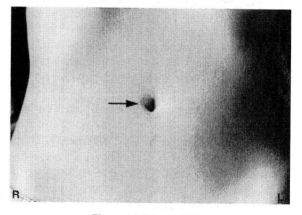

Figure 10.4 Lung Qi Xu.

2. The navel then should have a solid border with no interruptions or indentations, no flaccid or collapsed borders. It should not appear to

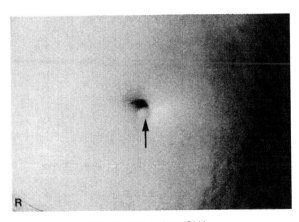

Figure 10.5 Kidney Qi Xu.

'look up or down' (as though it were an eye). The tissue around the navel ring, or border, should be firm, not dough-like. Weakness or flaccidity in the surrounding tissues is indicative of poor vitality, poor response and recovery.

3. The navel should not exhibit any surrounding puffiness or edema. Puffiness is indicative of Yang Deficiency. The most common place to find puffiness is inferior to (below) the navel; this is especially true in overweight people. In Chinese medicine, this sign is viewed as Spleen and Kidney Qi and Yang Deficiency with retention of Damp, generally summarized as Kidney Yang Deficiency (see Fig. 10.6). Occasionally some puffiness may be seen in the areas of the Lung or the Spleen, indicating Deficiency of the Lung Qi (Yang) and Spleen Yang.

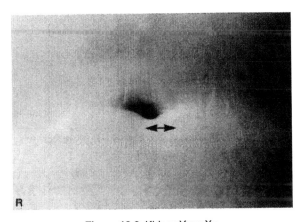

Figure 10.6 Kidney Yang Xu.

4. While the healthy navel should have full pulsation around it, it should not visibly pulse 'off center'. This is indicative of Spleen Qi Deficiency (because the navel pertains to the Spleen). The pulsation is relative to the strength of the person's constitution or vitality, so it has a range of appearances. Ideally, it is visible by simply looking down at the perimeter of the navel. If it is not apparent, it may also be viewed by bending down level with the abdomen and inspecting it, although in such cases it probably is not as full as it should be.

If any abnormally prominent pulsation is detected in the vicinity of the navel, particularly on both sides of the midline but also superior to the navel pulsation in the CV 9 (Shuifen) area, the possibility of an aortic aneurysm must be investigated. This is a potentially serious life-threatening condition necessitating immediate referral for Western medical evaluation.

Most abdominal aneurysms are asymptomatic or detected at incidental physical examination or sonography. However, they may present as an ache in the midline, lumbosacral pain or abdominal lump or the patient may have noticed a prominent abdominal pulsation. They take years to develop, but are fatal within minutes when they rupture. The most common cause is arteriosclerosis; patients with high Blood pressure are prone to developing abdominal as well as other types of aneurysms. The cause of death is often not revealed until an autopsy is performed. Figure 10.7 shows what an abdominal aortic aneurysm looks like.

5. The healthy navel should be 'tucked in'; that is, it should not protrude (see Fig. 10.8) which may indicate a 'connective tissue disturbance'. This is a broader designation than used in the West.

The term 'connective tissue' encompasses vascular tissue proper (areolar, white and yellow fibrous, reticular, adipose), cartilage and bone. Connective tissues are concerned primarily with supporting bodily structures and binding parts together. However, they are also involved in other functions such as food storage, Blood formation and defense mechanisms. The Japanese theory basically maintains that when immunity

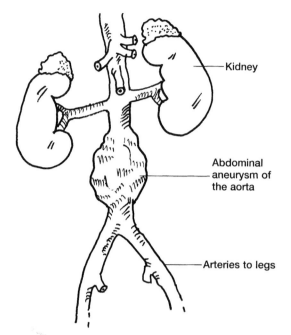

Figure 10.7 Illustration of an abdominal aortic aneurysm.

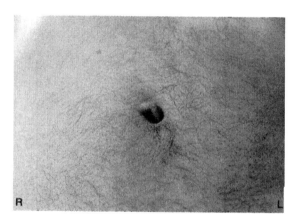

Figure 10.8 Protuberant navel.

is weak, these tissues become the battleground for pathologic activity. Thus from this perspective, connective tissue disease includes not only generally accepted illnesses, e.g. systemic lupus erythematosus, rheumatoid arthritis, etc., but also encompasses conditions resulting from secondary disease (e.g. interstitial inflammation, etc.) in connective tissue; for example, tendonitis, fibrositis, atopic dermatitis, kidney infection, etc.

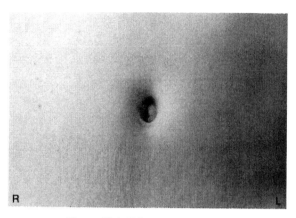

Figure 10.9 This navel is too wide.

In short, this may include any disease that may be a sequela to weak body immunity. A navel which is protruding (commonly described as an 'outie') is considered a reflection of weak immunity.

6. Likewise the navel should not be too wide (see Figure 10.9). Its clinical significance is the same as a protuberant navel; that is, weak immunity.

7. By contrast, if the navel is too tiny, narrow, long or deep (see Figs 10.10–10.13) it is indicative of decreased Qi flow to the Lower Jiao. In terms of Zang-Fu, this is indicative that the Kidney is not grasping Lung Qi. The shape of this navel may also be an inherited trait, in which case it signifies lack of fetal nourishment and thereby a constitutional weakness in the development of the child. This constitutional weakness would manifest as Lung Deficiency with systemic Qi Deficiency.

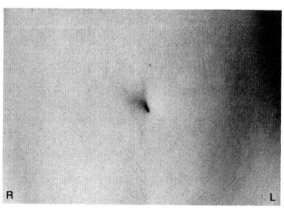

Figure 10.10 Navel too closed, too tiny.

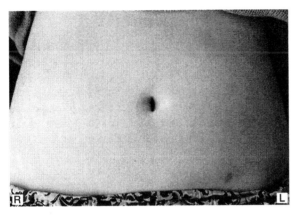

Figure 10.11 This navel is too narrow.

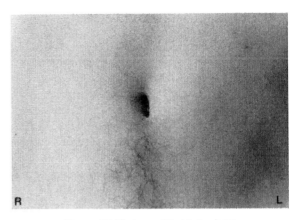

Figure 10.12 A navel that is too long.

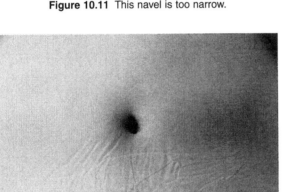

Figure 10.13 This navel is too deep.

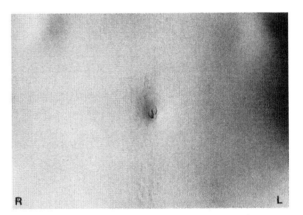

Figure 10.14 Navel is too shallow.

8. The navel should be deep, not small, flat or shallow (see Fig. 10.14). If it is not deep, it suggests insufficient vitality or, in Zang-Fu terms, Kidney Qi Xu.

9. The navel should be located on the midline of the trunk. According to the classical Chinese perspective, an 'off center' navel can indicate a structural and functional weakness (Deficiency) of the Spleen and Kidney (see Fig. 10.15).

10. When the healthy navel is palpated it should feel loose above and resilient below. There are several pathological findings that may be evident if these characteristics are reversed; that is, resilient above and loose below. This indicates Stomach Yin Deficiency and Kidney Qi Deficiency, respectively.

11. The area surrounding the healthy navel should not contain excessively hard or rigid

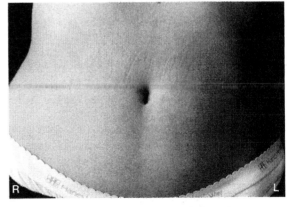

Figure 10.15 An asymmetrical navel.

muscles. The presence of such rigidity is usually a sign of Excess due to an underlying Deficiency, particularly if the rigidity is found inferior to the navel.

12. There should be no pain or reactivity (discomfort) associated with palpation of the healthy navel. Areas reacting to palpation with discomfort, tenderness or pain suggest internal organ problems. Abdominal guarding indicates emptiness of the Kidney, especially of adrenal function. Lack of any reactivity may be a sign of advanced Deficiency, meaning that the vital Qi is weak. For this reason, some elderly persons are less responsive to navel palpation. Additionally I have found that certain drugs, such as prednisone, may make the navel insensitive to palpation.

13. The area around CV 9 (Shuifen) (located 1.0 cun superior to the navel) should be slightly depressed and should not be tender. If it is, it may indicate an imbalance in the ability to eliminate water. A weak navel ring with a lack of pulsation suggests Spleen/Stomach insufficiency, possibly pancreatic insufficiency. Moderate pulsation may indicate general exhaustion and emptiness of the Liver and Kidney. A strong pulsation may indicate the possibility of an emotional disorder. And a big visible pulsation may suggest a possible aortic aneurysm (see above).

For clinical convenience this information is summarized in Table 10.1.

Table 10.1 Comparison of the healthy and unhealthy navel and its differential diagnosis

Healthy	Unhealthy	Differential diagnosis
1. Well shaped with strong surrounding tissue, with a slight depression above it. No interruptions, indentations. Not 'looking up or down'	Any other depression around the border, flaccid or collapsed borders. Appears to 'look up or down'	Deficiency (Xu) of the organ corresponding to that part of the abdominal map 1. Above = Spleen/Stomach Qi Xu 2. Left = Liver Blood Xu 3. Right = Lung Qi Xu 4. Below = Kidney Qi Xu
2. Firm navel border	Dough-like surrounding tissues, that is, the navel ring is weak, feels weak	Poor response and recovery
3. No puffiness	Puffy	Yang Xu generally seen in the Kidney area, i.e. below the navel
4. Full pulsation around navel	Pulsing off center or above	Spleen Qi Xu; possible aortic aneurysm
5. Tucked in	Sticking out	Connective tissue disturbance = weak immunity
6. Not too wide	Too wide	Connective tissue disturbance = weak immunity
7. Not too tiny, too narrow, too deep or too long	Tiny or narrow or deep or long	Lung-Kidney disharmony, insufficient oxygenation to the Lower Jiao. If congenital = lack of fetal nourishment
8. Not small, flat, shallow	Small or flat or shallow	Insufficient vitality
9. Centrally located on abdomen	Off center	Center of gravity off = Spleen/Kidney weakness
10. Loose above, resilient below	Tightness above and emptiness below	Stomach Yin Xu/Kidney Qi Xu respectively
11. Area surrounding navel is not hard	Hard rigid muscles around it	Excess may be due to an underlying Deficiency
12. Area without pain or reactivity	Painful, reactive	Reactive = internal organ problems Antagonistic resistance = emptiness of Kidney, especially adrenal function
13. Slight depression above navel in the area of CV 9 (Shuifen); no tenderness	a. Sensitive CV 9 (Shuifen) area b. Weak and lifeless c. Moderate pulsation d. Strong pulsation e. Big pulsing	a. Imbalance in eliminating water b. Spleen insufficiency, possibly pancreatic insufficiency c. General exhaustion and emptiness of Liver and Kidney d. Psychoneurosis (patient feels unhappy and fearful) e. Possible aortic aneurysm

Pregnancy of course is a condition that affects the entire abdominal and navel presentation and is not diagnosed according to the aforementioned criteria. It is not considered abnormal.

Figure 10.16 also delineates the characteristics of the healthy navel and helps to provide a picture of the features that need to be addressed. Practitioners can then consult Table 10.1 to find

Patient's name:_____   Date:_____

Major complaint and accompanying symptoms:_____

_____

Record the results of observation and palpation of the navel in the appropriate column

Healthy navel description	Healthy	Unhealthy
1. The navel is well shaped with strong surrounding tissue, a slight depression above it. No interruptions, indentations. Not 'looking up or down'		
2. It has a firm navel border		
3. There is no puffiness around it		
4. There is a full pulsation around it		
5. It is tucked in		
6. It is not too wide		
7. It is not too tiny, too narrow, too deep, or too long (specify)		
8. It is not small, flat, or shallow		
9. It is centrally located on abdomen		
10. It is loose above and resilient below		
11. The area surrounding navel is not hard		
12. The area surrounding the navel is without pain or reactivity		
13. There is a slight depression above navel in the area around CV 9 (Shuifen) and no tenderness upon palpation		

Other:_____

Drawing:

Tenderness – where? Describe:_____

_____

Ability to clear navel. What points had the most clearance value?:

_____

Treatment with what modalities:_____

_____

Effect on major complaint if any and/or reaction to treatment:_____

_____

_____

_____

Figure 10.16 Navel diagnosis form.

the meanings of the pathological presentations and use these to guide the construction of a treatment plan.

CLEARING THE NAVEL

The goal of treating the navel is to reduce any palpable tension in this area. Such tension can impinge on the function of the corresponding organs assigned to the *Nanjing* navel map. Record the results of the navel inspection and clearance on the form in Figure 10.16.

Clearing the navel entails the following specific steps.

● After navel inspection, palpate around and just beyond the borders of the navel – not directly on it, just as one would never directly needle the

navel because it is scar tissue. Palpate completely around the navel at a distance equal to that between the navel and KI 16 (Huangshu), approximately 0.5 cun around the navel, and hereafter called Japanese KI 16. With the fingers extended and slightly cupped, palpate around the navel in a clockwise direction at eight places (Fig. 10.17). Assign numbers to the positions as you palpate them and ask patients to tell you if they detect discomfort at any of those locations.

Tension at the navel can be very painful, so prepare the patient for this possibility. Observe the patient's facial expressions as you press at a 45° angle toward the navel as if you were going underneath it. Determine which positions elicit the most discomfort. The first time you palpate the navel, this area may be very uncomfortable and guarded. However, over time as the patient

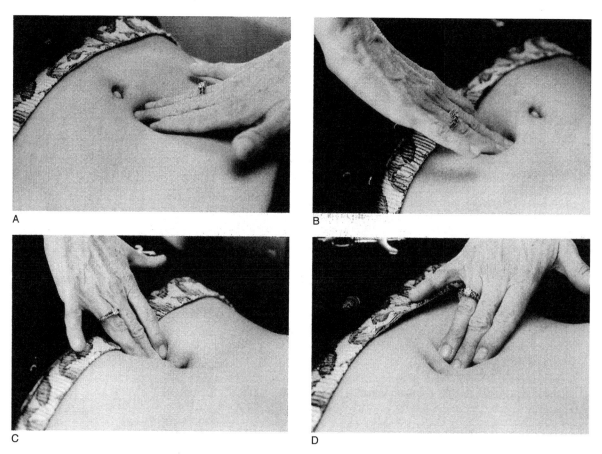

A

B

C

D

Figure 10.17 A–D: How to palpate the navel.

is treated and repalpated and treated, tension at the navel decreases which signifies overall improvement in health.

● The navel area, like the abdomen, basically presents in three ways.

1. It may feel tight or 'rock-like'
2. It may feel vacant (mushy or deficient)
3. Or it may simultaneously feel tight *and* mushy in the same point.

Regardless of the point's sensation proceed as follows.

● Apply deep dispersive pressure to KI 1 (Yongquan), bilaterally, one foot at a time. This point can be exquisitely tender. (I call it the 'raise the dead' point to emphasize its ability to move Qi and Blood.) After pressing this point for 3–5 seconds, recheck the painful navel area to see if it is less tender, more pliant, etc. However, if the tenderness has not been resolved by 80–100%, sequentially press the following additional points for 3–5 seconds: KI 6 (Zhaohai), KI 3 (Taixi) and KI 7 (Fuliu). I prefer the Japanese point locations for KI 6 (Zhaohai) and KI 3 (Taixi) (see Figs 8.8 and 8.16). Remember:

1. Japanese KI 6 is situated at one of the alternative Chinese locations; specifically, 1 cun inferior to the distal border of the medial malleolus. This is in contrast to the Chinese location, slightly less than 0.5 cun inferior to the medial malleolus. I find it by sliding up over the side of the foot, at the junction of what the Chinese texts refer to as 'the red and the white skin', inferior to the medial malleolus.
2. Japanese KI 3 is the same location as Chinese KI 5 (Shuiquan).

Kidney points can be effective for the clearance of the navel region because:

1. a very tender area is usually reflective of a long-term process and long term pathology tends to translate into Kidney dysfunction
2. if the area inferior to the navel is painful, this indicates Kidney involvement because this is the Dan tian region, where the root of the Qi, the energy of the Kidney, resides

3. the Kidney meridian traverses the area vertically adjacent to the navel at KI 16 (Huangshu).

● If these Kidney points do not sufficiently loosen up the area around the navel, press Liver 4 (Zhongfeng) bilaterally, also one point at a time. LR 4 is the Metal point on the Wood meridian and as such, is a clinically effective point for moving Liver Qi because Metal controls Wood. It is best at moving Liver Qi Stagnation in the Lower Jiao. Other points that may clear the navel are LR 5, LR 3 or LR 14 for tenderness to the left of the navel, SP 4, 6 or 9 for tenderness above the navel and LU 1, 2, LI 4, TE 3 or SI 3 for tenderness to the right of the navel. Note that these are the same points used to clear each of the sections of the abdomen, left, above and to the right.

● Procedurally, you can clear the navel every time you clear the abdomen which, as we have established, should be during every patient visit. It is easy to do and does not take that much time to accomplish. Additionally, it tends to be the most stubborn area to clear, largely because it reflects the root pathology so paying attention to it is beneficial in order to resolve tension. However, we should note that because it is such a tender place and because so many patients particularly dislike this part of the palpation, you do not need to do this every time if it interferes with the administration of the treatment plan. In such cases you can monitor the navel every six visits or so.

INTEGRATING THE NAVEL EXAM INTO THE TREATMENT PROCESS

Note that the points used to clear the navel are the identical points used to clear the Lower Jiao (KI 1, KI 6, KI 3, KI 7), as well as to the left of it (LR 5, LR 3, LR 14) and to the right of the navel (LU 1, LU 2, LI 4, TE 3, SI 3). The preponderance of the points pertain to the Kidney and in clinical fact these points provide the highest clearance value. However some new points are introduced, specifically LR 4, SP 6 and SP 9 with LR 4 being the second highest clearance point of the navel area.

TE = standard abbreviation of the World Health Organization (1989) for Triple Warmer.

If there is an overlap of points from the abdominal clearance (8.4) and the navel clearance (see Fig. 10.16) it is apparent that these are clinically significant points for the patient. This means that they can both be worked on by the patient at home and likewise may be needled or treated with moxa or the Tiger Thermie warmer in the office. These points can be used in and of themselves or as the skeletal outline of treatment. Additional treatment strategies are provided below that emphasize the importance and clinical efficacy of treating the navel.

Chinese navel treatment modalities

From the classical Chinese perspective, the use of the navel revolves around the treatment of Lung, Spleen and Kidney disharmonies. While this is not an exhaustive list, the conditions described in Table 10.2 represent the most common applications of navel treatment detailed in basic texts and/or which I have observed during my studies in China.

Indirect moxa (Jian jie jiu)

Applying moxa indirectly to the navel can be highly effective for allergic disorders including sinusitis, allergic rhinitis, sneezing, nasal congestion, rash, watery nose and eyes, hives, nasal itching and headache. Moxa promotes the circulation of Qi in the 12 regular channels, to tonify Deficiency and to dispel Cold and Stagnation of Qi and Blood.

Indirect moxa can be applied in the form of moxa rolls, a moxa burner, belly bowl, stick-on adhesive moxa, the Tiger Thermie warmer or other methods with which one is familiar. Indirect moxibustion can be applied for 3–5 minutes per treatment once a week. If self-administered, it can be applied daily. The course of treatment is dependent upon signs and symptoms.

In commenting on the use of the navel for allergic disorders, American author and practitioner Bob Flaws writes:

...the root of allergic diseases is mostly Qi vacuity, while evil Winds are the branch. In clinical practice it is the vacuity of the three viscera of the Lungs, Spleen

and Kidneys which is mostly seen. The ancients commonly chose the navel and the points around the navel to treat Lung/Spleen insufficiency diseases. The navel communicates with the five viscera and the six bowels and joins the channels and vessels of the entire body. Therefore, it is said in the *Yi Zong Jin Jian (The Golden Mirror of Ancestral Medicine)* that acupoint Shen Que (CV 8) is able to treat 'the hundreds of diseases'. Shen Que is capable of regulating the channels and vessels, Qi and Blood of the entire body. By stimulating Shen Que, one can course and free the flow of Qi and blood, regulate the internal viscera, and strengthen organic function. In terms of modern medical theory, stimulating Shen Que can regulate the nervous, hormonal and immune systems thus improving organ function and returning it to normal. (Flaws 1988, p. 2)

Clearly we can see from this passage that the navel is an optimum place to treat the root cause of much illness.

Moxa on salt (Geyen Jiufa)

Burning moxa on salt filled to the brim of the navel is a traditional Chinese technique. Salt is used for its ability to both insulate from intense heat, yet conduct a moderate amount of that heat. It is used for two major conditions: skin diseases and Yang Deficiency. For skin diseases that are associated with the Lung, treatment of the navel is quite effective.

Skin disorders – acne. One of the most basic treatment strategies in Chinese medicine uses Five Element theory, e.g. when an organ (associated element) is deficient, tonify the mother. In this case, Spleen (the navel) is the mother (the preceding element in the Sheng cycle) of Lungs. In Beijing, at the Beida and Hepingli Hospitals, I observed that skin problems such as acne are treated quite effectively with this technique. The frequency and duration of therapy vary with the presentation and severity; typically 3–5 cones of moxa are burned on the salt in the navel during daily treatment for 10 days and then monitored for improvement and/or continued treatment.

Yang Deficiency symptoms. Symptoms of Yang Deficiency include cold limbs, weak legs, soreness, vomiting and loose stools with undigested food. Moxa on salt is clinically effective and surpasses other techniques for these conditions.

Table 10.2 Moxa and cupping treatment modalities for the navel

Function	Treatment modality	Method*	Clinical condition
1. To promote the circulation of Qi and Blood in the 12 regular channels, to tonify Deficiency, to dispel Cold and Stagnation of Qi and Blood	Indirect moxa over navel	Moxa rolls Moxa box Belly bowl Stick-on adhesive moxa Tiger Thermie warmer Apply 3–5 minutes per treatment once a week. If self-administered, may be applied daily	For allergic conditions, e.g. sinusitis, allergic rhinitis, sneezing, nasal congestion, rash, watery nose and eyes, nasal itching, headache, hives
2. To deliver the therapeutic effects of moxa	Moxa on salt over the navel	3–5 cones of moxa burned on the salt in the navel daily if possible for 10 days or once a week for 10 treatments	a. For skin diseases, e.g. dermatitis, acne b. For Lung Deficiency (when an organ is deficient (LU), tonify the mother (SP-navel)) c. For Yang Deficiency symptoms d. To increase the will to live
3. To fortify the Yang and warm the Middle Burner	Moxa on ginger over the navel	Cut the uncooked ginger into slices one inch in thickness and perforate with tiny holes. Place ginger on the navel. Burn one cone of moxa on the ginger on the navel or points around the navel like ST 25, CV 6. Let each burn down completely; repeat for a total of four cones. Treat once a day for 10 days or once a week for 10 treatments	a. For Spleen and Kidney Yang Xu symptoms, e.g. loose stools with undigested food, constipation, painful menstrual periods and abdominal pain, to consolidate the stools, support assimilation of nutrients b. Allergic rhinitis
4. To strengthen the Spleen, Lung and Kidney	Cupping over the navel	Apply a single large-size cup daily for about 5 minutes. Do not make the cup too tight. Remove the cup and wait 2–3 minutes, then repeat again	a. For skin diseases, e.g. dermatitis, urticaria, atopic dermatitis b. To prevent miscarriage in patients with a history of miscarriage
5. For all of the above reasons	Clear by hand	Palpate around the navel at eight spots (N, S, E, W, NE, NW, SE, SW). Identify tender points. Press on clearance points one at a time in this order. KI 1, 6, 3, 7, LR 4. Check tender navel point after each clearance point. To reinforce clearance, needle navel points, or clearance points or both	All of the above

* With all of these methods, course of treatment is dependent upon presentation of signs and symptoms.

An example of a more esoteric application with this modality is treating the navel in patients who lack the will to live. This is viewed in Chinese medicine as Yang Deficiency. Such patients are depressed, lack the will to function and may be suicidal. In my clinical practice I use this as the method of choice when the patient's Kidney energy is very weak and when they are manifesting psychologically more than physically (although usually there are accompanying physical components such as extreme lethargy, digestive disturbances, sensations of cold and others).

Moxa on ginger (Gejiang jiufa)

Spleen and Kidney Yang Deficiency. The Chinese use of moxa burned over ginger (*Rhizoma Zingiberis Officinalis Recens*: Sheng Jiang) is a common treatment approach for Spleen and Kidney Yang Deficiency manifesting as loose stools with undigested food, constipation, painful menstrual periods and abdominal pain. The acrid hot nature of the ginger assists in fortifying the Yang of the body and warming the Middle Burner, consolidating stools and supporting assimilation of nutrients as well as providing energy to the Kidney to control the lower orifices. The use of moxa on ginger is also applicable for allergic rhinitis.

Cut the uncooked ginger into slices one inch in thickness and perforate with tiny holes. Place the ginger on the navel. Burn one cone of moxa on the ginger and repeat three times, for a total of four cones. Let each burn down completely. The skin around the navel should become flushed. Treat once a day for 10 days (which equals a course of treatment). One to four courses are generally needed depending on the patient's age, duration of symptoms, etc.

Systemic Cold with Yang Deficiency and/or Blood Stagnation. Using the insulation technique described above, perform the same procedure. Clinical manifestations include amenorrhea or dysmenorrhea due to internal Cold as well as abdominal pain and constipation due to Yang Deficiency. Treat according to signs and symptoms.

Cupping (Ba guan liao fa)

Threatened abortion. At inpatient hospitals in China, women with a history of threatened abortion or habitual miscarriages are commonly hospitalized for the duration of their pregnancy. To strengthen the Kidney energy and prevent loss of the fetus, they are treated daily with cupping directly over the navel with a single medium or large cup. This is a unique application of cupping and of treating a problem in pregnancy with Chinese medicine. While this is a powerful technique with which the Chinese have success, personally I have not used it.

Skin disorders – urticaria. Cupping the navel is also very effective for skin diseases such as urticaria or rashes due to Dampness. It is also an excellent therapy for children or those who suffer from intractable skin diseases such as atopic dermatitis or acne.

The cup can be applied daily for about 5 minutes. Do not make the cup too tight. Remove the cup and wait 2–3 minutes and then repeat once (Fig. 10.18). For convenience, patients can self-administer after brief training if they purchase a set of cups with a suction apparatus.

Again, the Lungs and areas they govern, such as the skin, are strengthened through treating the elemental mother, the Spleen, which corresponds to the navel.

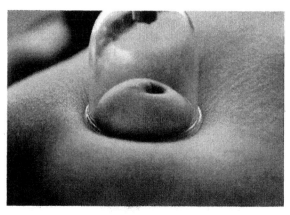

Figure 10.18 How to cup the navel.

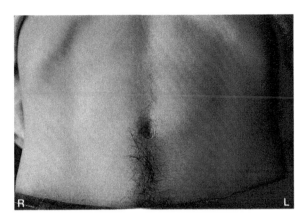

Plate 1 Basically this is a fairly healthy navel. There is some Lung Qi and Liver Blood Deficiency as indicated by the depressions on the right and left of the navel respectively.

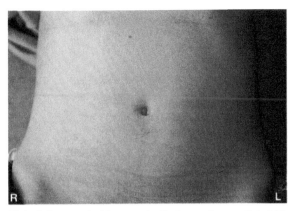

Plate 2 A somewhat tiny navel with depressions on the right and left. The diagnosis is insufficient vitality, Lung Qi Xu and Liver Blood Deficiency.

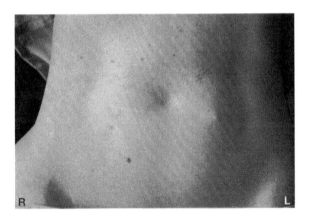

Plate 3 This patient has no navel. It was surgically altered when a cesarean section was performed. Note the puffiness in the lower abdomen, especially in the Liver area and lower abdominal quadrant, the diagnosis of which is Lung Qi, Liver Blood and Kidney Yang Deficiency. Interestingly, this patient has hepatitis C. Note the abdominal coloring is greenish, indicating Stagnation. There is also a cyst on the left-hand side. Patients who have their navels removed during an operation often suffer from multiple health complaints.

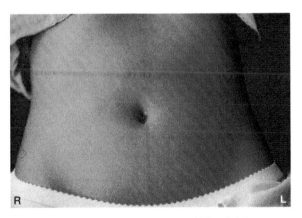

Plate 4 A fairly healthy navel which could be slightly more closed. Note the rays of sunshine within the navel, a good sign. Some Lung Qi Deficiency and Liver Blood Deficiency are present, as shown by the slight depressions on the right and left.

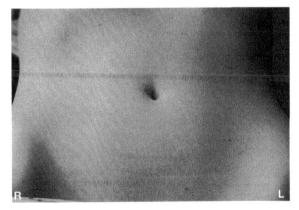

Plate 5 Pronounced Lung Qi Deficiency and Liver Blood Deficiency as shown by the depressions on the right and left.

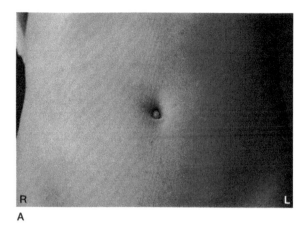

A

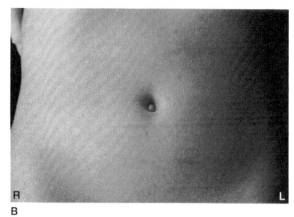

B

Plate 6 A, B: A protuberant navel (an 'outie'). The healthy navel is tucked in. This indicates a connective tissue disturbance.

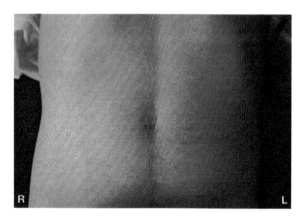

Plate 7 This navel has a laparoscopic scar within it. The navel should never be cut, as it is a forbidden point for needling. Overall, the diagnosis is a connective tissue disturbance, meaning weak immunity.

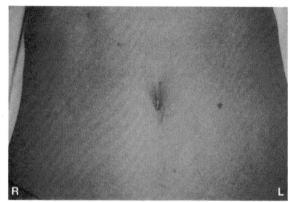

Plate 8 Another navel which has been cut by surgery and which has a significant scar within it. It is too small and not deep enough. This indicates weak vitality and can lead to a Lung-Kidney disharmony due to the scar.

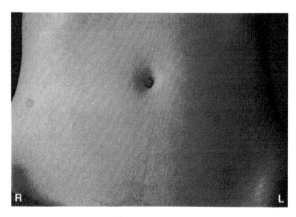

Plate 9 Lung Qi Deficiéncy as shown by the depression on the right.

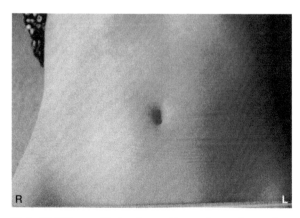

Plate 10 This navel is too tiny and has a depression on the right. This indicates insufficient vitality and Lung Qi Deficiency.

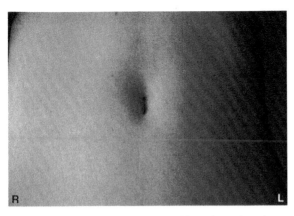

Plate 11 This navel is too narrow and long; it needs to be rounder and more open. This shape can lead to a Lung-Kidney disharmony.

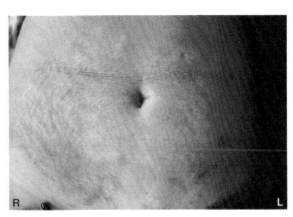

Plate 12 This navel is too closed which can indicate a Lung-Kidney disharmony. There is also Lung Qi Deficiency and Liver Blood Deficiency, as shown by the depressions on the right and left. The lower abdomen is very puffy, indicative of Kidney Yang Deficiency. Note the greenish-brown marks on the lower abdomen, indicating Blood Stagnation. The patient has a cesarean section scar in the pubic area. She has migraine headaches and multiple chemical sensitivity.

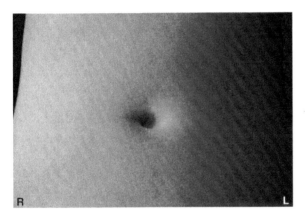

Plate 13 This navel is too open. In particular, the depression on the left indicates Liver Blood Deficiency.

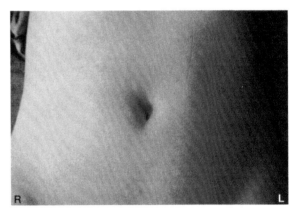

Plate 14 This navel is narrow and should also be more open. It can indicate a Lung-Kidney disharmony. It is more closed at the bottom, indicating a Kidney Qi Deficiency. There is also some Liver Blood Deficiency, as shown by the depression on the left.

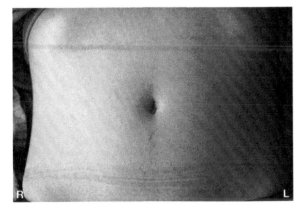

Plate 15 This navel is almost the opposite of Plate 14. The Spleen area is too closed, indicating Spleen Qi Deficiency. There is a depression on the right indicating Lung Qi Deficiency.

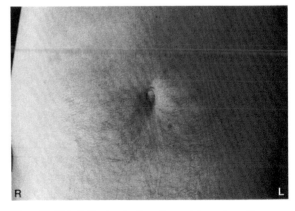

Plate 16 This is the beginning of a protuberant navel indicating connective tissue problems (weak immunity). The biggest depression is at the bottom, indicating Kidney Qi Deficiency. Note the pronounced reddish color of the abdomen, indicating Heat as the swelling in the Liver side of the abdomen (left). The patient has high Blood pressure and has a red face as well.

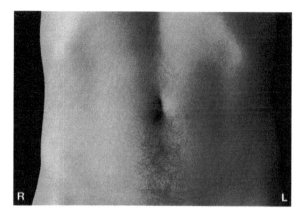

Plate 17 This navel is too narrow, indicating Lung-Kidney disharmony.

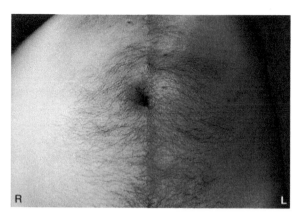

Plate 18 This navel is slightly small with a depression on the right pointing to Lung Qi Deficiency.

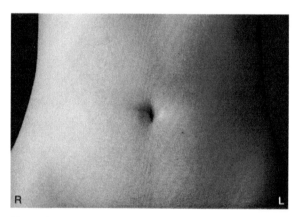

Plate 19 This navel is too narrow, indicating a Lung-Kidney disharmony.

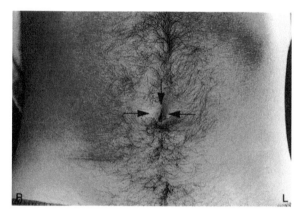

Plate 20 Narrow, asymmetrical navel (deviates to the patient's left). Lung Qi, Spleen Qi and Liver Blood Deficiency are indicated by the collapsed borders in those areas (arrows).

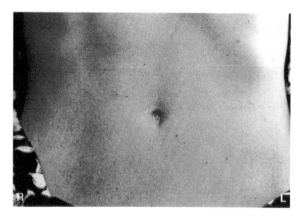

Plate 21 This navel looks downwards, indicating Kidney Qi Deficiency and some Lung Qi Deficiency due to the collapsed Lung border. Note the profuse red dots on the abdomen, indicating Blood Stagnation.

Japanese navel treatment modalities

Local needling

If navel tenderness diminishes significantly, the practitioner may either do nothing or reinforce the clearance by choosing one of the aforementioned points to needle, generally the ones that were most effective in reducing the tenderness. If navel tenderness does not diminish by 80% but the area is less tender, choose one or two of the tenderest points within the KI 16 radius and needle. Insert the needle(s) at a 15–45° angle toward the navel, to a depth of about 0.5–1.0 cun. Do not elicit *Da Qi* and do not use any other needling method. Simply insert, then withdraw and insert again. With this technique the needle is being used to mechanically break up any Stagnation.

The navel or Jing treatment

This is an excellent tonification treatment for patients with Lung, Spleen and Kidney disharmonies or for patients exhibiting many symptoms of Deficiency (weakness, fatigue, etc.) and involves treatment of eight points around the navel. These points correspond to the cardinal directions, (north, north-east, east, etc.) and, according to Dr Tran Viet Dzung, stimulate Eight Extraordinary Meridian functions. They are located at a distance equivalent to the KI 16 radius from the navel. The Kidney 16 (Huangshu) area is 0.5 cun around the entire navel. Dr Manaka says that Kidney 16 is the Front Mu point of the Kidney.

This treatment may use needles, the Tiger Thermie warmer, cups or a combination of these. If needles are used they are inserted to a depth of approximately 0.5 cun, sometimes up to 1.0 cun, on a 45° oblique angle towards the center of the umbilicus. No *Da Qi* arrival is sought nor should any manipulation of the needle be done. Needles are retained for 10–20 minutes. The more deficient the patient is, the shorter the retention time. This is a very powerful treatment due to the energetics of this area. Patients are characteristically guarded in this area so it is advisable to clear the navel before inserting the needles to avoid discomfort. Figure 10.19 shows the positioning of

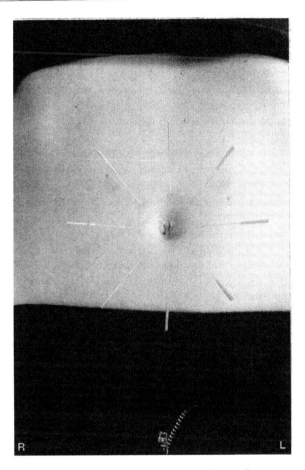

Figure 10.19 Needling the navel with an Extraordinary Meridian treatment.

the needles in this Eight Extraordinary Meridian style treatment.

An efficient method of treating the area of the navel is to cup or moxa the umbilical area. This treatment in effect mirrors the Jing needle treatment without the insertion of eight needles that can be bothersome to some patients. Use a glass or plastic suction cup and retain cup for approximately 10 minutes. Moxa in the form of the Tiger Thermie warmer, moxa box or belly bowl can also be employed.

Conclusion

In short, the classics remind us of a very basic and perhaps underused treatment strategy:

when an element or an organ is deficient, tonify the mother. For example, Spleen is the mother of Lungs and the grandmother of Kidney, making it a valuable choice for correcting pathologies that could result from disharmonies of the two latter organs, whether those disharmonies are symptomatic or preclinical, because this strategy addresses the root. Therefore treatment of the navel (which corresponds to the Spleen/Earth element) represents a very direct, efficient and effective strategy for bothersome, as well as serious, diseases. It seems that the proverbial notion of navel gazing is as old as the *Nanjing* itself and certainly merits further contemplation.

The following cases illustrate the value of the navel as a diagnostic and treatment site.

Case 10.1 Umbilical suppuration

An interesting case, which illustrates the relationship between the navel and the Lungs, involved an elderly gentleman whom I was treating for periodontal gum disease. We had very good results with this disorder primarily by the use of herbs as described in a previous report (Gardner-Abbate 1995c).

One day when he arrived at my office he exuded the overwhelming odor of mothballs emanating not only from his clothes but also from his skin and breath. The odor was much stronger, more noxious and pervasive than that caused by clothing stored in mothballs for the winter.

During the exam I discovered that his navel was uncharacteristically red, with a clear, thick discharge oozing from the center. Because the navel can indicate Lung pathologies and I knew that the camphor in the mothballs (Cinnamomum camphora: Zhang Nao) is acrid, hot and poisonous and can be paralyzing to the respiratory system, especially if ingested, I asked him about the mothball odor. He explained that he was having his home professionally treated because of a serious infestation of moths. His daughter had moved out of the house during this period because she didn't think it was healthy to be exposed to the mothballs at that intensity. Although the odor was making his wife sick, he didn't seem to mind the smell. I explained that I suspected that the suppuration of the navel was being caused by the camphor irritating his Lungs and recommended that he leave his house. However, this option was not of interest to him and within a month the oozing and redness ended as the smell in his home abated.

Case 10.2 Umbilical herniation

A 46-year-old male was overweight by about 100 pounds. His major complaint was lethargy. Additionally, he presented with other signs and symptoms of both Spleen and Kidney Yang Deficiency with Dampness, such as itchiness in the genital region, loose stools with undigested food, gas, abdominal distension and pallor. He overate and did not exercise. Abdominal inspection revealed an umbilical hernia located on the left of his navel in the Liver area, possibly due to the excess weight he was carrying.

A needle (#1 gauge, 40 mm Seirin with tube inserter) was inserted to a depth of 1.0 cun at the site of greatest herniation. After the needle had been in place for about 5 minutes, the herniation visibly decreased by about 75%.

The patient was told that he needed to lose a significant amount of weight through a combination of exercise and diet. While the patient was impressed with the needling results, he did not want to make either of these behavioral changes. Surgical repair of the herniation was advised.

NEW WORDS AND CONCEPTS

Aneurysm – a sac formed by a local enlargement of the wall of an artery caused by a disease or injury.

Birth Trauma Mu point – the navel.

Missing Organ Shu point – the KI 16 radius.

Umbilical herniation – a ballooning out of the intestinal wall within the peritoneal sac.

QUESTIONS

1. Using the Chinese medical concepts of Lung, Spleen and Kidney, explain why digestive problems, cold limbs, threatened miscarriage, allergic and skin diseases are all effectively treated through the navel.

2. Match the navel shapes listed in Column A with the corresponding diagnosis listed in Column B. Some answers may be used more than once.

Column A

1. Pulsing navel

2. Navel that is too narrow

3. Puffy lower border

4. Navel sticks out

5. Hard CV 7 area

6. Big pulsing at CV 9

7. No energy/depression at CV 9

Column B

a. SP and KI Yang Xu

b. SP Qi Xu

c. Potential aortic aneurysm

d. Insufficient oxygenation or Qi flow to the lower abdomen

e. Connective tissue disturbance, i.e. weak immunity

f. KI Qi Xu

---

3. What other name do the Japanese use for CV 8 (Shenque)?

4. What is the relationship between the navel's shape and underlying bodily energetics?

5. How is Heart pathology seen in the umbilical region?

6. What are the modalities that may be used in the navel treatment?

7. What do each of the directions around the navel correspond to in the navel treatment?

Clinical notes

Birth trauma

Some of the most important variables and their consequences are listed here to give the reader a sense of the significance of the birthing event.

1. Forceps used on the head and face can lead to the formation of scars and a sequel of problems due to scars; for instance, memory problems can develop due to scars in the head region.
2. Anesthesia administered to the mother can cause physiological problems for the child.
3. If the birth was premature, constitutional problems can result; for instance, respiratory function could be inherently weak because the Lungs are the last organs to develop.
4. Cutting the cord too close to the abdominal wall can lead to excess bleeding, small bowel obstruction or even possible death.
5. Whether the birth was vaginal or cesarean can create certain conditions surrounding the particulars of the delivery.
6. If the birth was a breech presentation some trauma may occur.
7. If the cord was prolapsed and wrapped around the baby's neck, insufficient Blood flow to the newborn may cause corresponding brain damage, lifelong handicaps, low birth weight, stillbirth or death.
8. A coiled cord can lead to flaccidity and prolapse and the problems connected to prolapse such as umbilical cord compression.
9. Umbilical cord compression can lead to heart rate deceleration, drop in Blood oxygen content and increase in lactic acid.
10. Finally, a variety of drugs such as high Blood pressure medication given to pregnant women can affect the unborn child.

How to use the Tiger Thermie and Lion Thermie warmers

The Tiger Thermie warmer, which I stress throughout this book, is the tool of choice for both applying moxa as well as mechanical or pressure therapy to points or areas. Brilliant in concept, it is weak in design as far as the comfort level of holding the implement goes. The photos throughout this book show how to use the Tiger Thermie warmer or its larger version, the Lion Thermie.

There are two basic ways to use it – deeply or lightly. In the first case, when treating a structure such as the navel, a scar or points located in fleshy areas, employ a brisk, flicking motion by pressing down and simultaneously turning or scooping out. Apply the moxa heat as close to each point as possible so that the entire area is covered. Go around the navel or scar for about 3 minutes or apply moxa to a specific point several times. Don't linger on any point or area too long unless you are using the moxa in a direct non-scarring method. In this case, hold the implement on the point until the person tells you it is hot. Each time they say this is the equivalent of a direct non-scarring moxa.

In more delicate regions such as the sinuses and the neck, apply a feathery, light style of moxibustion. Gently stroke the region by brushing the instrument on the affected area such as the orbit of the eye. Apply the warmer for about 3 minutes on average. Periodically check that the instrument is not getting too hot.

Patients love the Tiger Thermie warmer as its heat is soothing and relaxing. The item is inexpensive, easy to learn how to use and an excellent tool for self-treatment of many conditions including the prevention of disease. The Tiger Thermie warmer produces less smoke than the Lion Thermie warmer and I prefer it because of this feature. It is easier to hold and more applicable to the areas for which moxa is suited.

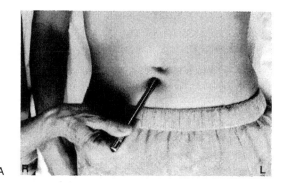

A

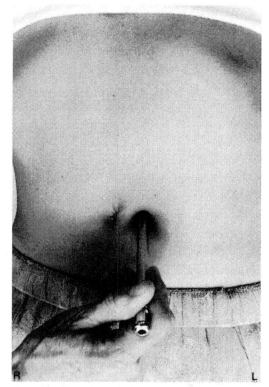

B

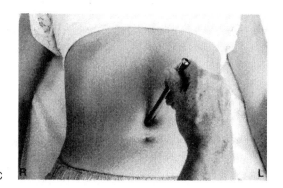

C

Figure 10.20 A–C: How to Tiger Thermie the umbilical area.

11

Contraindications and modifications to treatment

PART 1: ACUTE ABDOMINAL SYNDROMES

As I established at the beginning of this book, practitioners commonly think that the primary use of abdominal palpation and diagnosis is for abdominal problems. I hope I have demonstrated that this assumption is incorrect and that the use of abdominal diagnosis and palpation is for virtually every illness. In fact, it may not be possible to treat abdominal conditions, especially in their acute phase when they are at least very painful if not actually life-threatening.

This category of disease merits special mention to illustrate the applicability of the Japanese system to these problems. It is not the purpose of this chapter to differentiate any of these disorders from either a Western or a Chinese perspective. However, the fundamental thought processes about the way these problems are dealt with in the Japanese system are explained. In addition to this, basic charts are provided of some of the more pronounced symptomatologies of these problematic disorders so that appropriate referral and treatment can be made.

As we have seen, abdominal palpation and diagnosis are powerful diagnostic and treatment tools. They can be used to treat virtually any condition. Palpation discloses not only the patient's major complaint but also the fullness of their presentation. That pattern however, is reduced to its most common denominator, what we could call the root, the bottom-line picture of Yin, Yang, Qi and Blood and organ pathology if it is involved.

Some illnesses with abdominal symptoms are more easily treated by the Japanese system than others. As we have seen in the healthy Hara examination, the modified abdominal examination and the navel examination, if a patient has any articulated illness or the preclinical roots of any disorder, it will be disclosed through careful examination of the abdomen. Pathological abdominal findings derived from those examinations do not necessarily imply that the patient has any 'abdominal' problem although they may. Typical 'abdominal' symptoms include abdominal distension, gas, menstrual pain or fullness in the epigastric region. These symptoms are very well treated through the abdominal clearance protocol whether they are part of the major complaint or accompanying signs and symptoms of any other pattern.

THE ACUTE ABDOMEN

Abdominal pain is an ordinary human malady. It is a common accompaniment to many disorders, some of which are minor, acute and transitory while others are grave, chronic and even life-threatening. When certain patterns, generally of sudden onset, are characterized by severe or unrelenting pain, whether of a chronic or acute nature, that is localized or diffuse, the patient has an illness termed an acute abdominal syndrome. Abdominal pain is a significant abnormal symptom because its cause may require immediate surgical or medical intervention. The most common causes of severe abdominal pain are inflammation, perforation of an intraabdominal structure, circulatory obstruction, intestinal or ureteral obstruction or rupture of an organ located within the abdomen.

Abdominal pain accounts for about 40% of emergency room visits. The major acute abdominal syndromes include appendicitis, perforated gastric or peptic ulcer, strangulated hernia, small and large bowel obstruction, stomach ulcers, diverticulitis, cholecystitis, cholelithiasis, pancreatitis, ruptured abdominal aortic aneurysm, ectopic pregnancy, pelvic inflammatory disease, gastroenteritis and biliary or renal colic.

Skillful history taking as well as recognition of signs and symptoms are imperative in order to diagnose these illnesses although sometimes imaging studies with MRIs or CAT scans may be required. Information about the onset, duration and character, what makes it better or worse and location and symptoms associated with the pain is critical in making an accurate diagnosis. Since some causes are life-threatening, it is expedient to consider the worse-case scenario to systematically rule out possibilities. As with all illness, it is the task of the physician to differentiate the signs and symptoms of the disease in order to arrive at the correct diagnosis and treatment plan. Acute appendicitis should never be lower than second on your list with patients who have their appendix but interestingly, it is still the most common misdiagnosed surgical cause of acute abdominal pain (Trott et al 1995).

As Oriental medical physicians, we do not diagnose illness but rather differentiate its pattern. Therefore, it is important for us to recognize these symptoms and make an appropriate referral. It is possible that we will encounter these cases within our clinical practice but we generally have less opportunity to treat an acute abdomen since patients with this problem are more likely to seek emergency room medical care, as well they should. Because we do not want to run the risk of mismanaging their treatment we need to be aware of our limitations with such cases.

If you are confronted with patients who present with abdominal pain ask them to characterize the pain, its location, onset, duration, intensity and how it is impacting them. Western doctors as well as Oriental doctors find that abdominal pain, like all pain, is difficult to diagnose so as many factors as possible should be utilized to decipher it.

For handy reference, Table 11.1 summarizes the most common signs and symptoms of the more frequently encountered acute abdominal syndromes along with their etiology and standard Western plans. The practitioner is encouraged to consult other Western medical texts for more details on these diseases.

Table 11.1 Common signs and symptoms of acute abdominal illness and their Western etiology and treatment

Illness	Definition	Symptoms	Etiology	Treatment
Acute gastroenteritis	Inflammation of the stomach and intestines accompanying numerous GI disorders	Anorexia, nausea, vomiting, abdominal discomfort, diarrhea, abrupt and violent onset, rapid loss of fluids from vomiting and diarrhea, cramps, diffuse abdominal pain, fever, leukocytosis	Bacterial enterotoxins, bacterial or viral invasion, chemical toxins, miscellaneous conditions such as lactose intolerance	Bed rest, sedation, intravenous replacement of electrolytes, antispasmodic medication to control vomiting and diarrhea. Medication with an antitoxin if due to bacterial endotoxin. Bland diet
Acute cholecystitis	Acute or chronic inflammation of the gall bladder	Steady severe pain in the upper right quadrant of the abdomen (may refer to right shoulder), nausea, vomiting, eructation, flatulence, anorexia, sometimes fever and leukocytosis, history of fatty food intolerance, postprandial fullness, tenderness, muscle guarding, rebound tenderness. Gall bladder may be palpable, hyperbilirubinemia and bilirubinuria	Acute is generally due to obstruction by a gallstone that cannot pass through the cystic duct. Also may commonly result from chemical or bacterial inflammation of the gall bladder	Diagnosed through ultrasound. Surgery is the preferred mode of treatment
Chronic cholecystitis		Pain at night following a fatty meal	May be complicated by biliary calculi, pancreatitis or carcinoma of the gall bladder	Surgery is the preferred mode of treatment
Diverticulitis	Inflammation of one or more diverticula – small outpouches of the bowel lining that protrude through the muscle layer of the bowel	Steady, crampy pain particularly over the sigmoid colon in the lower left quadrant, leukocytosis, alternating diarrhea and constipation, chills or fever, rectal bleeding, tenderness, muscle guarding and rebound tenderness, nausea, mild vomiting, fever and leukocytosis. (Symptoms are similar to acute appendicitis but on the left side.) History of previous attacks, mass and tenderness in lower left quadrant	The penetration of fecal matter through the thin-walled diverticula causes inflammation and abscess formation in the tissues. With repeated inflammation, the lumen of the colon narrows and may become obstructed. They form in weakened areas of the bowels, usually the large intestine	Bed rest, intravenous fluids, antibiotics, nothing taken by mouth in acute phase. High-fiber diet, use of stool softeners. Surgery
Acute appendicitis	Inflammation of the vermiform appendix, a dead-end tube that leads from the cecum, where the large intestine begins, in the right lower abdomen. May rapidly lead to perforation and peritonitis	Epigastric or periumbilical pain eventually shifting to the right lower quadrant of the abdomen. Insidious to acute and persistent. Nausea, vomiting, anorexia, constipation (perhaps diarrhea), decreased or absent bowel sounds, tenderness, muscle spasm and rebound tenderness in lower right quadrant, fever, moderate to slight leukocytosis with neutrophilia. Patient keeps knees bent to avoid tension of abdominal muscles	Due to an obstruction of the opening of the appendix by a piece of stool, by a parasite or an infection	Surgery if necessary

Table 11.1 Common signs and symptoms of acute abdominal illness and their Western etiology and treatment (*continued*)

Illness	Definition	Symptoms	Etiology	Treatment
Acute pancreatitis	A rare condition in which pancreatic enzymes escape into pancreatic tissues and the pancreas becomes inflamed. Occurs suddenly and may be severe to life-threatening	Common in cases of cholelithiasis, variable pain, typically epigastric and radiating to the back, severe and constant pain that may last for several days or may be mild pain aggravated by eating and slowly growing worse. Becomes worse when walking or lying down. Lessens when you sit or lean forward. May be accompanied by prostration, sweating and shock, nausea, vomiting, abdominal distension and tenderness, elevated amylase levels, hyperbilirubinemia and hypoglycemia can occur. Fever, anorexia, swollen tender abdomen, increased pulse rate, person looks and feels sick. In some cases patient becomes dehydrated and has low blood pressure. Heart, lungs or kidneys may fail. Bleeding in the pancreas can occur, leading to shock or even death	Damage to the biliary tract by alcohol, trauma, infectious disease such as mumps, or certain drugs, or gallstones or common duct stones, prescribed drugs, surgery to the abdomen, or abnormalities of the pancreas or intestine	No food by mouth to prevent stimulation of the pancreas. Nasogastric suction to remove gastric secretions if vomiting. Usually gets better on its own. Other measures depending upon severity of signs and symptoms
Acute intestinal obstruction	Blockage of the intestine, either the large or small	Symptoms depend on the site and degree of obstruction. Diffuse pain, sudden onset, crampy abdominal pain, constipation, inability to pass gas, hyperperistalsis and borborygmus, vomiting, abdominal distension, high-pitched rushes	Two types: 1. Simple mechanical intestinal blockage of fluid, food, gas or digestive secretions 2. Strangulation or infarction	Treatment depends upon diagnosis. Most require surgery
Perforated ulcer	The penetration of a peptic ulcer into the wall of the stomach or duodenum and entry into an adjacent confined space or organ	Epigastric pain, history of ulcers, abrupt steady onset of pain, anorexia, nausea, vomiting. The patient likes to lie as still as possible as even breathing can worsen the pain. Abdomen is tender, rebound pain is intense, bowel sounds are absent or diminished	Rupture of a peptic ulcer	Acute abdominal surgery
Ruptured aortic aneurysm	Rupture of the abdominal aorta	Excruciating pain in epigastrium, lower abdomen and back, abrupt onset, sharp, severe pain, variable symptoms, hypotension or shock, abdominal aneurysm. Highly lethal	Familial inheritance, trauma, arteritis syndromes, syphilis and congenital connective tissue disorders	Surgical emergency

The acute abdomen and abdominal clearing

Acute abdominal syndromes have five major signs and symptoms in common. These are pain, distension, obstruction, vomiting and heat. When these symptoms appear as a group, do not clear the abdomen. Pressure should not be applied to the organs for they could be perforated, inflamed or severely obstructed. Palpation of the abdominal diagnosis points in such cases is contraindicated. However, treatment is not.

Treatment can be modified such that pressing the clearance points clears the abdomen. Sequentially treating the clearance points of each of the abdominal diagnosis points can assist the patient in the short term and should be used to ease the pain and even reduce some inflammation, obstruction, distension, vomiting or heat. Additionally the practitioner should refer the patient to a doctor or to the emergency room. It is more prudent to receive a diagnosis first from the physician most qualified to make it and then to evaluate the specifics of the illness before further treatment. The fact that the patient has an acute abdominal illness does not mean that they cannot be treated with Oriental medicine, but first we need to know what we are treating. Hence the necessity of diagnosis.

These rules of treatment of the acute abdomen are summarized below:

1. Treat the patient if there is no immediate life-threatening situation.
2. Do not press on the abdominal diagnosis points. Due to the nature of the pain, we already know that they are problematic.
3. Press on all the clearance points in the order of the abdominal clearing to achieve maximum result that is defined as a reduction in pain.
4. Expect these clearance points to be exceedingly tender since the person has an Excess condition. Remember, in general patients with excessive conditions have an aversion to touch.
5. Counsel the patients that these points will hurt but that your immediate goal is to reduce the pain such that they can seek further medical help.
6. Make appropriate written referral to a Western healthcare physician or emergency room if need be.
7. After the acute phase has been managed patients can then choose their preferred course of therapy. Invite them to return to discuss their treatment options.

Case 11.1 provides an illustration of how to treat a case of an acute abdomen using the clearance points. It is integral to understanding the strengths, limitations and modifications of using this Japanese style of treatment.

Case 11.1 The treatment of ulcer with clearance points

The patient was a woman in her early 40s who was a student at the college where I teach. One day after class she complained of excruciating stomach pain to the point where she felt she couldn't make it to her home. I was treating patients in the clinic that day and she asked if I could help her.

She had intense burning pain in the middle of the epigastric region that was so bad that she was lying on the table crying. I didn't know much about her except that she tended to worry, to be angry and had a pattern of irregular food intake. She couldn't seem to answer any questions about her condition because the pain was so bad. Clearly there was some Stagnation in the area that resembled Blood Stagnation.

Because direct palpation of the abdominal diagnosis points was contraindicated I proceeded to 'clear' her abdomen indirectly by pressing on all the clearance points in the order of abdominal palpation. They were all extremely painful since they were a reflection of her acute abdomen. The points that gave her the greatest relief were ST 34R, ST 44B but most notably SP 10L – points that indicate Middle Jiao blockage and Blood Stagnation. The clearance points helped with the pain to the point that she could go home with relative ease. Their effect was not permanent, nor did I expect that they would be. They did not get rid of her problem, which I suspected was an ulcer, but they significantly reduced her pain and made it possible for her to leave.

I recommended that she see a Western doctor as soon as possible to determine the etiology of her pain. The next time I saw her she reported to me that she had seen a doctor and was diagnosed with a duodenal ulcer. As a result of this she decided to change some of her food habits and to deal with the source of her stress and worry which was a relationship she was involved in.

If abdominal diagnosis and treatment, like other methods of Oriental therapeutics, are used preventively to harmonize the Qi and Blood and adjust the Yin and Yang, illnesses may not develop in the first place.

THE TREATMENT OF CANCER WITH ABDOMINAL CLEARING

The treatment of cancer is in some ways analogous to the treatment of the acute abdomen. It is a condition where we do not want to risk further harm to the patient, in this case by potentially causing metastasis of the cancer.

Information pertinent to abdominal diagnosis and treatment of cancer patients is virtually non-existent and so the information given below is derived from my knowledge of palpation and my clinical experience in the field of oncology.

While each case is different, at this point I have formulated the following ideas about the applicability of palpation to cancer patients.

1. If patients have malignant cancer and have not undergone surgery, chemotherapy or radiation, I do not perform abdominal palpation on them even if the tumor is not in the abdominal cavity. This is a conservative decision but one which may limit the risk of metastasis in the case of malignant cancer.

2. If the malignant cancer has been surgically removed and they are undergoing chemotherapy and/or radiation I still do not perform abdominal palpation on them. Some of the points in the abdominal clearance protocol may be needled based upon their energetics and the patient's presentation; however, I do not clear the abdomen indirectly using the clearance points as in the case of an acute abdomen.

3. My general rule of thumb is not to needle the abdominal cavity in the vicinity of where the tumor is or was.

4. If patients are in the recovery phase, meaning they have undergone the surgery and chemotherapy and/or radiation and may be on a course of drugs, I tend to treat them like any other patient in regard to needling the abdomen

or the treatment points. I do not use abdominal diagnosis as the basis of my diagnosis. Ultimately I work on strengthening their anti-pathogenic factor using some of the immunity protocols described in this book.

5. If the patient has survived the cancer for more than 5 years, abdominal diagnosis can be used as a method of diagnosis.

PART 2: THE LAW OF CURE AND THE CONCEPT OF THE HEALING CRISIS

In order to monitor the course of the patient's treatment and to evaluate therapeutic effectiveness, two more important topics need to be discussed here: the Law of Cure and the concept of the healing crisis.

THE HEALING CRISIS

A fundamental assumption of most therapies subsumed under the heading of natural medicines, such as acupuncture, herbology, naturopathy and all of the various massage techniques, is that the body tends towards balance and the result of that balance can be called health. When bodily energies become unbalanced they need to be corrected and hence all of the aforementioned medical systems, with their positive image of health based upon the healing capacity of the human body, attempt to redress those imbalances be they mental or physical.

Another operating premise of these types of medicine is that the body and the mind are an interrelated whole. Each is related to and reflects the other. Thus, all the body systems are intimately connected. Consequently, as disease progresses in a person it is not surprising that a change in one system may cause changes in another. Physical problems may precipitate psychological ones and vice versa. This is not to say that allopathic medicine does not see any connection between the parts of the body, for it does. However, it tends to see it more when entire systems are involved instead of what may appear to be isolated complaints. The body–mind interface is significantly less appreciated or understood.

Bodywork therapists in particular have been instrumental in raising the awareness of all practitioners on the intimate connection between chronic physical tension and armoring and chronic psychological defenses. Wilhelm Reich, founder of psychotherapeutic bodywork, discovered that patterns of chronic muscular tension were related to character structure. By character structure, he meant an individual's habitual attitude and consistent pattern of response to various situations (Frager 1980, p. 214). That tension is often a result of unresolved feelings accumulating in the body-mind and not being processed (Epstein 1994). As a result, when therapy of any sort is initiated to treat illness, we should not be surprised to see changes in other parts of the body, including the patient's emotional affect.

In Western medicine, these changes, if undesirable, are generally termed side effects. Most of them are adverse symptoms that result from drug use or other therapies. They are not considered beneficial to the organism but neither are they necessarily perceived as negative. Some of the mechanisms for adverse reactions are understood; others are not. It is not uncommon for patients to report that many side effects are worse than the original problem for which they sought treatment. However, they are part and parcel of most Western therapeutics. These unwanted side effects are simply the result of whatever intervention the patient is using. They are not what we refer to as a healing crisis.

In contrast to this approach, most naturalistic health systems tend to use medicines or therapies that minimize negative reactions. Most of the remedies they prescribe are natural versus synthetic ones. This is not to say that natural products cannot cause problems, for indeed they can. They may cause serious problems and even be fatal if used in the wrong dosage, are abused by patients, are misprescribed, self-prescribed incorrectly or inordinately relied upon. The responsible physician has the important task of seeing that these conditions do not ensue.

When a patient is under the care of a licenced practitioner, the provider must be able to recognize the signs and symptoms of recovery and decline so as to judge whether the diagnosis and therapy are correct for the course of the illness. Remember that a diagnosis in many instances is an educated guess, a tentative assumption based upon facts. The treatment plan and therapy, when put to the test, contribute to the overall assessment of the patient's diagnosis.

Not all healing involves a healing crisis. Most of it occurs silently without adverse signs and symptoms developing. But sometimes in the course of healing, due to the interrelatedness of organ systems, body parts and meridians, problems will surface. Because these changes typically may be disagreeable events, the patient may perceive that the treatment you have initiated is incorrect when in reality the fact that those changes do develop is proof that healing has been initiated. This sequence of events is what is termed a 'healing crisis'. It is a temporary exacerbation of symptoms that is required in order to bring about a desired therapeutic effect.

In homeopathic medicine, a healing crisis is called a homeopathic aggravation (Vithoulkas 1980, pp. 227–230). The proof that the remedy is working is the aggravation of symptoms that the patient develops. In other naturalistic forms of medicine, an aggravation of symptoms, and generally some form of discharge whereby the body attempts to purge itself of toxins, characterizes a healing crisis. These discharges take the form of a release of energy or tension on the physical, emotional, mental or spiritual level. While the discharges are often unpleasant to the patient, such as a productive cough, diarrhea, runny nose or an increase in sweating or fever, they are necessary in order to bring about resolution of the body's proper function. These styles of medicine, which assist in resolution, are the most beneficial therapies for the individual because they treat the root of the illness.

Cure is the restoration of mental, physical and spiritual balance to the person. Observers of the human condition over the centuries have noticed that healing or cure can be described according to various physical laws. These rules, called the Law of Cure, are summarized and discussed below. The healing crisis proceeds according to the Law of Cure. Recognition of the Law of Cure helps practitioners to assess whether a healing crisis is occurring or whether something has gone wrong with the treatment.

THE LAW OF CURE

The Law of Cure consists of three central tenets that aid the practitioner in monitoring the course of illness. They are listed below and discussed thereafter.

1. Disease and its symptoms move from within to without.
2. Disease and its symptoms move from above to below.
3. If symptoms recur, they will do so in reverse chronological order.

Disease and its symptoms move from within to without

Typically, in a healing crisis, the symptoms that the patient experiences move from internal to external. Such movement does not only refer to physical symptoms but to psychological ones as well. For instance, psychological symptoms (that could be thought of as internal) tend to lessen but physical ones (that could be thought of as external) could become aggravated in the course of the healing crisis. The change in mental symptoms is indicative that the spirit or vital energy of the patient has been contacted. Resolution of physical symptoms will follow. This is a positive progression of events. Acupuncture, in its theory of the Three Treasures, acknowledges this fundamental rule of cure when it claims that of the three treasures – Qi, Jing and Shen – the spirit is the most important level to reach to initiate changes in the rest of the organism.

What this theorem is asserting is that because of the body–mind connection, the change initiated on a deep level is advantageous and indicative that the healing process has begun. For instance, in the case of a patient who has insomnia due to inordinate stress at the workplace, as you attempt to treat the whole person through the abdominal presentation it would be good to see

the patient's emotional affect change first before the sleep pattern improves. The patient might now acknowledge frustration at work or suppressed anger or a desire to change the work situation as the abdomen is probed and cleared. As these feelings come to the fore they are not always pleasant to deal with and may be emotionally charged and temporarily worsened. However, they are a signpost to us that the root of the sleep problem has been uncovered and that it is likely to get better as the person comes to grips with the cause of the disorder as you treat what you feel in the abdominal examinations.

In another case not involving the psyche, we could see an increase in fever and sweating as we treat flu, for example. Instead of viewing this as abnormal or an incorrectly administered treatment, it can be the indication of a healthy immune system. It is a healing crisis, where there is a temporary aggravation of symptoms in order to bring about a desired therapeutic effect. It is also an example of illness resolving from within to without – the desired therapeutic effect is to expel the pathogen via the body's own natural defense systems of fever and sweat.

The clinical experience of Oriental medical physicians adds two theorems that are subsumed under this first rule of cure.

First, disease is getting worse if it progresses to a Cold symptom complex, indicating that the body's Mingmen is weak. We can likewise infer that the return of warmth is a positive sign. The healthy Hara examination can assess both of these patterns.

Second, if a condition progresses from Excess to Deficiency or to a condition of mixed Excess/ Deficiency, the antipathogenic factor is becoming weakened. Excess conditions, which are characterized by more virulent symptoms, are at least indicative that the antipathogenic factor is intact and engaged in fighting the pathogenic factor. Therefore, if the person moves out of a state of Deficiency to more excessive symptoms this can be considered a positive step. Likewise, performing the modified abdominal examination can show the practitioner Deficiency, Excess and combined Excess/Deficiency through the feel of the tissues. We prefer to feel tightness, or a combination of tight and mushy on the same point, than a sensation of emptiness. The tightness will in fact be relatively easy to clear. Diminishment of the vacancy will be a positive sign of augmentation of the body's Qi. It will take time to accomplish but it will happen as you employ this protocol.

Disease and its symptoms move from above to below

Healing should proceed from the upper part of the body to lower part. This is a primary treatment strategy whereby toxins and perverse energy are brought down from the upper parts of the body through the lower orifices, in the form of either removal or consolidation. Changes in urination and bowel movements or the menstrual cycle are good examples of this.

Let me provide an example. A patient complains of a frontal headache. You clear the abdomen and administer a treatment based upon your abdominal findings. When the patient goes home he has some copious bowel movements. Soon the headache is gone. The patient may not have seen the headache as connected to the stools and so he might think that your treatment caused him to have 'diarrhea' or more bowel movements than he is accustomed to or wants. But this is a proper sequence of events, a healing crisis if you will, the way to resolve the major complaint. The increased bowel movements stop within a few hours and the original complaint does not return.

If symptoms recur, they will do so in reverse chronological order

Symptoms may disappear in the reverse order of their chronological appearance. Older symptoms take more time to resolve than newer ones.

Let us look at another example of the healing crisis.

A patient had a history of painful menses for several years. One day the periods stopped and she was happy that she did not have the cramps and clots any more but she also knew that she was still in her menstruating years and that this cessation was abnormal. As you work on clearing her abdomen over the course of several weeks, she experiences cramps. When her periods are eventually reestablished, she initially has severe cramps and also large clots. The patient wonders if you have done something wrong to cause the cramps and clots. She needs an explanation for this occurrence. She does not understand that the cramps and clots are the mechanism by which the amenorrhea is being resolved. They should only be a temporary condition and this indeed is what ensues. Two months after menstruation resumes the clots and the cramps have totally disapperared and her period is normal.

Astute physicians must keep these principles in mind so that they do not panic and change their treatment plan and the patient does not think that the physician has done something wrong. Do not be tempted to suppress the illness. We must be well familiarized with the etiology and pathogenesis of illness, to recognize the pathologies of Yin, Yang, Qi and Blood and be aware of when a healing crisis might ensue and how it may progress according to the Law of Cure. Thus, we will see these occurrences as part of the healing process and can let the patient know that progress is being made. Accurate case history taking and understanding of these rules of cure are of the utmost importance.

As we have seen in previous chapters, palpation is unsurpassed in resolving bodily tension; hence its success in bringing about a solution to the person's problem but perhaps not without a healing crisis. As acupuncturist Stephen Howard (1995) reminds us, 'Every practitioner, in all traditions, has the potential to treat at every level depending on how the practitioner and the patient choose to frame the healing work they embark on together'.

Palpation is one such method which, through physical touch, imagery and conscious and unconscious prodding, can stimulate the body–mind interface.

Cases 11.2 and 11.3 provide additional examples of healing crises.

In conclusion, the practitioner must know how to gauge and register the information and problems encountered in clinical practice. Keep in mind that as sentient beings living in the world,

---

Case 11.2   Abnormal uterine bleeding

The patient was a 35-year-old woman with a major complaint of stress that she felt she internalized. Towards the end of her course of treatment with me for this particular problem, she experienced an abnormal uterine bleeding within her cycle. Following the expulsion of a large gelatinous mass, she said she felt 'a new freedom in her abdomen'. There were no other signs or symptoms to suggest that there were any other problems apart from this discharge. I advised her to see her gynecologist if any further bleeding occurred or if she was concerned about this; however, I also explained to her how I evaluated this discharge.

Because tightness in her abdomen had been her major complaint and my emphasis in treating her was on abdominal clearing, I did not feel this was unusual. Shortly after the bleeding, she claimed that she felt freed up from the stress which was her major complaint. Other signs and symptoms of tongue, pulse and palpation confirmed her verbal report. No further bleeding ensued and she no longer needed treatment for her major complaint of stress and she was released from my care stress free in body and mind.

Case 11.3   Palpation evoking prenatal memories

While I was teaching abdominal clearing to a class, a student in her 40s mentioned that she felt 'stuck' and volunteered for an abdominal clearing.

All her abdominal diagnosis points had a degree of pathology associated with them, which I don't remember and didn't record, as this was an in-class exercise. However, I do remember the following incident that occurred when I palpated ST 25L (Tianshu), the diagnostic point for Liver Qi Stagnation, Liver Blood Deficiency or a combination of both.

This point was tender when I went to clear it with the first and most important clearance point for ST 25L: SP 10L (Xuehai). SP 10 was inordinately tender and I was not even pressing as deep as one should on this point but the slow proper palpation of this point allowed me to stop at the depth she could sustain. When I palpated the point, she began to cry and uttered, 'All the blood, all the blood'. I stopped the abdominal clearing and asked her what she meant. She replied that she was back in the uterus and that 'There was all this blood'. She shook and cried on the table as her fellow students gathered around her.

At this point I immediately tried to bring her energy down and stabilize her by holding on to KI 1 (Yongquan). I attempted to guide her through her experience by saying that it was okay to feel this way and that the uterus was a safe place to be. But she surprised us by saying that it wasn't safe because she was feeling that she was the fetus and now had the knowledge that her mother wanted an abortion. (This case also shows that patients should be encouraged to interpret their own experiences, not have them interpreted for them.)

As I continued gently to hold this point, she started to calm down. She reported that she could understand the fear her mother experienced being pregnant and why she wanted an abortion. A peace seemed to descend over her with this realization.

Through this occurrence, which was extremely moving to all of her classmates as well as myself, we experienced on a very deep level the power of abdominal clearing. We saw first hand that a complaint of feeling 'stuck' in the lower abdomen was in its broadest perspective energetic and that an energetic complaint can have both physical and emotional correlates. At the end of this episode the student was very weak and shaken. Tiredness and disorientation were the residual effects of the process. A fellow student had to drive her home.

In a follow-up discussion with her several months later she revealed that she was feeling better about her relationship with her mother. She now felt separate from her whereas previous to the abdominal clearing she felt too connected to her. This feeling of separateness was functional for a person in their 40s. SP 10 still remains a tender point for her, a point perhaps with a message, and she says that she continues to treat it.

This is a very dramatic example of the power of SP 10 (Xuehai), a Sea of Blood point, which moves the Blood and disengages Stagnant Qi. Prenatal memory in this case was certainly encoded in the tissues affected by ST 25L and SP 10L. This case is also a good example of a healing crisis in which there is a temporary exacerbation of symptoms, particularly on a psychological or emotional level which shows that the root and the spirit have been reached through the power of touch, the power of the magic hand.

---

we are subject to things happening between treatments that may not be related to what was done in treatment. While a cause–effect relationship is sometimes difficult to establish, what occurs to a patient is not always due to the treatment. You need to ask yourself 'Are the symptoms the patient is experiencing part of a healing crisis or some other event?' The experienced physician will have more knowledge about the results to be expected from treatment.

As Fritz Frederick Smith MD, the developer of the Zero Balancing structural acupressure system, states:

In a healing crisis, ideally we do not treat the symptom; rather we let it run its course. But if the person must have assistance or treatment, the aim is to move forward through the problem and not eradicate its symptom per se. The problem should be understood in its proper context in the healing crisis. (Epstein 1994, p. 126)

Because a meridian-style acupuncture system, such as the Japanese system, can free up local blockages, it is an effective treatment strategy. Sometimes it precipitates a healing crisis. Sometimes it proceeds according to the Law of Cure. It is a direct way of establishing contact with a patient's spirit with its accompanying emotional and psychological components. This is what practitioners are attempting to reach and they need to determine if such energetic changes represent redirection, that is, a healing crisis, aimed at reestablishing the proper flow of Qi and Blood.

NEW WORDS AND CONCEPTS

Acute abdominal syndromes – a pattern of symptoms that is characterized by the acute onset of pain within the abdominal cavity.

Discharge – a sloughing off of pathological products such as mucus, feces, and other substances that the body needs to rid itself of.

Healing crisis – a temporary exacerbation of symptoms that brings about resolution of a health problem.

Homeopathic aggravation – the homeopathic term for a healing crisis.

Law of Cure – a maxim in naturalistic medicines that charts the progression of an illness from worse to better as it resolves itself.

QUESTIONS

1. What are the most common causes of severe abdominal pain?

2. Discuss the ways in which a practitioner could differentiate an adverse reaction (side effect) from a healing crisis.

3. Discuss the methods for gauging a patient's improvement (i.e. from month to month or week to week). Which method(s) do you feel is/are the most concrete for determining this (tongue, pulse, facial expression, etc.)?

4. Name five major signs and symptoms of acute abdominal syndromes.

5. Why did SP 10L in Case 11.1 so effectively help diminish the patient's stomach pain?

6. Match the abdominal condition listed in Column A with the differentiating signs and symptoms of that illness found in Column B (see p. 144).

Column A

1. Appendicitis

2. Cholelithiasis

3. Acute diverticulitis

4. Gastroenteritis

5. Pancreatitis

Column B

a. Acute colicky pain in the upper right quadrant that may radiate to the right scapula

b. Severe localized or diffuse abdominal pain, abdominal tenderness, often with abdominal distension, nausea, vomiting and diarrhea in the early stage

c. Pain in the epigastrium, cramps, diffuse abdominal pain, diarrhea

d. Severe abdominal pain radiating to the back, sudden onset, unrelieved by position changes, sweat

e. Lower left abdominal pain, tenderness, muscle guarding

The components of the Japanese physical exam and the treatment of disease

12

Physical examination IV: an introduction to the Japanese physical exam

AN INTRODUCTION TO THE JAPANESE PHYSICAL EXAMINATION

A fundamental tenet of this book has been that palpation plays a considerable role in both the establishment of a diagnosis and in treatment. In the acupuncture treatment system which I have described so far, I have proposed three physical examinations which all provide data about the patient. The fourth and final examination is a series of five bodily evaluations that collectively I have termed the Japanese physical exam. The significance of this examination and where it fits into the diagnostic and treatment system is introduced in this chapter.

Each distinct examination is performed to provide more data about the patient's health. The first three examinations, the healthy Hara exam, the modified abdominal exam and the navel exam, are relatively speaking energetic examinations while the fourth examination consists of inspecting some physical malformations. These deformations, some of which are subtle, are generally a result of underlying energetic changes that then precipitate physical changes. When form follows function more concrete manifestations ensue and problems are more substantive and therefore difficult to treat.

The components of the Japanese physical exam consist of examination of the inner thigh, scars, the sinuses, the neck and the back. The assumption of the Japanese physical exam is that all these areas are sites of important energetic functions and that if they are tense, flaccid or otherwise affected their function may be impaired.

Why these areas can become pathological, how to perform an evaluation of each of these areas and the clinical significance of each of their pathologies are discussed in subsequent chapters. In those chapters, separate evaluation forms for each of these parameters are included.

Ideally, the Japanese physical examination should be done the first time the patient is seen. It is analogous to asking all the questions. Realistically, however, this exam is usually conducted on the third or fourth visit because the first visit usually takes the longest amount of time. Another option is to administer one of the five subsets of the Japanese physical exam weekly sometime after the second visit so that the diagnostic and treatment protocol does not become overwhelming to the patient or the practitioner.

Because the components of this particular examination are actually physical changes in the person, they will take time to treat. The more items of this exam that the patient manifests, the more serious are the problems the patient has. These physical dimensions should be monitored and treated whenever the patient is seen in addition to pathologies which surface as a result of the modified abdominal examination in concert with the healthy Hara and navel diagnosis and treatment.

THE DIAGNOSTIC AND TREATMENT METHODOLOGY

Now that we have explored the historical and clinical reasons for the importance of palpation, the philosophical underpinnings of the process and the procedural methods and diagnostic significance of the abdominal findings, we can now start to synthesize the material.

My observation of practitioners exposed to what I have called the Japanese system is one of two reactions. They either reject it because they do not understand it or they become ready converts who throw away their previous treatment styles when they see it demonstrated because of the dramatic clinical efficacy of the system. This latter group may also think they have adopted a new system because they don't see the connection between their training and these new procedures.

Below, I explain how and why this system works through the simple organized presentation I use.

Overview: how to put it all together

The subject of this section is how to begin the treatment process. This is discussed below and its salient features are summarized in Box 12.1 at the end of the chapter to remind practitioners of the steps involved until they become an automatic operating principle.

Inquiry: the Five Preliminaries, the major complaint and the Ten Questions

The Five Preliminaries

The start of any therapeutic relationship begins with a diagnostic intake. Start by asking the patient what are called the Five Preliminaries, which cover:

1. the major complaint and its accompanying symptoms (which provide its differentiation)
2. the onset and duration of the major complaint
3. previous history and treatment of the major complaint, if any
4. personal medical history
5. family medical history.

This part of the interview process tells you what the patient's articulated concerns are, how they affect him, how they came about and have been managed and what is the wider context of the patient's experience. This is an extremely critical part of the interview which should not be skipped or glossed over for it is through the Five Preliminaries that the diagnosis – an educated guess, a tentative assumption based upon fact – is established. Later stages of questioning and physical examination are designed to back up that diagnosis and place it within the context of the person's energetic configuration.

The major complaint

The centerpiece of the Five Preliminaries is the major complaint, which is the reason why the patient seeks medical treatment. It is the articulation of the patients' awareness of their health. While patients may have other problems for which they may or may not seek treatment that are revealed in the course of the interview, the practitioner obviously must speak to the major complaint. A prime difference between allopathic and holistic practitioners is that as Oriental medical physicians, we must know how to treat that major complaint within the context of the whole person. This means performing minute questioning about the features of the chief complaint such as its onset, duration, previous history and treatment as well as executing the detailed physical examinations of tongue, pulse and palpation.

Certainly there are times when the major complaint is not connected to broader health issues, as in the cases of an acute sprain, traumatic injury, stomachache due to overeating or even a cold which the patient contracted due to unprepared exposure to wind. These conditions can be assessed for what they are and treated accordingly. However, many of the daily maladies that we experience as humans spring directly from our health, meaning our basic body energetics. The perceptive and classically trained practitioner looks at these energies from as many perspectives as possible in order to appreciate the complex interrelationships between the complaint and those energetics which are the underlying terrain.

In using the Japanese system, we are further able to discern those underlying energetics by the use of visceral palpation. As we have seen throughout this book, palpation reveals a more general, underlying, bigger picture of bodily energetics. It is the practitioner's role to interpret the bodily information derived from palpation in relation to the major complaint in order to formulate a treatment plan. These data may be framed less in Zang-Fu diagnostic language and more within the broad outlines of Yin, Yang, Qi and Blood. The practitioner may not even articulate a diagnosis but rather deal with the immediacy of the information produced through palpation. This is not to imply that the palpatory system is less astute or accurate, for as we have seen, it is grounded in the proven basis of the *Nanjing*.

While other practitioners of this style of acupuncture have produced abdominal maps that correspond to disease or organ patterns, I prefer not to codify an illness into such a pattern for several reasons. For instance, in the palpation system, the common cold frequently presents as tightness at ST 25 (Tianshu) on the right because that point is a reflection of the Lungs and our immunity. The cold, of course, is not isolated from the person who has developed it. Hence, while the main finding in a person with a Wind-Cold invasion may be tightness at ST 25R, just as that person may have a thin white tongue coat or a superficial tight pulse, additional findings should not be ignored, be they abdominal or any other that practitioners utilize as physical evidence to support their diagnosis and treatment plan.

In the web of diagnostic data, the major complaint is the focal point that brings the patient to you and that directs the treatment plan. As Oriental medical physicians we collect so much data in our search to understand the patient's bodily energetics that we must not confuse the forest with the trees. It is easy to become immersed in other pathology that we uncover that we might think is more significant than the patient's major complaint. Always keep in mind the major complaint – acknowledge it. Follow up upon it in each subsequent visit as the most relevant active problem, yet still treat the whole person with any subpathologies or patterns of disharmony the patient may evidence or report – what Western doctors tend to call 'passive problems'.

The Ten Questions

Next the Ten Questions, the traditional questions centered around temperature, perspiration, food/drink, appetite, stools and urination, pain, sleep, energy, exercise, reproductive/sexual history and emotions, are pursued. It is interesting to see that while the questions are so detailed and minute, they are essentially providing us with the bigger picture of Qi, Blood, Yin and Yang just like the abdomen does. They represent the broader context of the patient's health.

Prior to the interview phase, you can have your patient fill out various medical history and/or intake forms of your choice. I once thought that a comprehensive medical history intake form was the secret to being sure that all the questions were covered and I was constantly designing new ones. However, it didn't take long to see that patients appeared overwhelmed and confused, particularly by long forms. They tended to be succinct in their responses. Incomplete or contradictory information was frequently obtained the more detailed the questions were. What seemed to work best for me was to ask them everything personally. What individual practitioners do is up to them and their personal style. I found the forms got in the way of eliciting the information I wanted from the patients. I want their history to unfold before me in the way the patients prefer to tell their story.

Physical exams

Once the questions have been asked, we move on to those methods of diagnosis that center on the information obtained through the physical exam. Inspection, auscultation, olfaction and palpation are now performed to offer physical evidence to support the diagnosis. This is the stage where the four physical exams are performed to obtain physical verification of the evolving diagnosis, through looking, hearing, smelling and touch, to put us in contact with the living Qi of the patient.

Treatment

Treatment consists of several stages. It begins with abdominal clearing and then progresses to reinforcing with needles or other modalities and is further augmented by patient education. When a patient is first seen there are so many things that may need to be done that practitioners might not know where to begin. There is a lot to clear and a lot of tender points but over time, a pattern tends to emerge which is the underlying root. That root is usually a Deficiency. New things will come up based upon what patients are manifesting acutely (their condition), also referred to as the branch. Apart from the specifics of the treatment methodology, there are general guidelines

that should direct the practitioner in the treatment process. Each of these stages is described below.

Abdominal clearing by hand

Treatment begins once you start diagnosing and clearing the abdomen according to the modified abdominal examination. In the course of this process six major diagnosis points are felt and adjusted via palpation of the clearance points

Abdominal clearing dramatically removes Excesses and can begin the process of tonifying underlying Deficiencies as it brings energy to an area. As the abdominal diagnostic points are pressed and released, improved tone, removal of pain, tension, discomfort or emptiness confirms the diagnosis implied in the clearance or treatment points. If reactiveness diminishes during treatment, the healing power of the body has been activated. This is a positive sign and is of greater significance than what the patient reports. This is not to say that a major complaint, such as headache, no longer exists but rather that energy in the body has been so significantly adjusted that the headache too should be affected in time. It may be starting to abate as the abdomen, a reflection of the headache, is cleared.

Practitioners may use other indices that the treatment has indeed initiated the healing process, the change of pulse being the most common. As a practitioner, you must know that the healing has been put into effect. This may be confirmed by the patient's change of breathing, facial color or demeanor. On the surface these parameters may not seem so significant but in effect they are the most direct manifestations of the spirit being affected. Remember that the *Neijing* posits that the purpose of medicine is to effect a change in the person's spirit.

Most 'spirit connection' can be accomplished without the use of needles or palpation and if the practitioner is truly present for the patient, this will happen throughout the therapeutic relationship. This makes the definition of treatment very broad, exceeding the conventional definition of treatment. The Three Treasures diagnostic paradigm also reminds us that of the three treasures –

Jing, Shen and Qi – the spirit must be treated before Qi or Jing is regulated. Palpation is a very immediate, dramatic, objective and even visceral way of putting the patient and the practitioner in contact with the living Qi of the spirit and offers an index of how the healing process has been set into motion.

Point selection and treatment with needles or other modalities

It is impossible to provide the practitioner with the exact points for treatment because treatment is ultimately artistry. After all, each patient's spirit is unique and this is essentially what should be contacted in the healing process. This is what all the questions and all the physical examinations are about – an attempt to catch a fleeting glimpse of the ephemeral human spirit in its myriad manifestations.

If this treatment stance is adopted, the patient is treated as an energetic being and to a certain degree less as a physical one. The treatment is geared less towards indications, symptoms and physical manifestations of illness. For this reason it is not as important in the Japanese system to couch the diagnosis in the language of other diagnostic paradigms. In fact, some Japanese practitioners do not.

Now that the pattern of disharmony has been discovered on the abdomen and it is cleared as much as possible by hand, reinforcement of the clearance will help to hold the treatment.

Reinforcement is achieved through needling, Tiger Thermie warmer, moxa or other treatment modalities. Certain modalities are more indicated than others for specific conditions. For instance, moxa as applied through the Tiger Thermie warmer is soothing because it delivers the moxa in a pleasant warm fashion and is efficient because it can be used on so many areas without overheating the patient. Intradermals can be retained and worn by the patient as augmentation to treatment. Supplement the treatment with auricular acupuncture or herbal therapy that serve to further hold the treatment. Clinically, two discontinuous therapies combined together have a higher rate of clinical efficacy.

Regardless of which modality is employed, the selection of treatment points constitutes the next stage. How to synthesize these data is a complex task and practitioners have different opinions about it. Some claim that the clearance points that have the greatest clearance value should be needled. This rationale is certainly understood because of the clinical efficacy of those points. They serve to reinforce the action of the clearance protocol. Serizawa (1988) points out:

Since it is not practical or wise to treat all the reactive points with acupuncture and moxibustion, select ten to fifteen points for treatment which are most related to the problem or symptoms by traditional and anatomical correlation. The other reactive points can be massaged or treated more generally by the application of heat. The effect of a treatment is usually better when a selective approach is used in treating points. Treating the main reactive points usually has a positive effect on the body as a whole so that the lesser reactive points are normalized without specific treatment. The selection of points for treatment is a subjective process which very much depends on the practitioner's experience and skill in locating the most effective treatment points. (p. 110)

While I certainly agree with the stance that these treatment points have tremendous therapeutic significance for the patient, I employ a different methodology. My treatment plan tends to center around the following general guidelines.

● I prefer to assign the most painful clearance points to the patient to work on. The most reactive and painful points fall into the category of points expressing Excess – either real Excess or Excess due to an underlying Deficiency. Excesses can be treated relatively easily. Palpation is a physical modality uniquely qualified for resolving tension or tightness through a dispersive technique. Patients can press these clearance points on a daily basis, perhaps the equivalent of having daily treatments in China. Have them do this every day, about 3–5 times a day for about 3–5 seconds. This way they can also adjust the pressure so that they can build up to taking the proper stimulus. However, caution the patient not to do this too many times a day or to cause bruising. If the patient is not interested in self-treatment I definitely needle or treat the main reactive points.

• I mark the points on the patient with a sterile purple-marking pen that will not rub off unless alcohol is also used to swipe the points. Additionally I also draw the points on a prescription pad so the patient can consult the drawing. Writing the instructions on a prescription pad reminds patients that this assignment is part of their therapy and reinforces the body–mind energetic. I do not give them too many points to press so that they do not become overwhelmed with things to do.

• The points that I tend to needle are those that require tonification. They are the points that reflect the root pathology. A typical treatment may consist of 1–6 points dependent upon the pathology presented. If points require moxibustion I will usually perform that until I teach the patients how to treat themselves if they want to, usually with the Tiger Thermie warmer. These may be points that have had smaller clearance value yet contribute to the fine-tuning of clearing the abdominal points.

• My choice of a smaller number of points to needle centers around what I would call the root points or the common denominator of points that were most useful in every exam when clearing the thigh, the navel, the abdomen, scars, etc. For instance, KI 1 (Zhongquan) is a clearance point that is frequently found to clear the abdomen, the navel, the thighs and scars.

• Determining these root points is a distillation process derived from a synthesis of the diagnostic pattern that unfolds from the palpatory exams used in this work. The treatment points incarnate what I call the 'essence' or the 'spirit' of the person. I choose what I call the common denominator of the patient's presentation, be it a Yin problem, a Kidney problem or whatever. Ultimately, needle selection is a matter of artistry in the sense that the points each practitioner might select may be different. That artistry, however, is based upon a perception of the pattern within certain guidelines. As practitioners become more familiar with the material, that artistic agreement will become closer but probably never coincident. This is not unlike what occurs in the practice of Chinese medicine. There is no one way to do things and maybe not even a better way – just a way to try to help patients.

• It is rarely practical or wise to treat all the reactive points and, I would add, not even necessary because the abdominal clearing does so much. I treat few points with needles, generally about five points in my average acupuncture treatment, because fewer needles are more suited for Deficiency patterns and deficient patients. This minimal point selection is geared toward root treatment, nudging the basic bodily energetics back into alignment. Unilateral needling, which is common in this approach, facilitates reduction of the number of needles. Needles are selected according to the side of the body that each particular meridian may have an affinity for, as demonstrated in the pulse system. The use of moxibustion as delivered through the Tiger Thermie warmer is extremely efficacious and can be applied generously to many areas of the body, for instance, the sinuses, Naganos,* the neck and the navel in addition to some focused needling. Plus the patient can be instructed to use it.

In conclusion, when selecting points to needle, choose points that meet the following criteria.

• Points with which you can coordinate a relationship between your Chinese and Japanese diagnosis or points which can be supported in terms of your predominant diagnostic framework; in other words, points which make sense to you.

• From amongst the points you have chosen, determine how to needle them unilaterally to maximize your needling options.

• Choose only one set of distal Kidney points. For instance, select KI 1 (Yongquan), KI 6 (Zhaohai), KI 3 (Taixi) or others but not more than one set bilaterally. However, you could use a distal Kidney clearance point such as KI 1 with an abdominal one such as KI 16 or KI 27.

• From two to eight of the Confluent points may be selected. These points do not need to be

---

* The Naganos are a special group of four points located between the Large Intestine and Triple Warmer meridians. They begin in the Large Intestine 11 (Quchi) area and are about 1 cun apart as you move distally. See Section 5 where they are discussed in the point energetic section and illustrated in the point location section.

chosen as a Master/Couple set. These points constitute the skeletal outline of the treatment. Other points may be added for their clearance value or their therapeutic value.

These points with their appropriate needle methods are summarized in Table 12.1.

Patient education

It is my belief that while the needles are retained it is helpful to give the patient an image of what the needles are doing. A practitioner of any style, be it Five Element, Zang-Fu or Japanese, can offer the patient a guided image of what the needling is meant to accomplish.

An illness can be perceived differently according to the various diagnostic paradigms. It could be called a Water/Fire imbalance (Five Elements), a Kidney/Heart problem (Zang-Fu) or an autonomic nervous system disturbance (Japanese). Explain to the patient how the imagery of the diagnostic paradigm can be achieved through the points that are treated. Also let patients know how long the needles will be retained so they have a sense of the process.

You could also instruct patients to breathe deeply into their abdomen so that they can feel their breath inflating it, thus infusing it with life. And then, like a wheel, you want them to bring this energy back to the chest and to continue to circulate it in this manner. Have them clear their mind of any distractions or thoughts so that the mind is free and not working, a task that consumes Qi and Blood. Simply have them breathe or hold the image that you have imparted in front of them as the treatment commences.

Explain the clinical significance of the points to the patient, that is, what they do in the body. For instance, I reveal how stress can consume Yin and lead to Yang rising. This energy could produce the migraine headaches that they are experiencing. Therefore GB 41 (Zulinqi) could be tender because it regulates this function. I utilize treatment time by teaching the aforementioned information since my primary orientation as a practitioner is to teach patients about their bodily disharmonies.

Patients enjoy this procedure and when they return are good reporters of how the points worked or any problems they had in administering the treatment. As needed, new points can be added to their repertoire of clearance points and ones that are not needed can be abandoned. However, it is interesting to note that these points tend to stay the same for the individual throughout the course of treatment because the palpation process really does reveal root disharmonies.

Self-treatment by patients accelerates the healing process and allows the practitioner to spend less time on clearing and more on clarifying and treating the root which is usually an underlying Deficiency. The course of treatment in this system is exponentially faster because of the emphasis on treating the root of the disease. The practitioner may be better able to treat the root because needles, moxa or herbs may be required and the patient is not qualified to administer them.

Effect a change

A guiding principle in all medical approaches should be to do no harm. As practitioners, you have a responsibility to safeguard the vital Qi, the life force. Treat every patient to the best of your ability but in that quest, don't err on the side of doing too much in any one treatment or doing things you're not proficient with. Realize that you can't and shouldn't do everything in one treatment. The *Tao* advises doing things in small amounts and this protocol, with its minimum use of needles, does just that. As a result, after the treatment, a common reported finding is that patients feel balanced, rested and supported instead of drained, spacy or weakened.

Evaluate and continue to treat

Treat weekly according to the presentation or pattern that is the clearest. Repeat all the steps of the diagnostic and treatment procedure described above. There is no need to repeat the healthy Hara examination or the Japanese physical exam weekly. However, these should be spot-checked

Table 12.1 Needle schema for the abdominal clearance protocol

Diagnostic point	Clearance point	Needle method
CV 14/15 (Juque/Jiuwei)	PC 6 (Neiguan)	Left side Perpendicular, 0.5–0.8 in., get a little Qi
	LU 7 (Lieque)	Right side Oblique, needle with or against meridian, 0.3–0.5 in., get some Qi
	KI 6 (Zhaohai)	Right and left Japanese location (which is also Chinese location), needle parallel to skin in direction of meridian, 0.1–0.2 in. posteriorly horizontally
	KI 25 (Shencang)	Left Horizontally–transversely, towards lateral aspect of chest, very shallow, 0.3–0.5 in.
	CV 12 (Zhongwan)	Perpendicular, 0.3–0.5 in, get Qi
CV 12 (Zhongwan)	ST 34 (Liangqiu)	Right Obliquely in direction of meridian, 15° angle, 0.5–0.8 in.
	ST 44 (Neiting)	Right and left Sole of foot between 2nd and 3rd toes, perpendicular, 0.3–0.5 in., use Tiger Thermie or needle
	SP 4 (Gongsun)	Right and left Perpendicular, 0.3–0.5 in., or in direction of meridian
ST 25 (Tianshu) Left	SP 10 (Xuehai)	Left; more medial location, oblique to transverse, needle in direction of meridian, 0.5–0.7 in.
	TE 5 (Waiguan)	Right; perpendicular, 0.5–0.8 in., get Qi
	GB 41 (Zulinqi)	Left Chinese or Japanese (slide back until just before cuboid bone), needle in direction of meridian at a 15° angle, 0.3–0.5 in.
	LR 5 (Ligou)	Left usually Chinese (2) or Japanese locations Obliquely upward 0.3–0.5 in.
	LR 3 (Taichong)	Right and left Needle in direction of meridian, 0.3–0.5 in., no stimulation
	LR 14 (Qimen)	Right Obliquely toward lateral aspect, 0.3–0.5 in., no stimulation
ST 25 (Tianshu) Right	LU 1–2 (Zhongfu–Yunmen)	Area. Right and left Transverse, toward lateral aspect of the chest, very shallow insertion
	LI 4 (Hegu)	Right and left Perpendicular, 0.2–0.4 in., get Qi
	TE 3 (Zhongdu)	Right and left Transversely in direction of meridian 0.3–0.5 in.
	SI 3 (Houxi)	Right and left Obliquely upward 0.3–0.5 in. Under the bone. Get stimulus. Could do GB 41 (Zulinqi), TE 5 (Waiguan) if still not clear.
CV 4 (Guanyuan)–6 (Qihai)	KI 1 (Yongquan)	Right and left Perpendicular, 0.3–0.5 in., lift and thrust or Tiger Thermie
	KI 6 (Zhaohai)	Right and left Japanese location (which is also a Chinese location), needle towards ankle bone parallel to skin, shallow, 0.1–0.2 in.
	KI 3 (Taixi)	Right and left Japanese location near KI 5 (Shuiquan), needle towards heel, transverse, 0.2–0.3 in.
	KI 7 (Fuliu)	Right and left Transverse in the direction of the meridian, 0.3–0.4, in. upwards
	BL 62 (Shenmai)	Right Straight down from Chinese BL 62 (Shenmai) and back, transverse in the direction of the meridian, 0.2–0.3 in.
	KI 16 (Huangshu)	Right and left Obliquely towards the navel 0.5–1.0 in. or Tiger Thermie

TE = standard abbreviation of the World Health Organization (1989) for Triple Warmer.

occasionally to look for changes. The healthy Hara is the bottom-line diagnosis on the big picture of Qi, Blood, Yin and Yang so this will change slowly. But when it does you have succeeded in treating the root. The Japanese physical exam expresses physical changes that have come about as a result of substantial energetic imbalances so these too are likely to change slowly. When they improve, the functioning of the body is improving as well.

Box 12.1 summarizes this process from intake through to treatment.

Box 12.1 The diagnostic and treatment methodology

1. Conduct the interview, asking the Five Preliminaries and the Ten Questions.
2. Perform the physical examinations (inspection, tongue, pulse, olfaction, auscultation), and the healthy Hara examination, the modified abdominal exam, the navel exam and the Japanese physical exam.
3. Administer treatment.
   - Clear the abdomen by hand.
   - Reinforce the clearance with needles or other modalities to treat the root.
   - Augment treatment with patient self-treatment of points.
   - Effect a change.
4. In subsequent treatments, evaluate and treat in stages according to which pattern is clearest.

NEW WORDS AND CONCEPTS

Belly bowl – a Korean-style moxa instrument in which moxa is burned, generally directly over the navel. See Supplier section.

Five Preliminaries – the basic area of questioning in the patient interview prior to the Chinese questions referred to as the Ten Questions.

Jing Deficiency – a weakness of the essential substance of rarefied energy stored in the Kidneys and the Extraordinary Meridians.

Naganos – a group of four points located between the Large Intestine and Triple Warmer meridians. They are found at the lateral end of the elbow crease and proceed distally, about one fingerbreadth apart. They are indicative of the condition of the person's immunity.

Reactive points – points which are responsive to palpation; ah shi points, passive points.

Ten Questions – the multitudinous detailed Chinese questions pertaining to body temperature, perspiration, food/drink, appetite, stools and urination, sleep, energy, exercise, reproductive/ sexual history and the emotions.

Three Treasures – a particular diagnostic framework referring to the Jing, Qi and Shen.

QUESTIONS

1. What are the modalities through which reinforcement is accomplished?

2. What is the point selection geared toward and why and how would one select a smaller number of points?

3. Describe ways in which the practitioner can involve the patient in taking part in their healing throughout the treatment regimen.

4. What are the components of the Japanese physical exam?

5. Explain why the presence of any of the components of the Japanese physical exam would signify significant pathology.

6. Why will the components of the Japanese physical exam take longer to treat? How often should they be monitored and treated?

7. What are the Five Preliminary questions that are asked with regards to the main complaint?

While it is always important to treat a person's major complaint in the context of their whole clinical presentation, it is also important to familiarize yourself with important treatment of disease points which are valuable in the overall treatment. Match the following major complaints/illnesses with their treatment of disease points. To familiarize yourself with the treatment of disease points, see Section 5 and the indices at the end of the book.

1. Asthma, bronchitis
2. Ligament problems
3. Hip joint pain
4. Chest pain
5. Sciatica
6. Carpal tunnel syndrome
7. Sinus problems
8. Shock, trauma
9. Allergic reactions
10. Dysmenorrhea
11. Acute stomachache
12. Blood pressure disorders
13. Edema of foot

a. GB 1 (Tongziliao)
b. KI 1 (Yongquan)
c. LU 4 (Xiabai)
d. ST 44 (Inner Neiting)
e. SP 8 (Diji)
f. LR 4 (Zhongfeng)
g. LR 8 (Ququan)
h. LU 7 (Lieque)
i. BL 39 (Weiyang)
j. BL 66 (Zutonggu)
k. KI 6 (Zhaohai)
l. LU 5 (Chize)
m. BL 1 (Jingming) and BL 2 (Zanzhu)

13

Japanese physical exam 1: treatment of inner thigh compression

The first evaluation within the Japanese physical exam is that of inner thigh compression. This is an important topic that has implications for patients' health and their abdominal presentation.

The condition of the inner thigh is largely a reflection of underlying Blood vessels and meridians in that area which traverse to the abdomen. Hence, if there are problems with inner thigh functioning they can be diagnosed through abdominal palpation. Let us first investigate the significance of inner thigh pathology and its etiology and then turn to the diagnosis and treatment of inner thigh compression.

INNER THIGH PHYSIOLOGY AND PATHOLOGY

The inner thigh houses the greater saphenous vein, the longest vein in the body. It is the function of this vein, like all veins in the lower part of the body, to carry deoxygenated Blood from the lower extremities back into the inferior vena cava and thence to the heart for reoxygenation.

Several physiological facts contribute to the development of inner thigh problems. First, the venous system is under less pressure than the arterial system so that poor Blood flow can ensue. Coupled with this, veins in the legs, as in the entire body, are subject to the laws of gravity. Due to their location in the lower part of the body, they are more susceptible to impairment of their function. Inner thigh compression can likewise affect the return of Blood to the abdomen. The cumulative effect of these three conditions is that insufficient Blood returns to the upper part of the body and stagnant Blood in the lower part of the body and the abdomen can result.

The clinical symptoms of inner thigh compression are many. They include anemia, dizziness, edema of the lower extremities, varicosities, hypothyroidism, fibroid tumors, painful periods, PMS symptoms, ovarian cysts, endometriosis, high, low or labile Blood pressure and other vascular disturbances.

Inner thigh compression can arise from several causes. For instance, tight clothing, poor posture, scars or injury on the thigh, high-heeled shoes, childbirth, insufficient or excess muscular development – in short, anything that can affect the integrity of the inner thigh or the circulation of Blood in that area can impair the venous as well as arterial circulation of Blood in the leg. Avoidance of smoking or other drugs that increase the risk of clotting are appropriate prophylactic measures to reduce the risk of inner thigh compression.

As part of the Japanese physical exam, the inner thigh of both men and women should be checked to see if there is any involvement. Visual inspection is part of that examination, as is palpation. Remember that as part of the Japanese physical exam, inner thigh compression represents a physical, structural abnormality that is bound to have energetic counterparts. Checking the inner thigh and then correcting any problems associated with it will have beneficial results for the entire body.

When the inner thigh is healthy it should be firm and smooth, not soft, lumpy, mushy, nor hard, misshapen or edemic. Thighs that are soft and lack tone are indicative of Deficiency. Moderate physical activity is needed to maintain muscle tone and facilitate circulation. Apart from cosmetic reasons, firm thighs provide the appropriate degree of tension or tone to promote correct functioning of the underlying vessels, including the meridians. Thighs which are hard, knotted, lumpy or misshapen are pathological as well. They need to be free from tension so as not to impair functioning in that region. Interestingly, even athletes and dancers who may have firm, 'attractive' thighs may have pathological tension in the inner thigh area. Therefore, the thighs should be inspected and palpated to determine any possible inner thigh disturbance.

DIAGNOSTIC ASSESSMENT AND TREATMENT

Evaluation

Procedurally there are two avenues the practitioner may pursue to treat the inner thigh. These are discussed below.

First, the practitioner can clear the abdomen. If less than 100% clearance is achieved, the inner thigh can be checked since it is one of the components of the Japanese physical exam. After the thigh is cleared there should be significant improvement in the abdominal clearance points that were previously resistant to clearance. I prefer this approach to assessing the relationship of the thigh to the abdomen and the clearance points that are significant for treatment.

Another approach is to check the thigh first and clear it. Then you can proceed to clear the abdomen, which should be easier if the thigh pathology was reflected on the abdomen. With this procedure, however, you cannot ascertain the effects of the thigh on the abdomen because you don't know the original abdominal presentation. In any event the cumulative effect is the same; that is, you are clearing things as you encounter them. The thigh affects the abdomen and the abdomen affects the thigh. What is important is to appreciate the relationship between the thigh and the abdomen and the person's health.

1. The first step in inner thigh clearance is to reduce any tenderness in this area by hand. When palpating the inner thigh, have patients recline on their back with their legs separated and slightly turned out. Instruct patients on what you will be doing so that they understand why you are touching the inner thigh that is an intimate and guarded area. The thighs need to be visible so the patient should be wearing a gown. The gown should be properly draped over the patient to shield private areas and maintain modesty. Tuck it around the upper part of the thigh so that the complete thigh can be viewed.

2. Next, mentally divide the surface of the inner thigh into three lines running longitudinally upward from the knee to about 2 inches below the pubic region. The most anterior line above the knee is the Spleen meridian. The middle line is the Liver meridian and the posterior line is the Kidney meridian. Remember that the Spleen meridian moves anterior to the Liver meridian at SP 9 (Yinlingquan), whereas below the knee the Liver meridian runs anterior to the Spleen.

3. Now palpate these meridians at four points along each meridian, roughly equidistant from each other, starting at about 2 cun above the knee and moving in an upward direction towards the abdomen (Fig. 13.1). Since this is an area prone to tension as well as guarding, tenderness may be present so it is likely that patients will react. Prepare them for this by explaining the procedure and the expected sensations. As with all palpation, look at the patients while pressing on the points to see how they react to the palpation and to avoid causing unnecessary pain. In addition to a pain response, you may feel lumpy, knotted

tissue or soft flaccid skin that is indicative of the problems in the inner thigh.

4. Apply firm sustained pressure to each point, pressing down perpendicularly on it for about 2–3 seconds. Press slowly to the point of resistance in the tissue, just as in abdominal palpation. Determine which is the most tender point on each meridian. If the palpation process is too painful, stop. The patient's discomfort reaction provides you with the information that you need to know, which is that the inner thigh is congested. Do this procedure on each leg, beginning with the right.

Clearance

Now from amongst all three meridians, choose the most tender point. This is the point you will try to clear. The first clearance point is KI 1 (Yongquan) because of its powerful ability to activate the circulation of Blood. One side at a time, apply deep dispersive pressure to KI 1, rubbing it for about 3 seconds. This point will be tender if there is inner thigh tension. Now go back and check the most tender thigh point and see if there is improvement. Because of its energetics, KI 1 should significantly contribute to inner thigh clearance. Minimally, it should clear 50%. It is not uncommon for it to resolve the tenderness 100%.

The aim of the clearance procedure is always to reduce as many problems by hand, so if 100% clearance has not been obtained, move on to the next point which is LR 4 (Zhongfeng). LR 4 is the Metal point on the Wood meridian. Because Metal controls Wood it is the primary point to move Liver Qi Stagnation anywhere in the body, particularly in the lower abdomen. It is also an effective point for Blood Stagnation because the Blood follows the Qi. Again, press this point one side at a time for the standard palpation time and check to see how this contributes to the clearance of the inner thigh. It generally has considerable effect.

Because of their powerful energetics, KI 1 (Yongquan) and LR 4 (Zhongfeng) are effective for clearance of the whole inner thigh, not only if the tender thigh points were located on the Kidney or Liver meridians. Try to clear any residual

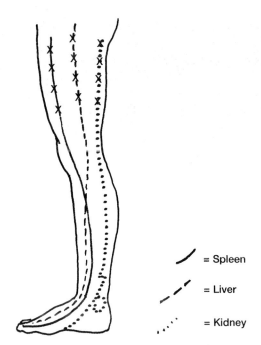

= Spleen

= Liver

= Kidney

Figure 13.1 Where to palpate the meridians of the inner thigh (x).

discomfort of the thigh with SP 6 (Sanyinjiao), KI 6 (Zhaohai), KI 3 (Taixi) and KI 7 (Fuliu). SP 6 is effective particularly for tenderness on the Spleen line but it can clear any thigh point. As group Luo of the Three Leg Yin, it has a powerful effect on the circulation of the three Yin meridians of the leg, which traverse the inner thigh. KI 6 will contribute to thigh clearance if Kidney Yin is present. KI 3 is better for Kidney Qi (Yin and Yang) and Kidney 7 is best for Kidney Yang problems.

Note that this process is applied to the most tender point. The assumption is that if the most tender point can be cleared sufficiently, normalization of other points will follow. If you want, you may check the other tender points but this step is not necessary.

Now that the inner thigh has been cleared by hand, the abdominal presentation should be improved if thigh tension was more than local. The clearance points of the inner thigh are important treatment points for the patient, who should be taught how to press these points on a regular basis to improve Blood flow through the thigh. The Tiger Thermie warmer can also be used on the clearance points for about 3 minutes on each point. These points can also be needled by the physician to consolidate clearance. For added effect, intradermal needles can be inserted into the clearance points and retained by the patient for appropriate retention times.

Figure 13.2, the thigh clearance form, is provided to assist the practitioner procedurally in this examination.

Kiiko Matsumoto claims that the simple kitchen rolling pin can also be employed to promote improved Blood flow in the inner thigh. She recommends rolling the device on the inner thigh for about 3 minutes per leg in an upward direction. Because imbalance of one part of the body is generally compensated for by a concomitant change in a related part, roll the outer thigh in a downward direction for the same amount of time. This mechanism can also assist in weight reduction, breakdown of cellulite, improved tone of the entire thigh as well as improved Blood circulation. Roll the inner thigh upward and the outer thigh downward to promote appropriate vascular flow.

Contraindications

Hydraulic and mechanical manipulations such as the rolling pin are contraindicated in deep vein thrombosis. Deep vein thrombosis (DVT) is a clinical condition in which a thrombus of fibrin, red Blood cells, platelets and granulocytes develops within a deep vein. There is a danger that the thrombus can become detached and then lodge in the lungs, particularly if the size of the embolus exceeds the lumen of the artery of the lungs. A detached thrombus is called an embolus. Emboli can range from 1.0 to 1.5 cm wide and can be 50 cm long!

Most thrombi first form in the deep venous system of the calf. The majority (80%) of these remain localized and eventually resolve on their own but approximately 20% propagate above the knee. Roughly half of these will become emboli, accounting for 95% of all clinically significant pulmonary thromboemboli (Catlett & Welch 1996). The most common sites for the development of DVT are the iliac and femoral veins of the lower limb. Other veins which can be affected include the posterior tibial vein and the profunda femoral vein (Fig. 13.3).

The occlusion of a vein in this manner produces clinical manifestations that include stasis symptoms (Box 13.1).

Superficial thrombophlebitis must be distinguished from DVT and cellulitis since both disorders are associated with warm, erythematous legs but are managed differently and have different clinical implications. In general, DVT is characterized by greater swelling than superficial thrombophlebitis and is much more likely to result in pulmonary embolism. Figure 13.4 shows the general routes of transmission of a thromboembolus.

As in any diagnosis, a thorough medical history is of critical importance. Establishing a family history of DVT is imperative. However, the incidence of DVT is difficult to diagnose by clinical history and physical examination. Minimal leg symptoms may be associated with extensive venous thrombosis and the classic symptoms of pain, redness and swelling of the leg can be caused by non-thrombotic disorders.

Patient's name:_____   Date:_____

Major complaint and accompanying symptoms:_____

_____

1. After abdominal clearing, what was the most significant pathology remaining that you were unable to obtain sufficient clearance on?_____

_____

_____

_____

_____

2. Circle the leg, meridian and point which was the most tender.

        Right SP 1 2 3 4

              LR 1 2 3 4

              KI 1 2 3 4

      Left SP 1 2 3 4

              LR 1 2 3 4

              KI 1 2 3 4

3. Record points used to clear the most painful thigh points.

Points	Degree it contributed to clearance
KI 1	
LR 4	
SP 6	
KI 6	
KI 3	
KI 7	

4. Describe the patient's reaction to thigh palpation, what you felt if anything upon palpation, presentation of patient's thighs. Then record the results of the thigh clearance/patient's reaction to thigh clearance.

_____

_____

_____

_____

_____

_____

_____

5. After the thigh clearance go back and check the points on the abdomen on which you did not obtain 100% clearance. Was there any change in abdominal presentation? Describe.

_____

_____

_____

_____

Figure 13.2 Thigh clearance form.

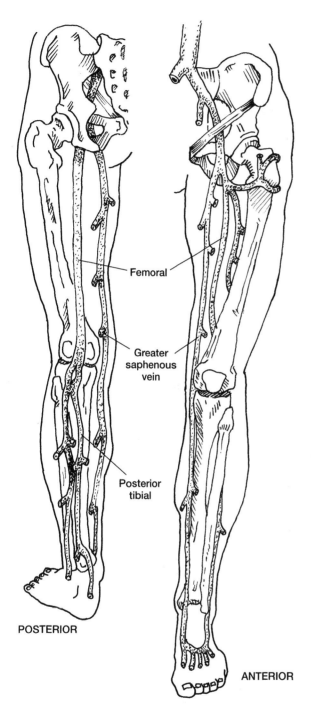

Femoral

Greater
saphenous
vein

Posterior
tibial

POSTERIOR

ANTERIOR

Figure 13.3 Problematic veins for acute deep vein thrombosis.

There are certain high-risk groups within the population for this condition, including patients with excess clotting disorders, patients who have injury or disease to the legs, patients who have had knee or hip surgeries such as total hip replacement, cancer and abdominal surgery. It is hypothesized that there will probably be an increase in the prevalence of DVT because the average age of the population is increasing. Older age is becoming less of a contraindication for surgery and many surgical patients, young and old, are being discharged from hospital before they are fully ambulant. Groups who are at high risk for thromboembolism are shown in Box 13.2 although this list cannot be exhaustive.

Because DVT may be clinically silent, meaning it is difficult to diagnose without instrumentation, the massage therapist or physician who uses mechanical stimulation, such as the rolling pin, or even deep palpation in the region of the inner thigh needs to be cognizant of common clinical manifestations of DVT as well as population groups who might have a tendency to develop this potentially life-threatening condition. However, it is important to reiterate that while there seems to be a correlation between certain overt signs and symptoms of stasis in the lower limb, without sophisticated instrumentation such as duplex ultrasonography, venography and CT venography (Baldt 1996), a positive diagnosis of DVT cannot be made. Symptoms include tenderness, pain, swelling, warmth and discoloration of the skin. Treatment includes bed rest and anticoagulant drugs to prevent movement of the thrombus towards the lungs.

NEW WORDS AND CONCEPTS

Cellulitis – inflammation of cellular or connective tissue which spreads through the tissue.

Embolus – a mass of undissolved matter present in a Blood or lymphatic vessel brought there by the Blood or lymph current. Emboli may be solid, liquid or gaseous and may consist of bits of tissue, globules of fat, air bubbles, clumps of bacteria and foreign bodies such as bullets. Emboli

Box 13.1	Possible signs and symptoms of acute deep vein thrombosis (compiled from Bell & Simon 1982)
Pain	Usually described as a constant dull ache of the lower extremity. May be inguinal and/or low back pain with iliofemoral thrombosis. Pain is aggravated by standing or walking, may be relieved by bed rest, and occasionally increased by coughing or sneezing
Unilateral swelling	Commonly absent in bedridden DVT patients but in others there is swelling of the ankle or calf or simply loss of the normal concavity distal to the malleolus
Warmth and redness	Patient may have sensation of warmth in lower extremity. Examiner may feel it with back of hand after legs have been uncovered for several minutes. Redness will be apparent in 20% of patients
Superficial venous dilation	On dorsum of foot and anterior tibia in 30% of cases
Dependent cyanosis	Bluish discoloration of foot or lower one-third of leg, relieved by elevation, may be present
Palpable thrombi	Presenting as a tender cord within the thrombosed vein. Palpable in only 10% of instrument-proven DVT cases, but almost certain indication of DVT (98% of positive palpation cases will have DVT)
Fever and/or tachycardia	May also be present

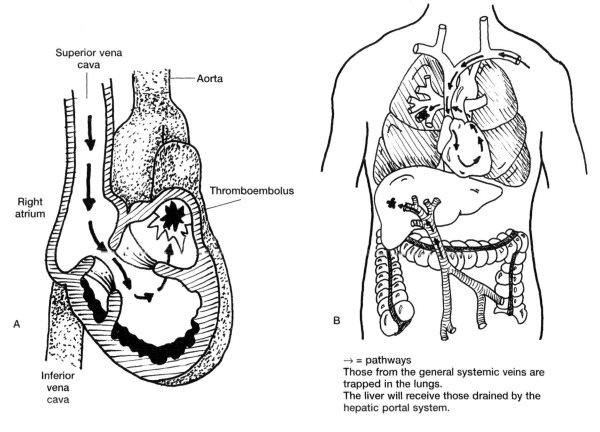

→ = pathways
Those from the general systemic veins are trapped in the lungs.
The liver will receive those drained by the hepatic portal system.

Figure 13.4 Thromboembolus and the principal pathways of transmission.

Box 13.2	High-risk groups for deep vein thrombosis
Immobilization	Patients with pelvic fractures, acute head or spinal injury, cerebrovascular accident, other disease or weakness, total hip replacement surgery; highest in the surgical population with lower extremity fractures
Age	Greatest frequency of pulmonary embolism (PE) occurs between 50 and 65 years of age. Up to 90% of fatal PE are thought to occur in patients over 50 years of age
Cardiac diseases	Especially atrial fibrillation, congestive heart failure (CHF) and myocardial infarction (MI)
Trauma	Up to 15% incidence of PE in accident victims. PE high in major burn victims, high-risk trauma patients and those with major orthopedic surgery
Obesity	Most for those whose weight is 20% over standard weight
Cancer	Especially lung, pancreas, stomach
Pregnancy and postpartum period	Due to venous stasis caused by an enlarged uterus, change in coagulation factors and Blood vessel trauma at birth
Oral contraceptives	Changes in coagulation factors
Some Blood and metabolic diseases	Such as carriers of thrombogenic mutation, hyperhomocysteinemia and vascular disease

may arise within the body or they may gain entrance from without. Occlusion from emboli usually results in the development of infarcts.

Superficial thrombophlebitis – inflammation secondary to thrombosis of the superficial venous system.

Thrombus – a Blood clot obstructing an artery or cavity of the heart.

QUESTIONS

1. How is a thrombus perceived in Chinese medicine?

2. Name the eight possible signs and symptoms of deep vein thrombosis.

3. Name nine possible groups who are at higher risk for venous thromboembolism.

4. How does a thrombus become an embolus?

5. How does a pulmonary embolus develop?

6. What are some of the ways to reduce inner thigh compression?

7. What are some of the clinical manifestations of inner thigh compression?

8. Using palpation, how would you make the diagnosis of inner thigh compression? Before clearing the inner thigh, specifically how would you rule out the patient's risk of releasing a thrombus of the deep veins during your procedure?

9. List/discuss the important energetics of KI 1 (Yongquan), LR 4 (Zhongfeng) and SP 6 (Sanyinjiao) which effectively enable them to clear the inner thigh.

10. Using both Western and Chinese theories of the inner thigh, explain the method of direction that is used when rolling the thigh with the rolling pin.

11. Try to explain how/why problematic veins for deep vein thrombosis primarily traverse the Yin aspect of the thigh/leg. In other words, why would deep vein thrombosis occur more on the Yin aspect of the body?

14

Japanese physical exam 2: clinical significance and treatment of scar tissue

WHAT IS A SCAR IN ORIENTAL AND WESTERN PARADIGMS?

This chapter devotes itself to the second physical evaluation within the Japanese physical exam, namely the treatment of scar tissue. This is a very important and perhaps underappreciated topic that merits consideration in a practitioner's treatment repertoire. Particularly within this book, with its emphasis on meridian energetics, we need to consider all factors, one of which are scars, that can influence the flow of Qi and Blood. The scar tissue that we are referring to here are scars formed on the surface of the body as a result of injury or operation; that is, not internal scarring of tissue. Chapter 10 on navel diagnosis and treatment also presented some information on scars since the navel is a scar.

First, we will look at the general ways in which scars are viewed in Western and Oriental medicine and then turn to their treatment.

Western perspective

A scar is the name applied to a healed wound, ulcer or breach of tissue. It includes malformations caused by incisions, cuts, burns, injuries or even cystic acne. Scars on the surface of the skin consist of essentially fibrous tissue covered by an imperfect formation of epidermis. The connective tissue corpuscles that wander into the wound in the course of its repair produce fibrous tissue and so at first it is delicate in texture and richly provided with Blood vessels. Accordingly, at this stage, a scar is soft and has a redder tint than the surrounding skin. Gradually this fibrous tissue contracts, becomes denser and loses its Blood vessels, so that an old scar is hard and white.

Scars, whether they are caused by accidents or by surgery, are unpredictable and disorganized in the manner in which they form. Increased vascularization and an increase in fibroblasts that synthesize collagen follow cutaneous wounds. Initially, excessive and unordered deposition of collagen fibers occurs but eventually, the collagen realigns and the scarring matures and becomes less noticeable.

The more severe forms of scarring are keloid and hypertrophic scars. They tend to be harder and non-elastic, have an inhibited range of motion and are raised and discolored, usually purple or red. With hypertrophic scarring, the collagen continues to be produced and fails to mature and reorganize. It stays within the border of the scar but is usually raised. Keloids tend to be hard, thick, bumpy and red and are often associated with pain, burning, itching, tingling, tightness and unpleasant pulling sensations. With keloids, the scar tissue continues to grow beyond the size of the initial wound or incision. Collagen is overproduced in response to severe skin damage. The more disorganized and imbalanced collagen becomes, the bigger and more discolored the scar will be.

The way a scar develops depends upon many factors, the most common of which are detailed below.

- The nature and severity of the original injury such as its location, size and depth.
- The surgeon's skill or the method of treatment or care, if any, that the scar received.
- How the person's body heals.
- The Blood supply to the area.
- The direction of the scar formation.
- The thickness and color of the skin.

All these factors contribute to the outcome of a scar and the potential degree of disturbance that it may cause. Thus, when a scar forms it can take on various shapes, colors, textures and height. Concomitant symptoms that may accompany initial unhealed scar formation include pain, itchy and burning sensations, tightness and localized obstruction, oozing or weeping suppuration. After the scar has completely healed, other symptoms may include numbness or tingling in the area, unpleasant pulling sensations, coldness, restricted range of motion, pruritus or other disagreeable sensations. One of the reasons why such symptoms arise is because contraction in the area of the scar may naturally develop and this contraction can cause tension and muscle and tendon restriction.

Oriental perspective

Within the system of Chinese medicine, channel theory postulates that scars may significantly block the normal flow of Qi and Blood within the major meridians, potentially reducing the overall vitality of Qi. Neither do the Japanese dismiss the clinical significance of scars in their body of medical information, due to their estimation of the relationship between form and function and meridian energetics that they share with their Chinese roots.

According to Oriental medicine, scars are potential organ–meridian disturbances. Because they are on the exterior, that is, the surface of the skin or in the musculature, they may interfere with the superficial flow of Qi and Blood in the meridians. Whether a scar is indeed an organ–meridian disturbance needs to be determined. There are several ways to decipher this, the most important of which is palpation.

THE TREATMENT OF SCARS

The allopathic community devotes a significant amount of attention and research to scars. They are addressed not only for cosmetic reasons or for the emotional pain of disfiguring scars but also to reduce pain, pruritus or restriction of movement caused by lesions close to joints. Some doctors have also observed that scars are a prime site for the subsequent appearance of skin cancers because scars have less pigment than the rest of the skin (Rosenfeld 1986, p. 305). As physicians, we are interested in treating scars for those reasons as well but have the additional perspective of considering scars significant because they can affect meridian energetics.

The next part of this chapter covers how to treat scars particularly with Oriental therapeutics. Supplemental information taken from Western medicine as well as other traditions is also provided to offer the practitioner a fairly comprehensive and practical treatment plan for scars.

Western treatment

In the Western medical community, the treatment of scar tissue has included low-dose radiation, excision surgery, scar revision, plastic surgery, cryosurgery and skin grafts. Other treatments include cortisone injections, laser surgery, pressure garments, scarabrasion, synthetic antibodies (to stop the action of certain factors which promote the regrowth of new skin), electrical stimulation and silicon gel sheeting. Apart from electrical stimulation and some methods of silicon polymer sheeting, evaluation of other methods has shown that most are invasive, expensive and usually ineffective. Of course, all the factors that influence scar formation also enter into the equation for scar healing and Western technology is making advances in this field almost daily.

The use of electrical stimulation and silicon sheeting has had excellent results in reducing the formation of hypertrophic scarring (Weiss et al 1989). It is also known to reduce the significantly increased number of mast cells that are associated with keloid and hypertrophic scarring (Hirshowitz et al 1993, Kischer et al 1978, Reich et al 1991). It has been particularly successful in the management of hypertrophic and keloid scars caused by burns, cuts, incisions and surgery.

It is believed that the static electric field in the polymer sheet that is in contact with the scarred area may be the critical factor in scar inhibition. It appears that the electrostatic ionic bonding process actually rebuilds skin from the inside out. The inherent flexible nature of its ionic bonds provides a consistent matrix for balanced fibroblast activity. This facilitates realignment and normalization of the collagen molecules. The electrostatic ionic bonding process simultaneously helps degrade excess amino acids and polypeptides on collagen molecules usually associated with exaggerated scarring. The body naturally dissipates the old built-up collagen and the scar eventually softens, flattens and shrinks. Color normalizes, redness diminishes and any unpleasant appearance or sensations are greatly reduced. The reason why I have included this explanation of the mechanism by which it is believed to work is because I would hypothesize that needling has a similar effect.

The thin, pliable, comfortable silicon sheet is simply placed over the scar and secured with medical tape. It can be worn daily for 2–9 months depending upon the severity of the scarring. A typical sheet usually remains effective for one year. The sheet is durable and washable. In between use it can be stored in a clean zip-lock bag. It is an interesting adjunct to scar treatment that the Oriental physician might want to investigate since it is easy to do, extremely effective and not incompatible with the principles of Oriental medicine. The sheeting (ReJuveness) is available from RichMark International Corporation (see Supplier Section on p. 305).

Oriental treatment

As we have seen, in Oriental medicine, scars are viewed as potential organ–meridian disturbances. Because of this feature, no scar should be discounted because of its possible effects on the functioning of the body. When performing the interview, patients should be asked if they have any scars. Then, when a physical examination is performed, the scars should be inspected and then evaluated, particularly scars which are the result of surgery, large scars and scars which are 'troublesome' to the person, meaning they associate some unpleasantness with them such as burning or numbness. However, no scar should be ignored. The scar evaluation process is summarized below.

Scar assessment

1. Begin by inspecting each scar. Look at its size, height and location in relation to meridians,

shape, texture and color. In general, the bigger and more discolored the scar, the more likely it will be tender upon palpation. Usually when scars are unreactive they are pale, soft and flat, not hard, raised, red, purple or dark. Still, all scars should be checked to determine their involvement in the person's health.

2. Scar location is a critical variable relating to the effects that a scar might cause so check the locations of all scars. Areas with important energetics such as the lower abdomen, the neck, face, head and spine can have profound implications if the person has significant scars. While acupuncturists see this problem from an energetic perspective, the Western medical community acknowledges this fact as well through the explanation that scarring can inhibit nerve root Blood supply. For instance, there is general consensus that postoperative scarring after diskectomy in the lower lumbar region is an important cause of treatment failure because it can interfere with the function of delicate spinal nerves by decreasing Blood supply and increasing neural tension. So for patients with back pain, check for scars in the back area. Their treatment can greatly help the patient.

3. Scars are evaluated by palpating around their borders. Press on the immediate perimeter of a scar at an angle as if going underneath it. Never palpate directly on top of a scar, just as you would never needle into scar tissue because of its dense unorganized matrix. Tenderness at the scar indicates tension which is indicative of obstruction in the flow of Qi and Blood. Perception of weakness, emptiness or numbness that the practitioner might feel or that the patient may report indicates Deficiency in that area.

The treatment of scar tissue

Oriental medicine holds that acupuncture and electroacupuncture are acceptable methodologies in the treatment of scars. As with simple acupuncture, the treatment of scars with injection therapy and liniments are possible options. Injections work in part because they stimulate Qi flow strongly as they physically break up contracted tissue. Problematic old scars can be viewed as manifestations of Blood Stasis so they

should be treated by blood-moving herbs such as Catharmus, Ligusticum or Salvia that can be found in various liniments and injections. Tenderness of the scar or any abnormal feeling can be released or treated by clearing the scar by hand, by needles, intradermal needles, moxa, liniments and injection therapy. Scars can be treated with these modalities to reduce their bulk and their adhesion to fascial membranes (Skardis 1995).

If you are using this information in conjunction with the Japanese system outlined in this book, take the following steps.

1. Conduct the healthy Hara examination to see what it reveals.
2. Clear the abdomen and the navel region to treat the whole person energetically at the root level.
3. Clear the inner thigh to promote Qi and Blood flow to the entire body.
4. Scars can now be inspected, palpated and cleared. Scar clearance can resolve local problems as well as improve abdominal presentation. If there was any area on the abdomen that was not sufficiently cleared, see if treating the scar improves abdominal clearance. Even if the abdomen was not affected by a scar, it is still important to clear scars for optimal health and Qi and Blood flow.
5. The various modalities with which to treat scars are described below and summarized in Box 14.1.

1. Clearing the scar by hand. It is impossible to describe how to clear each tender point in a scar by hand because of their individual characteristics. If you have understood the thought processes outlined so far, you should have an idea of how to do this; that is, by selecting points based upon their unique energetics that move Stagnation or tonify underlying Deficiency. The points in the abdominal clearance protocol are amongst the most important points for achieving these results. In particular, KI 1 and LR 4 are two major points that have good effect in treating scars because of their ability to move the Blood and Qi. Palpate in the same manner as you

---

Box 14.1 Methods of treating scars

1. Clear by hand – think of which points might work.
2. Clearing by needle – retain needle for 5 minutes, repeat 2–3 times; only treat two tender areas at a time.
3. Implanting intradermals – retain 3–5 days. Insert at one or two tender areas around the scar.
4. Liniments – choose Chinese liniments that you prefer.
5. Moxa methods – use the Tiger Thermie in particular for about 3 minutes around the scar.
6. Injection therapy – to break up bloating or tension.
7. External moisturizers and massage – use vitamin E, aloe vera or other topicals.
8. Vitamins and foods – especially those rich in vitamin C.
9. Silicon sheets.

---

would in clearing the abdomen, the thigh or the navel. If these don't work, inspect the area where the scar is found and *think* about how it needs to be treated.

For instance, an appendectomy scar in the lower right quadrant might be cleared by the same clearance points as ST 25R (Tianshu). Likewise, a scar caused by a cesarean section which traverses the Ren channel might be cleared by the same clearance points of other points on the Conception Vessel line such as KI 1 (Yongquan), KI 6 (Zhaohai), KI 3 (Taixi) or KI 7 (Fuliu). If these don't work, other clearance points such as those for the Stomach and Spleen could be implicated if they too were severed. If you can't figure how to clear a scar it can always be treated locally with needles or some of the other methods which follow. Always try to clear scars by hand to minimize the use of needles. Both old and new scars can be treated in this manner. Procedurally, the following steps are involved in clearing the scar by hand.

- Palpate around the scar to determine its reactivity.
- Palpate the points that you think might be clearance points.
- Go back and repalpate the scar point to see if it has improved.
- Try to reduce as much scar tension as possible by hand by using additional clearance points.

- If the tension diminishes, you can end the treatment there or explain to the patient which clearance points were involved so that they can work those points by hand or with a Tiger Thermie warmer.
- You may choose to needle those clearance points for added effect.
- As a rule of thumb, any new scars can be worked on approximately 3 weeks after they develop. Wait longer with patients who may have poor healing capacity such as diabetic or immunocompromised patients. Strict asepsis of needles should always be enforced but practitioners must assiduously remind themselves of this when needling scars so that pathogens, which might cause infection, are not inadvertently introduced under the scar.

2. Clearing the scar by needle. If insufficient clearance has been gained by clearing the scar by hand, the actual tender scar points may also be needled. Pick from amongst any tender points the two most painful and needle them. Insert the needle at an angle as you go under the scar. This angle may range from 45° to a transverse direction depending upon the shape of the scar. Do not look for Qi nor tonify or disperse. Use the needle as a mechanical instrument to break up any tension by using a lift-and-thrust or in-and-out method. Retain the needle for 5 minutes and repeat 2–3 times in this manner and then withdraw.

My predilection is to use the thinnest needles available such as a #1 Seirin in order to subtly reestablish even the most minute of energetic pathways. However, if the tissue is dense and fibrous, thicker needles such as a #5 may be used. Needles may be inserted in several places but ideally in no more than two places per session. Figure 14.1 shows how to needle scar tissue.

Because energy can be trapped in these regions or even be empty, the 'release' of a scar can cause appreciable energetic disturbances as energy is unblocked and reestablished. Patients should be advised of possible reactions, which could be subsumed under the blanket of a healing crisis, although it may be impossible to predict the precise symptoms. Case 14.1 illustrates this point.

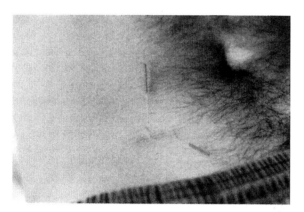

Figure 14.1 How to needle scar tissue.

This case illustrates a number of points that demonstrate the effects of scar treatment.

● The treatment of scars can cause physical and energetic changes. Some of these changes, that is, the negative ones, fall into the domain of what could be called a healing crisis. These potential effects should be explained to the patient and are viewed as a positive effect in which the Qi and Blood flow is readjusting itself. In this case, the patient felt a little spacy.

● The practitioner should direct the treatment plan, not the patient.

● Monitor treatment time. Twenty minutes was too long for the patient, hence the spacy feeling.

● Also practitioners needs to curtail their enthusiasm in doing too much in any one treatment. Stick to the major complaint – in this case the neck tension, which required further care and had been responding favorably to treatment.

3. Implanting intradermals. For scars which are small, particularly hard to clear, stubborn or related to other health complaints, intradermals are a useful treatment modality because they can be retained. Insert an intradermal needle such as a Spinex intradermal underneath the scar. You can use 3–6 mm intradermals depending on the width of the scar. Secure the intradermal with new adhesive tape. Consider the area where the needle is placed so that it will not cause any discomfort; for instance, an intradermal implanted around the waist could be bothersome because of

Case 14.1

A student learning this material was required to treat a patient for at least 3 weeks using the information given in this book. The following case is a synopsis of those treatments.

The patient came into the clinic with a major complaint of neck tension and some mild discomfort of the right shoulder and wrist. She was also recovering from a cold that exacerbated her asthma and bronchitis that she had had for a number of years.

First, the abdomen was cleared and it resolved about 80% through palpation. Since the neck was the area of the major complaint, it was inspected. The physical exam revealed that she had a scar on her right shoulder about $3\frac{1}{2}$ inches long and about 1 cm wide at its widest point. Palpation revealed that the tenderest points around the scar made the neck feel better so the student decided to treat the scar. Two needles were inserted at these points and retained for about 20 minutes. After treating the scar, both the student practitioner and a student observer noticed that the scar was less lumpy although it still showed purplish areas. The patient also felt that the scar was smoother.

The following week the patient reported that after the first treatment, her right shoulder felt less tense. Her asthma slowly improved all week. This week the patient pointed out a knotty scar about 2.5 cm in diameter on the right side of her forehead about 1 cm lateral to the center of the eyebrow. Additionally, she had another scar below this one – a thin straight line about 1 inch long centered over the right eyebrow. The patient requested that these be treated too.

As is normal when abdominal palpation is used as a method of diagnosis and treatment, the abdomen cleared much more easily than the previous week. The student then decided to treat the scar on the face. Two needles were inserted at the most painful places and retained for about 20 minutes. Following the treatment the patient said she felt a little spacy.

The next week the patient's asthma was much better. The neck still felt a little tender. For about 4 days following the treatment she had a frontal headache which she thought could be related to the scar clearing.

Two treatments later, the headaches had subsided, the asthma was much improved but the neck pain continued. (Note that it had not been treated beyond the abdominal clearance. The shoulder scar, which released the neck, had not been treated further since the student started treating other scars.) There appeared to be some further reduction in the size of the knotty scar on the forehead. The student did not follow up further since the term ended.

the need to bend. Have the patient retain the intradermal for 3–5 days depending on the comfort level of the needle or exposure to water or humidity so that infection does not occur. Proceed cautiously, inserting in only two tender areas around the scar. Have patients return to the office to have the intradermals removed or show them how to remove the needles. In this case provide patients with written instructions so they do not break or bend them. Figure 14.2 shows how to implant intradermal needles into scars.

4. Liniments. The application of liniments around the scar can also be effective in reducing its tension and restoring the proper flow of Qi

Figure 14.2 How to implant intradermal needles into scars.

and Blood. My liniment of choice is Zheng Gu Shui because of its ability to penetrate so deeply to the bone layer and to move Blood Stasis, promote healing and stop pain. Other similar liniments such as Tieh Da Yao Gin could be substituted, as their energetics are virtually identical. Liniments can be applied to the affected area on a daily basis. Do not apply to mucous membranes, close to the eyes or to open cuts or wounds or to scars that are unhealed. Apply the liniment generously with a cotton ball or a cotton swab around the borders of the scar as well as on top of it. Allow it to dry completely as it will stain clothing. Discontinue if irritation develops.

In the Chinese repertoire of external applications, Ching Wan Hung and Wan Hua have been shown to improve scar healing caused by burns or otherwise, particularly by influencing scar shape, size and color. Ching Wan Hung promotes circulation of Blood and Qi, cools Heat, stops pain and promotes tissue growth. It is a topical ointment for burns and scalds with excellent results. It reduces pain, swelling and blistering and can be used topically for hemorrhoids, bedsores, acne, sunburn and heat rashes (Fratkin 1986, p. 143). Wan Hua, another Chinese liniment, activates Blood Stagnation and hemostasis. It is excellent for burns and traumatized areas. Apply once a day to the diseased area with a cotton swab and cover loosely as it will stain clothing.

5. Moxa. Moxa, due to its powerful ability to gently penetrate to the meridian level, is an effective treatment modality. It not only warms but also invigorates the flow of Qi and Blood. Moxa is particularly efficacious when administered in the Tiger Thermie warmer because this instrument has the unique ability to deliver the moxa's heat and the therapeutic properties associated with it as well as to serve as a mechanical tool to break up obstruction. Do not apply the Tiger Thermie on top of the scar but rather apply pressure to the skin around the border. The entire border area can be treated so this is a very effective method to treat the entire scar. Results similar to those obtained from needling can be achieved and healing crises can ensue. Patients can be instructed on how to treat their own scars in this manner.

6. Injection therapy. Injection therapy is a modern Oriental treatment modality that is applicable to scars. Many physicians claim that injections yield dramatic and utilitarian results. When a liquid substance is introduced under a superficial scar or within a deeper scar the liquid bloats or balloons the scar tissue and mechanically breaks it up. An additional effect of injection therapy comes from the action of the substance injected, such as homeopathic preparations like Silica, Calcarea, Corydalis, any Chinese injectable or even bee venom. Saline is a common injectable which achieves good results.

7. External moisturizers and massage. Lubrication of the wound in the early stages of healing with various emollients has been shown to reduce scar formation. The most powerful of these are vitamin E, wheatgerm oil with vitamin E, cocoa butter, almond oil and vitamin C. With the application of these products, scar narrowing and a return to normal color have been known to occur. Choose these products in their purest form possible, such as D-alpha tocopherol vitamin E, without chemical additives. Massaging the healed skin with a moisturizer is one of the most effective things you can do to eliminate or reduce the size of a scar.

For burn scars, aloe vera assists in reducing inflammation and swelling by inhibiting the action of bradykinin, a peptide that produces pain in injuries like burns. It also inhibits the formation of thromboxane, a chemical detrimental to wound healing.

8. Vitamins and foods. Foods high in vitamin C, such as broccoli and citrus fruits, and foods rich in zinc like roasted pumpkin and sunflower seeds, peanuts, lean beef and dark turkey are correlated with faster healing and can be incorporated into a healthy, well-rounded diet.

In summary, physicians who have patients with scars should keep all these procedures and outcomes in mind for the benefit of the patient's health. The treatment of scars is an automatic consideration for a practitioner who appreciates the clinical utility and power of meridian therapy. The form in Figure 14.3 has been devised to assist you in evaluating and treating scars. It is also included in the Form section at the end of this book.

NEW WORDS AND CONCEPTS

Cryosurgery – the process of using liquid nitrogen to freeze skin growths, particularly cancers or scars.

Hypertrophic scar – a raised scar with characteristics similar to a keloid scar except that it forms within the borders of the original wound.

Keloid – a thick, fibrous scar that grows beyond its original wound borders.

QUESTIONS

1. What are the Chinese and Japanese theories on scars? Use these theories to explain the signs and symptoms of troublesome scars.

2. What are some of the symptoms that may accompany initial unhealed scar formation? List symptoms that may occur after a scar has completely healed.

3. Using Oriental medicine, what parameters are inspected in assessing a scar?

4. Once a scar has been inspected and palpated, what modalities may be employed to clear it?

5. What is the recommended number of needles or intradermals that should be used per treatment of an individual scar?

6. What are the major contraindications when treating scars?

7. According to allopathic medicine, scars are

Patient's name:_____Date_____

Major complaint and accompanying symptoms:_____

_____

The Scar – Inspection

1. Description (shape, size, color, texture, height, or any other sensations associated with it):_____

_____

_____

_____

_____

_____

2. Location:_____

_____

_____

_____

Palpation

3. Sensation upon palpation:_____

_____

_____

_____

Treatment

4. Treatment (which modalities used and why):_____

_____

_____

_____

_____

5. Result of treatment of scar (changes in color, size, shape, texture, height, accompanying sensations, other):

_____

_____

_____

6. Effect on major complaint if any:_____

_____

_____

_____

_____

7. Other comments:_____

_____

_____

_____

Figure 14.3 Scar treatment form.

primary sites for developing skin cancer. Explain this. How might this be explained using Oriental medical theory?

8. What points do you think could clear each of the scars shown in Figure 14.4?

9. How would you interpret the patient in Case 14.1 developing a frontal headache after a scar treatment on her face?

10. In general, what category of Chinese herbs may be used in the treatment of scars?

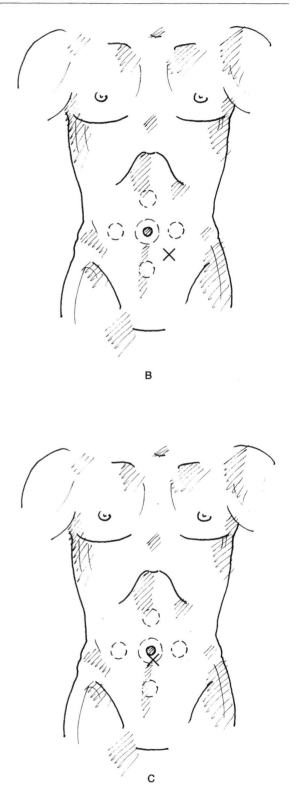

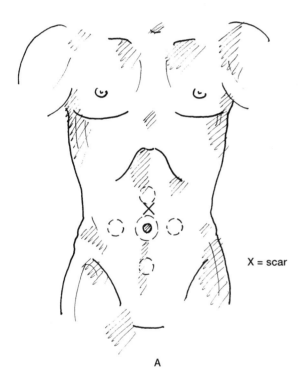

X = scar

Figure 14.4

15

Japanese physical exam 3: treatment of the sinuses

An estimated 35 million Americans suffer from respiratory problems in the form of sinusitis, allergic rhinitis and hay fever and 50 million may experience asthma or allergies. Over $1.5 million is spent in both prescription and non-prescription medications by desperate patients willing to try anything to escape the noxious symptoms associated with these disorders. While many of these medications are useful in managing these miserable symptoms, they are not effective in addressing the root of such disorders.

Both Western and Oriental medicine have theories explaining how these conditions develop. Within the system of Oriental medicine there are effective treatment approaches with acupuncture and herbs that can assist the patient. In this chapter unique Japanese treatment strategies are presented within the context of abdominal diagnosis and treatment for the care of these problems.

ANATOMY, PHYSIOLOGY AND PATHOLOGY

The sinuses are a collection of cavities surrounding the nose and within the forehead. Their function is somewhat debatable. They may be shock absorbers or have something to do with the resonance of the voice. They are lined with the same kind of membranes found in the nose. The sinuses drain into the nose through passages no wider than the lead in a pencil. When air and mucus get trapped inside the sinuses, pressure and pain can result. This can happen whenever nasal membranes swell and block the tiny passages to the sinuses.

Sinus infection or sinus inflammation presents with mucus, pressure and pain in the cheeks and forehead and often a low-grade fever. It usually begins with a cold or flu in which mucus gets trapped in the sinuses and then bacteria proliferate.

The signs and symptoms of chronic sinusitis are less overt. There are several causative factors of this variety of sinusitis. They include an anatomical obstruction such as a deviated septum and engorgement of nasal Blood vessels triggered by pollution, weather changes or allergic factors.

Sinus problems are more than pervasive within the population and their symptoms persistent to a point that exceeds aggravation. Any or all of the following features may characterize these illnesses: a runny or stuffy nose, postnasal drip, scratchy throat, swollen glands and cough. The patient additionally may experience red, itchy, watery eyes, ear pressure and pain, headache, low-grade fever, shortness of breath, fatigue and general lassitude, facial, cheek, eyelid and neck pain or a heavy feeling in the head and neck. These symptoms may be of an acute nature, such as seasonal allergies, or they can persist all year round.

Some of these symptoms are produced by exposure to pollens, air particulates, mite dung, household products; in fact, almost anything can be a causative factor. The essential allergy plan in Western medicine takes this into account and includes the following recommendations.

- Avoidance of the allergen.
- Desensitization of the patient through allergy shots.
- The treatment of symptoms through medications.
- Coping strategies such as keeping windows closed during windy, high humidity or high pollen count days, avoiding outside activities and other similar behavioral patterns.

It is commonly held, at least within holistic circles, that it is not so much the noxiousness of the pathogen that is the stressor as the state of the person's immunity. The symptoms listed above represent a hypersensitivity of the person to the pathogen that creates inflammation and the corresponding disorders of rhinitis if the nasal passages are affected, sinusitis if the sinuses are involved or hives or eczema if the skin reacts. Immunity is affected by inherited Qi and so rhinitis (or hay fever) is often an inherited condition. The major symptoms testify that the Liver, Lungs and Kidney are involved. In Oriental medicine the ideal treatment plan is, as always, to treat the root and hence allergy sufferers tend to receive excellent results when the root, that is one's immunity or antipathogenic factor, is treated comprehensively.

The sinus area in Chinese medicine belongs to the Lungs. Hence any sinus problem can be perceived as a Lung problem. As we recall from Zang-Fu physiology, the Lung is the Master of the Qi. If Lung Qi is weak the Lungs may not be effective in descending the Qi or descending and dispersing the Fluids which then accumulate in the nose so that pressure and tension develop in the nasal area. If an allergen is responsible for the sinusitis, the Liver and the Kidney may be involved as well. The individual's hypersensitivity to the pathogen may be more problematic than the strength of the pathogen.

The Liver plays a critical if understated role in immunity. As we know, it is the function of the Liver to promote the free flow of Qi, thereby harmonizing the patient's internal and external environments. When this patency is aggravated by a pathogen, Liver Qi Stagnation ensues. When the Liver energy is stagnant, it manifests as excessive energy. From a Five Element perspective, when Wood energy, in this case Liver, is excessive, it counteracts on the element that normally controls it, that is Metal, and the organ of the Lungs. Hence, symptoms of rebellious Lung Qi can ensue such as coughing, sneezing, stuffy or runny nose and other respiratory symptoms. This excessive Wood energy additionally draws from its mother, the Water element or the Kidney, thereby depleting Kidney energy.

If the patient has a diagnosed problem of rhinitis (the common term is hay fever) and sinusitis, these illnesses are indeed more than aggravating. They have a profound impact on the health of the person because of the involvement of various organs. However, the patient may also have what could be called a preclinical sinus problem.

The role of the sinuses as related to the health of the body deserves special consideration. As such sinus inspection and palpation merit attention. As we have seen in previous chapters, palpation can point to the more preclinical possibilities of sinus and hence organ dysfunction so that a potential problem can be dealt with. Sinus problems, if left untreated, are not only problems in and of themselves but can lead to other problems such as Blood pressure problems, memory disorders, neck problems and others because of the role of the Lung in providing oxygenation or Qi flow to the entire body.

SINUS EVALUATION AND TREATMENT

Questioning

The first step in assessing a patient's sinus health is to ask if the person has any sinus problems or if there is a history of them in the family. The sinus problem could be part of the major complaint or a component of the medical history. If patients have no sinus problems in either their personal or family medical history, the sinuses may not influence their health. However, as part of the complete Japanese physical exam, we should check for these pathologies.

The clinical or preclinical manifestations of sinus problems can include the following.

- A deviated septum (Fig. 15.1).
- Broken or floating facial capillaries or a puffy cheek area.

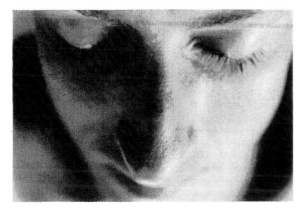

Figure 15.1 Deviated septum (deviates to the patient's right).

- Tenderness in the sinus area.
- A reddish coloration in the glabella region (at Yintang).
- A tight sternocleidomastoid muscle.
- A tight KI 16 (Huangshu) area (around the navel).

Figure 15.2 conveniently lists these pathologies, what they are indicative of, how to treat each of them and allows for any other notes you may want to add. Figure 15.3 depicts these pathologies.

Clear the abdomen

As always, this is an integral treatment approach to treat the whole person.

Physical exam

Conduct a complete sinus exam. This is described below.

Deviated septum

The septum is the structure that divides the nasal passages. A deviated septum can cause health disorders because as a physical malformation it may obstruct the entry of air or Qi to the Lungs, thereby resulting in many clinical disorders which may have the symptoms of systemic Qi Deficiency. A deviated septum can also arise from physical problems such as a broken nose or even through birth trauma. The septum can also deviate due to internal disorders of the Lungs such as nasal polyps or the use of drugs or inhalants that are directly introduced into the nasal passages. Regardless of its etiology, the significance of a deviated septum is that it can lead to insufficient oxygenation of the Lungs and thereby the rest of the body. It can also allow local infection to develop or persist, as in the case of sinusitis. It can cause problems such as poor memory, headaches, depression, migraines, asthma and many other health disorders.

To ascertain if the septum is deviated, look at the alignment of the septum and the size of the nostrils as patients recline on their back. The nostril is generally smaller on the side towards which the septum deviates. A deviated septum

Patient's name:_____ Date:_____

Major complaint and accompanying symptoms:_____

_____

_____

Check off any of the signs and symptoms the patient may have under the appropriate column.

Signs/symptoms	Etiology and diagnosis	Needle techniques	Observations	Abnormal	Normal
1. Sinus problems or history of same	Weak Lung function, broken nose, birth trauma, etc.	Consult specific manifestation described below and treat			
2. Deviated septum	1. Same as #1 plus lack of free flow of Qi and Blood in the local area leads to insufficient oxygenation. 2. Local infection 3. Trauma – birth, broken nose 4. Drugs	Palpate between nose and facial bones; needle at 45 degree angle transversely towards the lateral aspect of the face or apply Tiger Thermie to the area. Retain 10–20 minutes.			
3. Floating facial capillaries (engorgement of nasal Blood vessels) on orbital ridge of nose or below eye and/or puffy cheek	Focal infection, Heat in the Blood or Heat and Blood Stasis. Can be due to inverted postures, hot water, LR Heat, coffee, alcohol, weather, pollution	Needle transversely towards lateral aspect of face or bleed locally. Relieves hemostasis, invigorates Qi and Blood. Can add LI 4 and LU 7 for facial edema			
4. Tenderness in sinus areas (ST 2, GB 1, Yuyao, BL 2)	Preclinical or clinical sinus problems	Needle perpendicularly or transversely toward the lateral aspect or apply Tiger Thermie moxa around the orbital area for about 3 minutes			
5. Red coloration in the glabella (Yintang) region	1. Pituitary gland reflex can lead to thyroid problems, insomnia, infertility or memory problems 2. Heat in Blood, HT or SP 3. Serious, chronic sinus infection in cavity	Needle or bleed or intradermal Yintang. Can add SI 3			
6. Tight sternocleidomastoid muscle	Particularly posterior SCM = weak immunity or autonomic nervous system problems	See neck protocols ST 9R: use KI 6, ST 9L use KI 7 then TE 5R, GB 41L for both Needle ST 9 for 1 min. Massage works just as well 1. To treat muscle as a whole: KI 6, KI 7, TE 5, GB 41 2. TE 16 Check – turn head a. ST 25R may clear neck. Why? Neck could = pathogen and ST 25R treats LU and immunity b. Naganos 3. ST 9 – TE 3 releases carotid compression			
7. Pathology at the KI 16 area (or ST 25R)	1. Kidney disorders, Front Mu of the Kidney (according to Dr. Manaka) – Kidney is the root of the Qi 2. KI 16 = SP is mother of LU and grandmother of KI	See navel protocols in Chapter 10			

Treatment with additional points:
GV 4 = Tonifies Source Qi – needle 45° upward or Tiger Thermie.
ST 44 = Water point of ST – needle perpendicularly or Tiger Thermie or massage deeply.
TE 3 – Loosens carotid compression to release SCM/compressed carotid. Needle obliquely or proximally.

Figure 15.2 Sinus evaluation form.

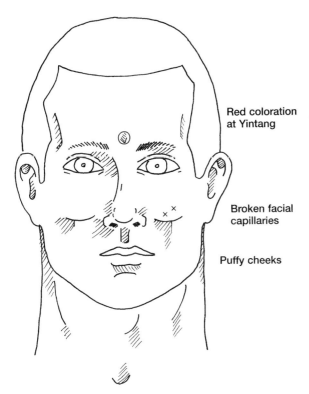

Red coloration at Yintang

Broken facial capillaries

Puffy cheeks

Figure 15.3 Sinus pathologies.

can be subtle or severe. The more deviated it is, the more it needs treatment.

To treat a deviated septum, palpate the border of the nose starting slightly lower than the inner canthus of the eye and down to the lateral border of the ala nasi. Use your index finger to reach this space between the nose and the facial bones. Mentally divide the area into four spots and as you press on each area, count from one through four and have the patient report the most tender points to you. Do this on each side of the nose. Choose the most tender point on each side and record.

Two treatment approaches are possible – needles or moxa – and potential realignment of the nose and resolution of the infection can result. If you choose needles, select a #1 sterile needle and puncture the most tender points on each side of the nose at an oblique to transverse angle towards the lateral aspect of the face (e.g. away from the nose and the eyes). The purpose of the needling or the moxa is to loosen the tension and treat the local infection if there is any. Retain for 20 minutes.

Warming the area with the Tiger Thermie warmer is also effective in treating this condition, particularly if there are several tender areas on each side of the nose. This is also less traumatic than facial needling which can be tender. Patients find the Tiger Thermie warmer in this area very soothing and efficacious (Fig. 15.4). Apply the moxa for about $1-1\frac{1}{2}$ minutes on each side of the nose in a gentle stroking motion. An Israeli study documents an 88% improvement in the symptoms of allergic rhinitis when treated with moxibustion (Sternfeld et al 1992). Moxa has the unique ability to perform the following functions:

- raise and maintain the white Blood cell count
- increase the movement of white Blood cells to the diseased area
- promote the white Blood cells' capacity to attack.

There are varying degrees of deviation of the septum from the most obvious to the subtly preclinical and both should be treated. The more pronounced the deviation, the longer it will take to remedy the problem and the more symptoms the person will have. Treatment can be expedited by teaching the patient how to moxa the nasal area with the Tiger Thermie warmer. Deep breathing exercises are helpful in improving oxygenation of the Lungs. Ayruvedic medicine recommends that the patient should not sleep on the side of the smaller nostril because this can lead to further obstruction.

Broken facial capillaries or a puffy cheek area

Broken facial capillaries are small spider-like capillaries found in the sinus areas that are engorged with Blood. Particularly, they are found on the orbital ridge or on the nose itself. They are typically red, sometimes reddish-purple or purple in color signifying Heat, Heat and Blood Stagnation or Blood Stagnation respectively. They are minimally indicative of stasis and sometimes of a local infection.

Broken facial capillaries can be caused in several ways, some of which are related to problems with

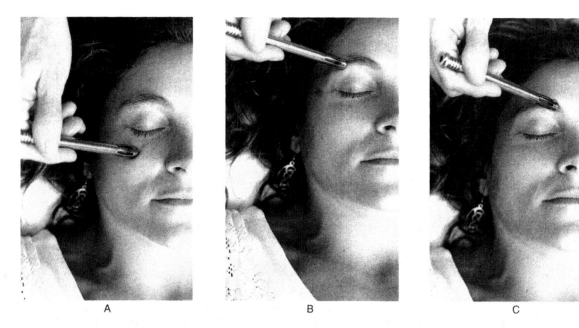

A   B   C

Figure 15.4 A–C: How to use the Tiger Thermie warmer on the sinuses.

the Lungs. Pollution, weather changes or allergic reactions can trigger their development. Very hot water applied to the face can cause this damage as well as inverted yoga postures such as headstands. In such cases these behaviors should be modified. Internally, Heat in the Liver can produce these symptoms too. According to Five Element theory, when the Liver is excessive it counteracts on what it normally controls, which is the Metal element and the Lung in particular. In the case of excessive Liver Heat, such as heat generated by alcohol, the Liver counteracts on the Lung, thus forming broken facial capillaries in the area of the nose, the highly vascularized external manifestation of the Lungs. To prevent this development, monitor alcohol, coffee and energetically hot and spicy foods that introduce excess Heat into the Liver.

If treatment is required, its aim is to dissipate the local Heat and the Stagnation. Bleeding the broken capillary does this relatively easily. In each treatment, bleed one or two capillaries at a time. Select the worst ones, meaning the biggest or the most discolored. Quickly and precisely insert a sterile #1 needle superficially into the capillary. A retention or non-retention method may be used but when the needle is withdrawn a

small amount of Blood should be expelled. If the needle is retained, insert it subcutaneously towards the lateral aspect of the face. Absorb the Blood and close the hole by pressing on the point for 5–10 seconds with a dry, preferably sterile cotton ball. This technique not only resolves the hemostasis and releases the Heat but invigorates the circulation of Qi and Blood. These vessels can also be cauterized by a dermatologist with similar result. Whether acupuncture or a cauterized needle is used, the capillary may fill up again. It can be treated 2–3 times in the manner described above but if the capillary becomes engorged again, the method is not working and should be discontinued.

Due to advanced Stagnation and Heat or Lung Qi Deficiency, the patient's cheeks typically present as puffy. The additional needling of LU 7 (Lieque) and LI 4 (Hegu) in the standard manner can assist in circulating energy to the face to reduce the facial edema.

Tenderness in the sinus areas

Because of the clinical significance of the sinuses in Chinese medicine, tenderness should be checked for in the areas around the sinuses. Start below the inner canthus of the eye below BL 1 (Jingming) and palpate the natural curvature of the infraorbital ridge, going from Bitong through ST 2 (Sibai), over to the outer canthus, up through the eyebrow area, through Yuyao and ending at BL 2 (Zanzhu). Do this on each side of the face.

Choose the most tender points on each side of the face. Needling of these points may be done in the standard manner of needling in the facial area, which is transversely towards the lateral aspect. If several points on each side are tender, you can use the Tiger Thermie warmer. Patients love this treatment and it is also a technique which they can learn and thus expedite therapeutic resolution.

Red coloration in the glabella (Yintang) region

Chinese medicine reminds us that when color organizes itself into discernible shapes rather than appearing diffusely, severe disorders may be present. In the case of sinus problems, a reddish coloration in the region of the glabella or Yintang area has a correlation with the condition of the sinuses. Specifically, a reddish coloration signifies Heat in the sinus cavities, usually of a chronic nature. Yintang also reflects the condition of the pituitary gland due to its proximity. The presence of pituitary hormones can heat up the blood. In Zang-Fu terms, this Heat in the Blood can also be called 'Heat in the Heart and the Spleen' because these organs dominate and control the blood. This condition can cause problems such as insomnia, thyroid problems, fertility problems and more.

This presentation is relatively rare but you will see it. Using a #1 needle, puncture subcutaneously downward through the glabella region. Obtain little to no Qi and retain for about 10 minutes. Patients like this point which produces a calming to invigorating reaction. The point can also be implanted with an intradermal needle so that the condition can be treated on a sustained basis. Additionally SI 3 (Houxi), Master of the Governing Vessel channel and the pituitary gland reflex, can also be needled to further influence the pituitary gland. Bladder 1 and 2 can be massaged or needled since they are also reflexes

of the pituitary gland. This is a very effective method of treating the sinuses.

A tight sternocleidomastoid muscle

Because of the interrelatedness of body parts, neck problems, specifically neck tension, can contribute to sinus problems and vice versa. A tight sternocleidomastoid (SCM) muscle needs to be cleared to effectively treat the sinuses if they are tender. This evaluation has several parts.

1. First, standing behind the patient, position your hands on his neck and apply light pressure with your middle three fingers to the surface of the SCM. Feel both sides simultaneously and check the tone of the muscle for resilience. It should not feel tense, tender or mushy, tight or loose, stringy or flaccid.

2. Next lightly palpate ST 9 (Renying), one side at a time, particularly feeling for tenseness or the patient reporting that it feels tender.

3. Finally, with the patient's head turned comfortably to one side, palpate down the posterior border of the SCM muscle. The Japanese call this entire area the TE 16 (Tianyou) area. Make sure that you are on the posterior border of the SCM. Frequently I find that practitioners are palpating between the sternal and clavicular heads of the SCM. This is not only incorrect diagnostically but is also dangerous when we move into the treatment phase.

Divide the length of the muscle into four points and gently palpate each point to a depth of about a half an inch. Count from one to four to demarcate the points and then have the patient report to you any tenderness. This is usually an extremely painful area so keep this in mind so you will be sensitive to the patient. Look at his reaction to your palpation. If it is too painful, stop the process. You know then that the neck has some pathology. Repeat this entire process on each side of the neck.

4. Once the neck pathology has been determined it can be treated. The tight SCM muscle in

---

TE = standard abbreviation of the World Health Organization (1989) for Triple Warmer.

general or ST 9 in particular is considered to be due to an imbalance in the autonomic nervous system which is composed of sympathetic and parasympathetic branches. In Oriental medicine a sympathetic nervous system imbalance is viewed as due to Kidney Yin Deficiency. Likewise, a parasympathetic nervous system problem is due to Kidney Yang Deficiency. (More will be said about this in the next chapter on the treatment of the neck.)

5. To treat the tight ST 9 on the right, KI 6, the primary point for Yin Deficiency in the Japanese system, is pressed bilaterally, one side at a time just as you do for the abdominal, navel and thigh clearances. Go back and recheck ST 9R. If its pathology is due to Yin Deficiency, KI 6 should clear it. If KI 6 does not appreciably reduce the tightness at ST 9R, press on TE 5R and then GB 41L. These two points are used like KI 6 as clearance points and are pressed the same way they are used in the abdominal clearance protocol. They should resolve residual discomfort at ST 9R.

6. ST 9 on the left is treated with KI 7, the tonification point that increases Kidney Yang. Press on it bilaterally, to the same depth and for the same amount of time as is done in the abdominal, navel and thigh protocols. It is generally successful in remediating a tight ST 9L problem. If it does not help appreciably, also press on TE 5R and GB 41L as you do for the right side.

7. To provide added reinforcement to the neck clearance, all the aforementioned points may be needled to their standard depths as summarized in Chapter 8. If ST 9 does not improve, it too can be needled. Carefully insert the needle perpendicularly to a depth of 0.3–0.5 in. Watch your depth; do not manipulate, lift or thrust. *This point can kill* as it is directly over the common carotid artery. Retain for one minute and remove. Gentle massage performed by the patient can have the same beneficial result.

8. To treat the tender posterior border of the SCM muscle, two options are available. The first and perhaps most appealing to patients is to gently apply the Tiger Thermie warmer for approximately 3 minutes to each side. Stroke the length of the muscle's border in segments of perhaps a third. Do not press deeply. The neck is a very vulnerable and delicate structure. Again, make sure that you are on the posterior border of the SCM, not in between the sternal and clavicular heads of the SCM as moxa here is dangerous. This treatment has tremendous efficacy in relaxing the entire muscle and removing tension. Patients love this treatment.

9. Another option is to treat the TE 16 area. The clearance points for this are a special group called the Naganos, named after Japanese practitioner Nagano. These points are also referred to as the Japanese equivalent of the LI 11 and 10 areas. These points are found by sliding over the ulnar bone beginning at the elbow crease and moving distally a length of four fingerbreadths. Press on these points to a depth of about 1 inch and number them from one to four as you move distally. They are almost always extremely painful. If the points are too painful to press, discontinue the Nagano palpation and simply use the information that they are very painful. After you press on these points on one arm at a time, go back to the tender TE 16 point and it should have cleared significantly. Do the same thing on the opposite arm.

10. For further reinforcement, the Naganos can also have the Tiger Thermie warmer applied to them. In this instance, the instrument is pressed moderately deeply into the points in what I call a dredging motion. Do this on all four points on each arm, moving from the LI 11 area to approximately LI 9. Move from point to point then go back to the first point and repeat until the time is up.

Pathology at the KI 16 (Huangshu) area

Like any disorder, sinus problems are not isolated events. They may be reflected on the abdomen in the modified abdominal exam at the ST 25 area on the right (Lung, Immunity and Triple Warmer reflex) or the KI 16 area. Remember, as we saw in Chapter 10, the KI 16 (Huangshu) area pertains to the Spleen. The Spleen is the mother of the Lungs and according to classical literature, the best way to treat the Lung and hence a sinus problem is through tonifying the mother of the Lungs, the Spleen. Review Chapter 10 on treatment strategies for the navel, which also address the Lungs. Dr Manaka contends that KI 16 is the real Front Mu point of the Kidney. Treating KI 16 strengthens the root Qi of the body, which Oriental practitioners believe is the causative factor of allergic and sinus problems. This point can be needled or the Tiger Thermie warmer applied to it, as was discussed in Chapter 10.

CONCLUSION

Abdominal clearing should always be used as part of the treatment of sinus problems and then the specific treatment of disease or clearance points for the sinuses can round out the therapy. Powerful supplemental points for this condition include GV 4 (Mingmen) which strengthens the immunity by tonifying Source Qi; ST 44 (Inner Neiting), the Water point of the Stomach, to cool Stomach Heat that may develop due to Liver Heat; TE 3 loosens carotid compression and allows for improved circulation of Qi and Blood between the upper and lower part of the body.

Needle GV 4 at a 45° angle upward to a depth of about 0.5 cun or apply the Tiger Thermie warmer for about 2 minutes. Warm the area by moving the Tiger Thermie on the point but don't linger on the same place. Needle the Japanese ST 44 perpendicularly 0.3–0.5 in. or massage deeply or apply heat with the Tiger Thermie warmer. Patients can be taught to rub Japanese ST 44 because of its benefits. Puncture TE 3 obliquely in the direction of the meridian, towards the wrist, 0.3–0.5 in. Case 15.1 provides an application of the material presented in this chapter.

Case 15.1 Treatment of allergic rhinitis with the sinuses and the Tiger Thermie warmer

The patient was a 35-year-old woman with two major complaints – arthritis in her big toes and the base of her thumbs and 'miserable' airborne allergies, notably to ragweed, especially in the spring. The toe pain was so bad that she found it difficult to bend her toes or even stand. They hurt on a daily basis and were exacerbated by damp. The allergies were characterized by a runny nose, red nose and eyes, itchy ears, sneezing, difficulty breathing, fever, hoarseness, tightness in the chest and tiredness to the point of exhaustion and irritability. She also had allergies to sugar and molds, including penicillin. The allergies were so pronounced that she had to wear a facemask. Allergies ran in her family on the side of her father and her paternal grandmother. She had asthma as a child. Her maternal grandmother had adult-onset diabetes. We will see that these problems were intimately related and hence easy to correct.

Physical examination revealed that the tongue was red and thin. The coating was dry and thick and yellow in the back. The Lung had a depression in it and there were red dots on the tongue as well. In Japanese acupuncture an enlarged big toe, what might be called a bunion, indicates weak Spleen function in metabolizing sugar. As a result bunions appear on the big toe, on the Spleen meridian, specifically SP 2 (Dadu) and 3 (Taibai), the Fire point and the Earth point of the Spleen respectively. Energetically, sugar is Hot so it appears on the big toe pathologically as a reflection of the Heat in the Spleen.

The first treatment centered on the toe pain since this was her articulated priority. The abdomen was cleared and the toes treated with Zheng Gu Shui and the Tiger Thermie warmer at SP 2 and 3. At the time of the next treatment which was one month later (because she had gone on vacation), her toe felt better but her allergies were making her super-irritable and exhausted. I showed her how to use the Tiger Thermie warmer on her sinuses, navel, Naganos and toe during that treatment. One week later when she came in, she reported a 'feeling of well-being' with using the Tiger Thermie warmer and her feet felt good; she could bend her toe. The treatment of the sinuses, Naganos and the navel was designed to support her immunity so she would be less allergic to ragweed and sugar. It also worked on her toe problem because the sugar had actually caused the bone deformity of a bunion.

Since she lived over an hour away she could not come to my office every week so she was instructed on how to use the Tiger Thermie warmer between visits. The next time I saw the patient her Lungs felt better but she still had some allergy symptoms. Two weeks later, the toes continued to improve. Her Lungs felt good to the point where she was able to work 5 hours in her garden with no mask. Her energy was good. The tongue was of normal color and it had less coat.

One month later on the last day of treatment, her Lungs felt 'great' and her energy was good. Her foot was less sore and she was less allergic to sugar. She still had some normal allergy symptoms since this was the height of the fall allergy season but she felt they were tolerable. Due to money constraints as well as traveling complexities, she was released from my care but instructed on how to continue to treat herself which is what she wanted to do. After only eight treatments over a 4-month period, she was ecstatic with her progress and her ability to care for herself.

NEW WORDS AND CONCEPTS

Allergies – an altered or heightened response of the immune system toward an otherwise harmless substance.

Pituitary gland reflex – SI 3 (Houxi) and Yintang are acupuncture points which can indicate the health of the pituitary gland.

Rhinitis – inflammation of the mucous membranes of the nose, usually accompanied by swelling of the mucosa and a nasal discharge. There are many varieties of rhinitis such as acute, allergic, atrophic or vasomotor.

Sinusitis – inflammation of one or more of the paranasal sinuses.

QUESTIONS

1. Give two areas on the abdomen where Lung pathology is likely to be reflected.

2. What does red coloration in the glabella region represent and what disorders can result from this?

3. In the treatment of sinus problems, what is the direction of needling in the facial area?

4. What factors do you think may be responsible for the prevalence of respiratory illness in the West today?

5. What problems can result if sinus conditions are left untreated?

6. What is the purpose of needling and moxa for a deviated septum?

7. What is considered the sinus reflex point?

8. Match the following classic Lung functions with the symptoms that would result from disruption of Lung function. More than one answer is possible.

Functions

1. Master of the Qi

2. Disperses and descends the Fluids

3. Opens to the nose and is reflected in the mucous membranes

4. Governs respiration

5. Controls the Liver (Wood)

6. Regulates the Wei Qi

7. Governs the skin

Symptoms

a. Inflammation of the mucous membranes of the nose and sinus cavities, stuffed nose

b. Fatigue, general lassitude

c. Watery eyes, runny nose, postnasal drip

d. Shortness of breath

e. Rebellious Lung Qi, i.e. coughing

f. Eczema, hives

g. Hypersensitivity to allergens, low-grade fever

h. Broken facial capillaries

16

Japanese physical exam 4: treatment of neck tension and tonsillar treatment

TREATMENT OF NECK TENSION

The neck is an extremely delicate structure, easily subject to stress. It bears about one-tenth of the body's weight or about 8 lbs on average, so it must be strong. Balancing strength with flexibility is an equally delicate task. The health of the neck is critical to the health of the rest of the body yet neck tension is a common human problem. Many acupuncturists commonly report that they feel inadequately trained when faced with this disorder. The purpose of this chapter is to explore the functional role of the neck in the human body, how to evaluate it through palpation and then to outline its treatment, particularly with Japanese techniques.

The evaluation of the neck is the fourth part of the Japanese physical exam. Its treatment, like that of any part of the body, can be done in any of the following circumstances:

- whether it is part of the major complaint or one of the accompanying symptoms of the major complaint
- if it is subpathology revealed by the patient in the course of the interview
- whether it is uncovered in the course of the evaluation of the entire person as the fourth component of the Japanese physical exam.

This approach applies to the evaluation of any body part prone to tension

Generalized neck evaluation and treatment

1. If neck problems are part of the major complaint the first step is to evaluate the neck by

conducting a physical exam. Practitioners may use any neck protocol they are familiar with or may adopt the one outlined later in this chapter. Evaluation precedes treatment. If the neck is not part of the major complaint but is a subpathology gleaned from the interview or discovered as part of the Japanese physical exam, it should still be addressed because the Japanese physical exam consists of physical parameters reflecting energetic functions that should not be ignored because of the significant role those body parts play.

2. Next, the abdomen is cleared by hand to treat the whole person. Depending on the significance of the neck problem, that is, whether it has local or systemic effects, is a Qi, Blood, Yin or Yang problem, it may appear under some energetic guise on the abdomen. Clearing the abdomen is always the core treatment strategy.

3. After the abdominal clearing, go back and check the neck to see if there has been any improvement. The abdomen generally has a good effect upon the neck since the neck disorder may be reflected on the abdomen. However, abdominal clearing may not be sufficient to treat the neck entirely, particularly if the person's problem is chronic in nature.

4. The navel, inner thigh and sinuses should also be examined and cleared as much as possible by hand.

5. At this point, treatment-of-disease points or neck protocols may be needed, some of which include clearing the neck by hand. Treatment-of-disease points are any points that have known clinical efficacy for a certain condition. You may select these from your education or experience or use the treatment-of-disease points consonant with the Japanese acupuncture system. The type of neck problem the person has dictates which points to select. These points are listed in Figure 16.1 and explained later in this chapter.

6. Reinforcement follows clearance. Reinforcement can be done with needles or any other preferred modality from the composite of points derived from all the previous examinations. Selection of points is a product of the data gained from these examinations, which indicate the person's entire presentation. Try to choose the points which have a common denominator in

terms of energetics. Treat according to which pattern is clearest.

Before becoming more specific about treatment, let us review the anatomy and physiology of the neck.

Neck anatomy

Anatomical review shows us that the neck houses many structures vital to health. Passing through the neck region are the cranial nerves, important Blood vessels such as the subclavian, common carotid and vertebral arteries along with the internal jugular vein. Endocrine and lymphatic glands are also located there. The neck is an important transit zone for vessels linking the brain and the heart as well as those for local head and neck supply.

Healthy neck tissue and musculature needs to be soft for the flexible functions the neck assumes, strong to hold the head erect, and with sufficient tone to promote proper functioning of the structures within it. Yet it is particularly prone to stress. Compression of the neck can influence the functioning of all these tissues. Australian acupuncturist and author David Legge (1990) summarizes in his book, *Close to the bone*:

Excessive muscle tension can be a problem. The neck is an area of the body that is vulnerable to physical attack. When threatened it is a common reaction to tighten the posterior neck muscles, pulling our heads closer to our shoulders, reducing the exposure of the back of the neck and increasing rigidity. This response can become chronic leading to shortening of the posterior neck muscles and a contraction of their associated connective tissue. (p. 97)

In Chinese medicine neck problems are essentially viewed as being due to derangement in the flow of Qi and Blood through the channels that traverse the area. Several major channels suffuse the posterior aspect of the neck: the Bladder, the Gall Bladder, Small Intestine, and Governing Vessel channels. The Large Intestine and Stomach channels are represented on the front of the neck. The Bladder channel is susceptible to Wind invasions, the Gall Bladder channel to Wood imbalances and the Governing Vessel channel to spinal problems which have numerous etiologies but essentially come down to trauma, energetic or organ dysfunction. The Stomach channel reflects disharmonies in the autonomic nervous system and the Triple Warmer to pathogenic invasion as well. The Large Intestine reflects thyroid pathology.

The common denominator of all neck problems, regardless of their diversity, is a derangement in the flow of Qi and Blood. As a result, many emotions can be associated with the neck, because emotions are just Qi that is out of balance. According to his experience Legge believes that the underlying cause of neck pain is anger. Although there is a strong relationship between the neck and the Wood element I have not seen it as the only clinical option. When tension comes about, its physiological correlate of irritability and anger can ensue and concomitantly if anger or irritability is a predominant emotion neck tension can develop. I have seen this as an association with neck problems, especially chronic ones. However, fear and grief can also be stored at this level. If pain is a component of the neck problem, it frequently has an emotional association.

In this chapter neck problems are not differentiated as they are in standard acupuncture textbooks under headings such as torticollis, cervical joint degeneration, whiplash or others. Rather, the Japanese pathologies are couched in Western terminology for, as I mentioned in Chapter 2, the Japanese tend to name problems more from a Western perspective than a Zang-Fu one. These problems will be discussed below and are summarized in Figure 16.1. Figure 16.2 depicts the areas of the neck that are evaluated.

Specific neck evaluation and treatment

The patient should be lying in a supine position with his face up, hands and legs outstretched in a relaxed position with the mouth slightly open and no pillow under his head. The following steps are then undertaken to specifically evaluate each neck pathology.

Evaluation of the sternocleidomastoid (SCM) muscle

1. Standing behind the patient, apply light pressure with your middle three fingers along the surface of the patient's SCM muscle on both sides simultaneously and evaluate the muscle tone for tension, tenderness or mushiness. This muscle should not feel tight or loose, stringy or flaccid but should have firm and resilient muscular tone. Serizawa (1988, p. 107) points out that many people show a discrepancy between the muscle tone of the SCM of either side. This can be due to habitual or postural reasons. This seems to be an accurate finding. Record your own subjective feelings and ask the patient to report to you what he feels.

2. Next, lightly palpate the anterior border of the SCM muscle, specifically at ST 9 (Renying). ST 9 lies directly over the common carotid artery, at the bifurcation of the internal and external carotid artery, and the carotid sinus. Prominent modern acupuncturist Bunshi Shirota describes the following physiological functions of ST 9.

The carotid sinus is the dilated portion of the internal carotid artery which has special parasympathetic nerve endings. The carotid sinus is thought to have the therapeutic effect of regulating the autonomic nervous system (the parasympathetic and sympathetic) through the autonomic fibers of the ninth cranial nerve (glossopharyngeal). It has a direct effect in lowering essential hypertension and has a broad range of clinical applicability. (Serizawa 1988, pp. 120–121)

More recent research supports the role of ST 9. Authors report the use of ST 9 because it promotes Blood flow to the head. It is also able to regulate body functions to achieve harmony of Yin and Yang and regulate Qi and Blood and smooth their circulation (Lushang & Fei 1997).

Like Shirota, it is my observation that tension or Deficiency at ST 9 means that there is an imbalance in autonomic nervous system functioning. Tension on the right signifies a sympathetic nervous system problem and on the left a parasympathetic disturbance because the right is Yin and the left side is Yang. Kiiko Matsumoto claims that this same finding pertains to the diagnosis of the SCM muscle itself.

The aim of treatment is to reduce any tension perceived in the muscle because tension makes

Patient's name:_____   Date:_____

Major complaint and accompanying symptoms:_____

_____

_____

Check yes if the neck area is normal, no if it is not.

Area of the neck to examine	Clinical significance	Yes	No	Treatment
1. Evaluation of the sternocleidomastoid muscle (SCM):				With palpation, needles, intradermals, or moxa
a. muscle itself	Right side = sympathetic nervous system disharmony; Left side = parasympathetic nervous system disharmony			For R use KI 6; for L use KI 7; for both use TE 5R, GB 41L Can also use TE 3R or bilateral
b. ST 9 area	Same as above plus possible thyroid problems – see #4			Same as above or needle or massage ST 9
c. posterior border (TE 16 area)	Immune system response (overworked or active battle)			Moxa Naganos or moxa local TE 16 area with Tiger Thermie
2. Scalene muscle evaluation:				
a. height of muscle (GB 21 area) (scalene compression of underlying Blood vessels and nerves)	a. Tight, hard, rock-like = scalene compression b. One side hard/thick, one side soft/thin = scoliosis			Needle LU 7, massage, intradermal Needle LU 7, massage, intradermal
3. Supraclavicular fossa evaluation:	This can lead to Blood Stasis pattern in the occipital region			
a. brachial plexus involvement	Sends Qi and Blood to the musculature of the upper limbs			Tiger Thermie or needle ST 12* or massage
b. vertebral artery	Sends Blood to the brain, head			Tiger Thermie or needle ST 12* or massage
c. subclavian artery	Source of Blood flow to the upper limbs			Tiger Thermie or needle ST 12* or massage
d. left ST 12	Heart Qi Xu			Tiger Thermie or needle ST 12* or massage
e. right ST 12	Spleen Qi Xu with Damp, right lymph duct congestion			Tiger Thermie or needle ST 12* or massage
4. Thyroid evaluation	KI Qi, Essence, Yin Xu, with Fire. Hypothyroid = KI Qi or Yang Xu; Hyperthyroidism – KI Yin Xu with Fire			Check ST 9, LI 18, and height (top) of SCM muscle, KI 3
5. Fat pad at GV 14	Adrenal exhaustion (severe KI Yang Xu)			Needle GV 14 or moxa Can add GV 4, KI 6, KI 16 or KI 27
6. Blood Stasis patterns in the occipital region	Blood Stagnation			Bloodletting techniques, see Table 16.1

*Remember, when needling ST 12, position patient in the lateral recumbent position. Do not obtain Qi.

Figure 16.1 Neck evaluation form.

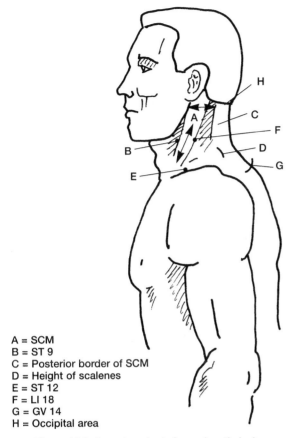

A = SCM
B = ST 9
C = Posterior border of SCM
D = Height of scalenes
E = ST 12
F = LI 18
G = GV 14
H = Occipital area

Figure 16.2 Areas to palpate for neck pathologies.

those systems go into overdrive or become dominant. Deficiency means that these systems are not performing their normal function. As we saw in Chapter 7, stress can affect both the sympathetic and parasympathetic nervous systems.

3. Tension at ST 9 on the right or the entire right SCM muscle is treated by palpating KI 6 (bilaterally) and then repalpating ST 9 to see if there is any appreciable change. KI 6, as we have seen, is the point of greatest Yin in the body. When Yin is deficient a sympathetic nervous system response is evoked. ST 9 on the left or the left SCM muscle is treated with KI 7. KI 7, the tonification point of the Kidney, benefits Kidney Yang in particular and assists in restoring balance of the parasympathetic nervous system.

If clearance is not achieved with these points, TE 5 on the right and GB 41 on the left should be palpated (the choice of which side to needle is connected to the energetics of the meridian). They have the effect of balancing the nervous system. This is partly summarized in the visual image of the way the Yangwei and Dai channels work together, like a spiral, to adjust the Qi and Blood of every part of the organism. These points may be needled according to the methods described in Chapter 8 or intradermal needles implanted to reinforce the effect. Additionally, ST 9 itself can be needled. Exercise extreme caution by slowly and shallowly inserting a #1 needle into the point about 0.3–0.5 in. or just above the arterial wall. Do not pierce it. *This point can kill.* The needle will pulsate or tick due to its proximity to the arterial wall. Retain the needle for no longer than one minute, then withdraw and massage the point. Massage in place of needling works just as well and is my preferred method of treatment. Patients generally seem more comfortable with this technique.

4. With the patient's head turned comfortably to the side, now palpate approximately four areas down the posterior border of the SCM muscle for muscle tension. Derive your own diagnosis from palpation and have the patient report which point is the most tender. This area usually feels rock-like and is extremely painful to the patient.

This area in Japanese acupuncture is considered the TE 16 area. TE 16 (Tianyou: Heaven's Window) is a reflex point for infection or the battle between the antipathogenic factor and any pathogen at the level of the throat. Tenderness here signifies either an active battle going on between these two forces or the fact the immune system is overworked. ST 25R on the abdomen is indicative of this pathology and when it is cleared, it may release the neck. In feeling TE 16, if you start to palpate it and it is too tender, just stop the palpation. It doesn't matter which discrete points hurt, they are all indicative of the same thing. These points can be extremely tender even in the person who does not have an active throat problem. It is not uncommon to feel this area as hard or like cement.

TE = standard abbreviation of the World Health Organization (1989) for Triple Warmer.

5. This tenderness can be treated very effectively and efficiently by pressing the Naganos which are another group of points diagnostic of immunity. Their locations and treatment techniques are described in Chapter 15, p. 184. The Naganos can be needled or treated with the Tiger Thermie warmer to reinforce neck treatment. The direct application of Tiger Thermie moxa to the posterior border of the SCM is very beneficial to the patient; the warmth of the moxa is relaxing and soothing. Patients love this treatment and can be taught to do it themselves. It loosens up tense neck tissue and has a positive effect on the underlying structures and energetics of the area. Figure 16.3 shows how to use the Tiger Thermie on the posterior border of the SCM.

6. The patient with either articulated neck problems, such as subluxated vertebrae, swollen glands, tendency to catch colds or have throat problems, or weak immunity in general will benefit from the periodic application of the Tiger Thermie warmer's moxa to this region of the neck. The points in the TE 16 area can be needled if they are stubborn and persistent and do not respond to the Tiger Thermie warmer. Insert the needle perpendicularly 0.3–0.5 in. Remember, an important rule of treatment is to avoid needling into tense, tight tissue, so the Tiger Thermie warmer is again the tool of choice to loosen tightness and confer the therapeutic effects of moxibustion. If you needle into the loosened tissue, obtain no Qi but use an in-and-out method to break up the obstructed, knotty Qi. The point tends to feel sticky.

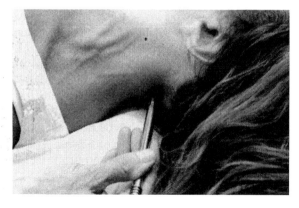

Figure 16.3 How to use the Tiger Thermie warmer on the posterior border of the SCM.

Evaluation of the scalene muscles

Now, with a grasping method (similar to loose pinching), feel the size and consistency of the shoulder muscles. They should feel firm but not hard or rock-like nor thin and soft. Occupational, postural or other pathological factors may account for their presentation. If one side is thick and hard and the other is thin and soft, scoliosis is a possibility. Tightness of the scalene muscles can cause compression of underlying nerves and blood vessels. LU 7 (Lieque) is the primary treatment point to open scalene compression because the Lung meridian runs through the shoulder. Check the alternative location of LU 7 as well which was described in Chapter 8, p. 86. Because of its size, the patient frequently reports no sensation when you palpate it. However, when the point is rubbed and then the shoulders are checked it has shown therapeutic result. Lung 7 can be massaged, or needled or an intradermal needle can be implanted into it for added effect. Needle the point proximally towards the shoulders 0.3–0.5 in.

Evaluation of the supraclavicular fossa

The supraclavicular fossa is also an area subject to tension due to the common effects of postural strain, tension and occupational stress. Specifically I am referring to that triangular area formed between the sternal and clavicular heads of the SCM right above the clavicle. This area in Japanese acupuncture is called the ST 12 (Quepen) area. It corresponds to the Chinese ST 12 location but is a little more medial and up to an inch above the traditional point location.

ST 12 is a highly important point for both diagnosis and treatment because of its clinically significant energetics. Notably all the Yang meridians meet there with the exception of the GV and BL channels. A number of important anatomical structures are directly beneath the point such as the brachial plexus, the vertebral artery, the subclavian artery, the right lymphatic duct and the aortic arch. These structures enter into the formation of the diagnosis. Apart from signs and symptoms, some of which may be preclinical, it may not always be possible to determine what specific problem the ST 12 area denotes exclusively through palpation. Questioning, along with other signs and symptoms, will contribute to the diagnosis. In any event, our aim is to eradicate the tense configuration at ST 12. Figure 16.4 illustrates the anatomical structures lying beneath ST 12.

Prior to palpation inspect the ST 12 area. If it looks narrow due to the shape of the shoulders it may be difficult even to get into the point to palpate. It can be a small space if the shoulders are slanted upward which is not the normal direction that the shoulders should go in. Using the index finger, press perpendicularly downward into the point, one side at a time. Because the point is prone to constriction, explain to the patient prior to palpation that this point may hurt. Patients call it an 'icky' sensation. It can feel

this way because of the downward method of palpation and the number of important structures that are found beneath it.

One structure includes a network of nerves in the neck called the brachial plexus. These nerves supply the musculoskeletal structures of the upper limb. The brachial plexus is buried among the deep muscles of the neck, the clavicle and the axillary space below the shoulder. Palpation of nerves can produce this disagreeable feeling. If the brachial plexus is involved the person may have numbness and tingling of the upper limb, nerve problems in the arm such as carpal tunnel syndrome or other similar problems such as repetitive motion syndromes.

In the Japanese system, ST 12 is the most effective point for these disorders. The source of this syndrome is generally not viewed as repetitive

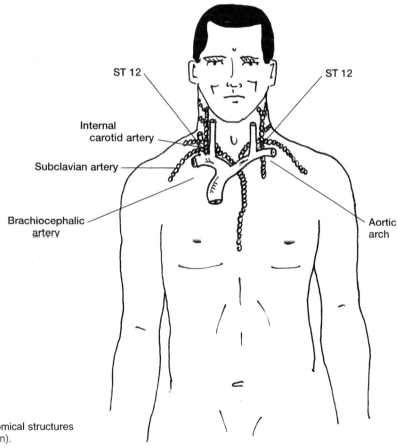

Figure 16.4 The anatomical structures beneath ST 12 (Quepen).

local motion of the wrist but rather the postural stress and muscular compression of the neck caused by performing those movements.

Another structure beneath the ST 12 area is the vertebral artery. The vertebral and internal carotid arteries are the sole supply of Blood and oxygen to the brain. They originate from the brachiocephalic artery on the right side of the body and the aortic arch on the left. If the vertebral artery is impaired it can lead to insufficient Blood flow to the brain. Vertebral artery problems can lead to memory problems, dizziness, empty, lingering headache and other similar symptoms.

Tenderness at this point may also be due to the involvement of another artery – the subclavian artery that runs deep and behind the clavicle which is the source of Blood flow to the upper limbs. Blood from the subclavian artery travels to the axillary artery, then to the brachial artery which finally bifurcates into the radial and ulnar arteries. Proper subclavian artery performance is imperative for the health of the limbs. If compressed, it may cause numbness and tingling and muscular atrophy and motor impairment of the upper limbs along with other similar problems.

Tenderness at ST 12 on the left side can also be caused by weakness of the Qi of the Heart. Relatively speaking, the energetics of the Heart are more left sided. As we have noted, the origin of the common carotid and subclavian arteries on the left side of the neck is different from the right. On the right side, the common carotid and subclavian arteries come off the brachiocephalic artery. On the left side the common carotid comes off the aortic arch stemming from the Heart; hence it indicates Heart problems.

If the energy of the Heart is weak it may reflect at this point. Search for corroborating signs and symptoms to support the diagnosis. For instance, for a patient with tenderness at ST 12L, ask 'Heart Qi Xu' questions such as 'Do you have any problems with memory, concentration, palpitations, chest pain or tightness?'. Energetic signs may support this too such as a pale tongue tip, a weak Heart pulse or tenderness at CV 14.

In contrast to this, tenderness at ST 12R indicates right lymphatic duct congestion because the right lymphatic duct is only on this side. The same approach can be used to ask the 'lymphatic questions' such as 'Do you have any problems digesting fats?' which signifies possible right lymphatic duct congestion. Such congestion can be due to failure of the Spleen to transform and transport Dampness.

Regardless of which scenario is occurring – brachial plexus involvement, vertebral or subclavian artery problems, Heart Qi Xu or right lymphatic duct congestion – the first aim of treatment is to lessen the tightness at ST 12. This can be done in three major ways – Tiger Thermie, needling or massage. My method of choice is to loosen this area with the Tiger Thermie warmer. It is soothing and efficacious without being invasive. Needling can also be done. If this is opted for, position the patient in the lateral recumbent position. The needling of ST 12 is not effective in any other position. One side at a time, cautiously insert a #1 needle perpendicularly towards the neck (or the spine), 0.3–0.5 in., not downward, which is the area over the apex of the Lungs and the transverse cervical artery. Do not obtain Qi, simply insert and retain for about 5 minutes. Or you can gently massage the affected area for about 5 seconds. Figure 16.5 shows how to use the Tiger Thermie warmer on ST 12.

Thyroid assessment

The health of the thyroid gland can also be determined by palpation of the neck. Part of this can be picked up by the pathology of the SCM muscle, specifically at ST 9 (Renying) below which is the superior thyroid artery. Tenderness at ST 9 and parallel to it, between the sternal and clavicular heads of the SCM at LI 18, may indicate an imbalance in the thyroid gland. Gently palpate both sets of points one side at a time and see if you feel tightness or if the patient reports tenderness. Additionally check the top of the SCM muscle for the same reactions.

Even though a patient does not have a Western medical diagnosis of a thyroid problem there are many patients who have what I would call 'preclinical' thyroid problems – perhaps as much as 25% of the population. When I use the term 'preclinical' I am not implying that at some point in

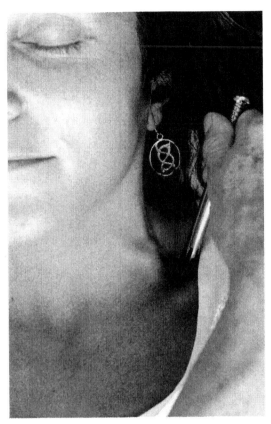

Figure 16.5 How to use the Tiger Thermie warmer on ST 12 (Quepen).

the future the person will develop a diagnosed thyroid problem; rather, I am referring to early energetic disturbances that are the roots of possible problems. They are energetic versus organic problems. The neck can be a useful place for the determination of this type of thyroid problem.

Treatment of the thyroid begins with KI 3 (Taixi), the Shu stream and Source point of the Kidney which regulates Kidney Yin and Yang. Remember, Japanese KI 3 has the location of Chinese KI 5. Needle the point perpendicularly 0.3–0.5 in. or with the needle directed proximally. Moxa with the Tiger Thermie warmer is applicable. Apply moxa to this point for about 3–5 times with a rubbing contact lasting about 10 seconds each time.

The function of the thyroid gland is to produce hormones that stimulate the metabolism of every cell. Similarly the Kidney can be viewed as the basis of all the functions in the body. The major clinical manifestation of an underactive thyroid, either diagnosed (called hypothyroidism) or preclinical, is fatigue. Many patients with the diagnosis of chronic fatigue actually have an underactive thyroid gland and that underactivity is usually diagnosed with medical tests. However, this preclinical problem can be established by the neck evaluation coupled with other supporting signs and symptoms such as fatigue, unexplained weight gain, feeling cold and other symptoms of Kidney Qi and Yang Xu.

Hyperthyrodism is a condition caused by excessive secretion of the thyroid gland, which increases basal metabolic rate, causing an increased demand for food to support metabolic activity. Hyperthyroidism would be diagnosed as Kidney Yin Deficiency with Fire. Signs and symptoms include weight loss, increased nervousness and increased heart rate.

See the Clinical notes at the end of this chapter for more information about the thyroid gland.

The fat pad at GV 14

In cases of severe Deficiency of Kidney Yang, an abnormal neck pathology can develop, that of a fat pad at GV 14 (Dazhui). Dazhui is the point of greatest Yang of the body. When the Yang is severely deficient, this Deficiency presents as a fatty pad at that point. The fat accumulation is evidence of the failure of the Yang of the Kidney to dominate water metabolism problems. The fat is water tied up in the form of Damp or fat.

With the patient in a sitting position, inspect GV 14 which is directly below the spinous process of C7. The fat pad extends around this point in an oval shape, seen visually as a distinct mound. Further confirm this by using a grasp palpation method.

Patients who have this problem have other signs and symptoms of Kidney Yang Xu such as excess weight, respiratory problems, loose stools with undigested food, lethargy, poor skin color, gas, abdominal distension, low Blood pressure, cold feet and others. Patients who have had a history of asthma or bronchitis may now suffer from adrenal insufficiency. Of all groups they tend to have this fat pad most of the time. Patients with hypothyroidism frequently have this pad.

There is also what I call a preclinical fat pad that appears in its formative stages. The texture of the skin here is commonly thick or fatty. It is more characteristic of patients with a lesser degree of Kidney Yang Deficiency than the more overt presentation that patients with adrenal exhaustion have.

Another disorder in which the fat pad develops is Cushing's syndrome.

Cushing's syndrome is a disorder in which the face becomes fatter than usual, usually round and red. The body also becomes fatter, and often a pad of fat develops between the shoulder blades, making them look round-shouldered. At the same time muscle tone is lost from the arms and legs; they will feel weak, tired, their skin may become thinner and bruises sometimes appear spontaneously on the arms and legs. The bones become thin and fracture easily. Cushing's syndrome is uncommon. It sometimes occurs in people on a long-term corticosteroid treatment. (Clayman 1994, p. 564)

Regardless of the diagnosis, to treat this problem, grasp the area and insert a fine needle subcutaneously through the pad, needling downward. Do not come out the other side. Do not obtain Qi but use a lift-and-thrust technique to simulate the point. Retain the needle for 10–20 minutes. You may also use the Tiger Thermie warmer around the borders of the area. Apply the warmer for about 3 minutes, using a moving technique. The area should get mildly red.

You can supplement this treatment by applying moxa to GV 4 (Mingmen, the Gate of Life) which is a primary point to tonify Kidney Yang. Mingmen may be needled in the standard way but the application of moxa is preferable for Yang Deficiency. Moxa can be applied to the needle or the Tiger Thermie warmer can be used similar to how it is used on GV 14.

Other supplemental points include KI 6 (Zhaohai), the point of greatest Yin and hence an indicator of stress because stress consumes Yin, KI 16 (Huangshu), which strengthens the source Qi of the Kidney, and KI 27 (Shufu), the parathyroid reflex point. Figure 16.6 shows what the fat pad at GV 14 looks like and Figure 16.7 shows

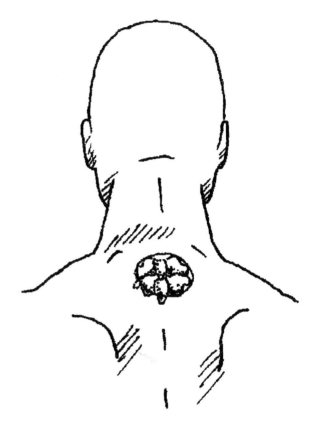

Figure 16.6 The fat pad at GV 14 (Dazhui).

how to needle it. See Section 5 for the needling methods of these points.

Blood Stasis patterns in the occipital region

The last neck pattern, that of Blood Stasis, is also seen on the back of the neck in the occipital region. It presents as a bruise or birthmark-like shape, red to reddish purple in color, at the base of the skull, in the BL 10, GV 20, GV 15–16 area. It should always be considered notable because of the clinical significance of Blood Stasis.

The etiology of the Blood Stasis characteristics can be due to any of the reasons in which Blood Stasis comes about. A congested ST 12 area can also lead to Blood Stagnation in the occipital area because the occipital artery, which comes off the

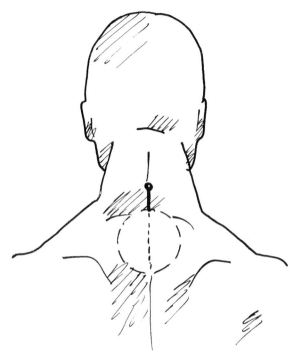

Figure 16.7 How to needle the fat pad at GV 14 (Dazhui).

Case 16.1   The management of chronic neck pain

The patient had a major complaint of headaches for a duration of 8 years. She compiled a headache management plan to help her cope with them since she did not want to take non-steroidal antiinflammatory drugs (NSAIDs) such as aspirin or common substitutes as she had already ineffectually pursued that route for several years.

The patient was generally able to correlate the headaches with specific factors so these are addressed within the plan. Nine times out of 10 she was aware that neck tension precipitated them so strategies for helping the neck needed to be included. Most of the features incorporated into the plan also represent a sensible approach for health maintenance in general such as the need for enough food and rest.

Headache management plan

1. Maintain regular sleeping hours.
2. Eat enough and frequently enough to avoid low Blood sugar.
3. Avoid foods that trigger headaches such as coffee, chocolate, nuts, citrus and MSG (monosodium glutamate).
4. Get massage as often as possible to dispel bodily tension.
5. Receive regular chiropractic treatments when the neck cannot be managed through tension reduction or tension reduction exercises.
6. Apply Zheng Gu Shui to the neck to move stagnant Qi and Blood.
7. Exercise to de-stress; consciously keep the shoulders and ribs from becoming elevated such that neck tension develops, and watch posture.

common carotid artery, runs backward to the scalp under the cover of the SCM muscle. It can also come about due to high Blood pressure as well as emotional lability. Blood Stagnation at the base of the occiput is dangerous because it may lead to insufficient Blood flow to the head with symptoms such as facial numbness, facial paralysis, deviation of the eyes and mouth and possible stroke.

In the case of Blood Stagnation in the occipital region, the Stasis should be broken up. Table 16.1 summarizes the methods of resolving this configuration (Gardner–Abbate 1996, p. 125).

Case 16.1 illustrates the relationship between chronic neck tension and stress headaches and how a pain management plan can be devised to control the effects of stress.

TONSILLAR TREATMENT

As we continue to explore the topic of neck treatment, a specialized area that deserves to be explored is the tonsillar treatment. This is a Japanese-style treatment with Chinese roots that utilizes acupuncture and moxibustion for immune enhancement. It is included in this book because of the emphasis of meridian therapy on treating immunity.

In this chapter, possible 'immunity' treatments are presented. Not only is this effective Japanese-style strategy discussed, in the Clinical notes I have included Chinese approaches that I learned on one of my externships to China. They are similar in their overall outcome as well as in the sense that the Kidney is perceived as the root of the Qi. However, there are differences that deserve to be explored.

All these treatments can be used in the following ways:

● by themselves

Table 16.1 Bloodletting techniques for Blood Stasis patterns in the occipital region

Instrument	Method
Plum blossom needle	Quickly and vigorously tap the skin of the affected area so that a slight amount of Blood is released. Carefully absorb the Blood with a sterile piece of gauze and dispose of it properly. Reusable or disposable plum blossom needles may be used. Sterilize or dispose of properly.
Bleeding needle	With a specialized bleeding needle (tri-edge needle) repeatedly pierce the affected area. If this needle or a medical lancet is used, more Blood will be extracted because of the size of the needle tip. Use the same quick and vigorous insertion technique, but pierce less frequently over the same skin area if you want less bleeding.
Filiform needle (common acupuncture needle)	Quickly and vigorously pierce the affected area. Repeatedly release small droplets of Blood as with the plum blossom and tri-edge needle techniques. Use a #28 or #30 gauge needle. Some patients tolerate the repeated insertion of this needle better than the piercing done by the plum blossom needle, which can be aggravating because of the number of needles in its head. It is also less painful than the lancet or a tri-edge needle because of its smaller tip. This is my preferred method of bloodletting.
Shoni-shin needle	This small plastic pediatric needle can also be substituted for any of the previous techniques. The clinical utility of this needle, apart from its effectiveness, is that it is plastic and disposable, whereas the reusable plum blossom needle needs to be sterilized before reuse. Also, the patients can keep the needle and treat themselves. (Note: Before disposal of the shoni-shin needle, please sterilize.)

- as the skeletal outline of any treatment approach
- after an abdominal clearing that may suggest their employment
- in the case of a diagnosis of weak immunity
- preventively to keep the antipathogenic factor strong.

This treatment is fully discussed by Japanese practitioner Kiyoshi Nagano (1991) in his article 'Immune enhancement through acupuncture and moxibustion: specific treatment for allergic disorders, mild infectious disease and secondary infections' and paraphrased below.

According to Doctor Nagano, when evil Qi invades the body, the tonsils, whose job it is to fight pathogens (antigens), produce antibodies. The tonsils are the first defense against pathogens so if the tonsils have been removed or if the tonsillar function is weak, these pathogens are not destroyed. The initial focal infection can go deeper into the body by way of the Blood vessels and other routes, thereby producing secondary infection. Additionally, the byproduct of the fight between the antibodies and the antigens can produce secondary inflammation.

Secondary infections can lead to autoimmune disease, allergic illnesses, chronic pain, mild infectious disease and secondary disease originating from the gums, sinuses and tonsils. The tonsillar treatment is directed toward the treatment of these secondary disorders. Through needling, acupuncture stimulation not only gives good symptomatic relief in inflammatory disease but also suppresses the underlying process of disease by several mechanisms that are listed below.

- Suppressing increased vascular permeability
- Suppressing histamine release
- Enhancing phagocytic activity
- Increasing release of morphine-like substances

The specific mechanism by which the tonsillar treatment works is to strengthen immunity by activating the functions of the bone marrow, white Blood cells, spleen, tonsillar tissue, lymph nodes, thymus and lymph tissue. Dr Nagano maintains that this treatment is not effective for hepatitis or AIDS patients. I have not used it for any of these conditions although I would still recommend it as a potential treatment strategy that deserves consideration.

The tonsillar treatment consists of a total of seven points. They are TE 16 (Tianyou) bilateral, KI 6 (Zhaohai) bilateral, LI 10 (Shousanli) (the Naganos) bilateral and GV 14 (Dazhui). The

Table 16.2 Analysis of point function in the tonsillar treatment

Point	Functions
TE 16 (Tianyou)	The evil Wind reflex, infection reflex, adenoid reflex: dispels Wind, eliminates Damp. Frees the channels. Diagnostic point for lymphatic glandular exhaustion which indicates the weakness of the immune system.
KI 6 (Zhaohai)	Adrenal reflex point – strengthens the adrenals, nourishes the Yin, calms the mind, benefits the throat, cools the Blood.
LI 10 (Shousanli)	Upper He (sea) of the Stomach. Powerful Qi and Blood tonic. Boosts immunity and fights off evil Qi.
GV 14 (Dazhui)	Point of greatest Yang in the body – meeting of all Yang channels. Evil Wind reflex. Adrenal exhaustion reflex. Relieves the exterior, opens the Yang, clears the brain, calms the spirit. Increases white Blood cells. Strongly tonifies Wei Qi.

cumulative effect of this point prescription is to boost immune function. In Table 16.2 I have provided an analysis of the points employed in this formula so that the user can appreciate the energetic interplay of each point and its contribution to the overall goal of immune enhancement. Figure 16.8 outlines the tonsillar treatment for the convenience of the practitioner and Figure 16.9 gives an appreciation of the relationship of the Naganos to the Large Intestine meridian.

The tonsillar treatment can be used 1–2 times per week with moxibustion administered every day for 1–4 months. The most realistic and efficient use of the moxa is for the patient to use it daily in the form of the Tiger Thermie warmer. The use of moxa is critical here due to its known therapeutic advantages that include the following actions:

● its ability to raise and maintain the white Blood cell count
● its ability to increase the movement of white Blood cells to the diseased area
● its capacity to promote the white Blood cells' ability to attack.

Dr Nagano maintains that the daily application of moxa is the key to cure. Additionally, specific treatment of disease points can be added to the core formula depending upon the presentation of the complaint. In his article, Dr Nagano outlines the specific treatment of several common and difficult-to-treat conditions for which the tonsillar treatment, supplemented with other points, can be used. Such conditions include the common cold, allergic rhinitis, chronic sinusitis, prostatomegaly, herpes zoster and others.

One of the conditions Dr Nagano covers is allergic rhinitis, a problem that many millions suffer from. Allergic rhinitis can be differentiated as an immune hypersensitivity that can lead to more serious problems such as bronchial asthma or even meningitis. The treatment of allergic rhinitis in traditional Chinese medicine calls for the use of moxibustion. The Tiger Thermie warmer can be used to accomplish this objective.

Israeli researchers have demonstrated the positive effects of the application of moxibustion therapy in the improvement of allergic rhinitis symptoms (Sternfeld et al 1992). In their trials they found that when moxa sticks were held 2–3 cm above the skin in the nasal area for 2–3 minutes, they obtained an 88% improvement in the symptoms of allergic rhinitis – an impressive result.

It is my experience that application of moxa with the Tiger Thermie warmer parallels the methodology and results of this study due to the fact that the moxa is applied even more directly than smoke through a metal instrument which is efficient in conducting heat. It is also non-invasive, soothing to the patient and does not produce much smoke close to the eyes, nose and mouth. A fascinating treatment of allergic disease, specifically allergic rhinitis, is found in Chapter 10, on the navel (p. 126). Figure 16.10 shows how to use the Tiger Thermie warmer on the Naganos.

NEW WORDS AND CONCEPTS

Adenoid – lymphatic tissue.

Patient's name:_____   Date:_____

Major complaint and accompanying symptoms:_____
_____

1. How did you use this treatment?

   On its own ☐

   As the skeletal outline to treatment ☐   list other points_____

   Preventively ☐

   For immunodeficient symptoms ☐

2. How do you feel this prescription might benefit the patient; that is, what is the rationale for the treatment?
_____
_____
_____
_____

3. After abdominal clearing what was the most significant pathology on which you obtained less than satisfactory clearance?
_____
_____
_____
_____

4. Describe the tenderness of the tonsillar points upon palpation.

   TE 16R   _____
   TE 16L   _____
   KI 6R   _____
   KI 6L   _____
   LI 10R   _____
   LI 10L   _____
   GV 14   _____

5. Describe fully the method administered (moxa, needles, including depths of insertion, retention time, etc.)
_____
_____
_____
_____
_____
_____

6. Describe the results of treatment (changes on the difficult point(s) to clear on the abdomen (recorded in #3), how patient felt, problems you had, assessment of treatment, changes in major complaint, accompanying symptoms, etc.).
_____
_____
_____
_____

Figure 16.8 Tonsillar treatment form.

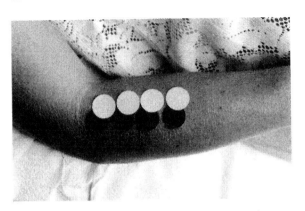

Figure 16.9 The locations of the Naganos in comparison with the points on the Large Intestine meridian.
Light = Chinese LI 11–8, dark = Japanese LI 11–10 areas (Naganos).

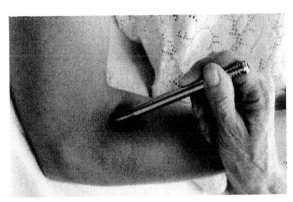

Figure 16.10 How to use the Tiger Thermie warmer on the Naganos or any fleshy point.

Adrenal exhaustion reflex – points of the body such as TE 16 that may become tender or pathological due to the sequelae of adrenal exhaustion.

Antigens – substances which induce the formation of antibodies. An antigen may be introduced into the body or it may be formed within the body. Examples are bacteria, bacterial toxins and foreign Blood cells.

Bloodletting – Chinese bleeding technique such as with a tri-edge needle performed for various therapeutic purposes.

Cushing's syndrome – a syndrome resulting from hypersecretion of the adrenal cortex in which there is excessive production of glucocorticoids.

Evil Wind reflex – points of the body that may become tender or pathological due to an invasion of an 'evil Wind', that is, any stressor that invades the body.

Flat palpation – a method of palpation where the muscle under examination can be pressed against the underlying bone. For example, the way LI 4 (Hegu) is palpated.

Grasp palpation – a method of palpation used when it is possible to grasp the muscle between the thumb and the forefinger, such as the SCM muscle.

Lymphatic duct congestion – impairment of the right lymphatic duct system, resulting in poor lymphatic drainage. It is reflected at ST 12R.

Lymphatic glandular exhaustion – Dr Nagano's theory of systemic deficiency or weakness due to weak or exhausted lymphatic glandular function.

Mini-thread moxa – very small moxa pieces the size of threads.

Nei Gong – internally cultivated Qi Gong.

Plum blossom needle – a seven star-style hammer used in Chinese treatment modalities to invigorate the flow of Qi and Blood and break up Stagnation.

Secondary infections – infections that develop secondarily to an original focal infection that was not completely destroyed.

Wei Gong – externally applied Qi Gong.

QUESTIONS

1. What effects does moxa have on white Blood cells?

2. List some of the difficult-to-treat conditions that the tonsillar treatment can be used for. How is the tonsillar treatment also a preventive treatment?

3. What two points in the tonsillar treatment can be used to calm the spirit? What two points do this in the immunity treatment for cancer patients?

4. What areas or points of the body are reflective of lymphatic glandular exhaustion?

5. What aspects of thyroid function can be subsumed under Kidney energetics in traditional Chinese medicine?

6. What are the appropriate needle techniques and safety considerations for ST 9 (Renying) and ST 12 (Quepen)? What methods(s) can be used on these two points instead of needling?

7. What important anatomical structures lie beneath ST 12? Explain why ST 12 on the left would be indicative of Heart problems (use both a Western allopathic and a traditional Chinese explanation).

8. Why is ST 12 considered the most effective point for carpal tunnel syndrome in the Japanese system?

9. What is the primary point to open scalene compression?

10. What method(s) should be employed in the treatment of tight tense tissue?

11. Define neck tension in Chinese medical terms.

12. Discuss the mechanisms by which anger could result in neck tension.

13. What is considered the thyroid reflex point?

14. Match the following neck pathologies with their related symptoms.

1. Fat pad at the GV 14 (Dazhui) area
2. Tenderness at ST 12 (Quepen) on the right
3. Tenderness at ST 12 (Quepen) on the left
4. Brachial plexus impairment or subclavian artery compression
5. Vertebral artery compression
6. Tension at ST 9 (Renying) on right
7. Tension at ST 9 (Renying) on left
8. Tenderness at the TE 16 (Tianyou) area

a. Numbness and tingling of upper arm
b. Memory problems, dizziness, empty lingering headache
c. Lymphatic duct congestion
d. Fatigue, low Blood pressure, hypothyroidism, cold limbs
e. Sympathetic nervous system problem
f. Palpitations, chest pain
g. Parasympathetic nervous system problem
h. Alternating chills and fever, sore throat

Clinical notes

A word about the thyroid gland

The thyroid gland, one of the body's seven endocrine glands, is located just below the larynx of the throat with interconnecting lobes on either side of the trachea. The thyroid is the body's metabolic thermostat, controlling body temper-ature, energy use and, in children, the body's growth rate. Of the hormones synthesized in and released by the thyroid, T3 (triiodothyronine) represents 7%; T4 (thyroxine) accounts for almost 93% of the thyroid's hormones active in all the body's processes. Iodine is essential to forming normal amounts of thyroxine. Thyroid-stimulating hormone, or TSH, secreted by the pituitary gland in the brain regulates the secretion of both of these hormones. The thyroid also secretes calcitonin, a hormone required for calcium metabolism. Hyperthyroidism refers to an overactive gland while hypothyroidism indicates an underactive thyroid.

Recommendations to prevent adrenal exhaustion (Balch & Balch 1990)

1. Avoid alcohol, caffeine and tobacco; these substances are highly toxic to the adrenal gland and other glands. Stay away from fats, fried foods, ham, pork, highly processed foods, red meats, sodas, sugar and white flour. These foods put unnecessary stress on the adrenal glands.
2. Consume plenty of fresh fruits and vegetables, particularly green, leafy ones. Brewer's yeast, brown rice, legumes, olive and safflower oils, nuts, seeds, wheat germ and whole grains are healthy additions to the diet. Eat deep-water ocean fish, salmon and tuna at least three times a week.
3. Take positive action to relieve stressful situations. Moderate exercise helps to stimulate the adrenal glands. Steps must be taken to protect these glands or they can become exhausted.

Immune deficiency diseases – a Chinese perspective

According to classical Chinese literature the Yuan Qi originates between the two Kidneys and circulates to the organs and the meridians via the San Jiao, the ambassador of the Yuan Qi, and through the Eight Extraordinary Meridians. As we know, defensive Qi (Wei) originates from the Middle Jiao but as the ancient texts say, the Lower Jiao confronts the pathogenic factors. Hence immunity is related to Yuan Qi and Wei Qi. It is also connected with Qi and Blood, the building blocks of health.

Qi Gong masters believe that Yuan Qi, the primary Qi, plays the most important role in immune problems. They administer their stored Yuan Qi, through the process of Wei Gong (or externally applied Qi), to their patients and believe it can strengthen the patient's immune system.

Wei Gong protects the Qi on the outside of the body. It is stored in the channels and thus in the winter these masters can wear thin clothes because they are full of Qi. Qi Gong masters believe they can augment their Yuan Qi. They collect it from the universe and from the Qi of the Stomach and the Spleen, yet they don't eat too much; they pay more attention to cosmic Qi. This Qi from the universe is stored in the form of Essence and the Essence is given out in the form of Qi by way of Wei Gong. Qi Gong masters recommend the practice of Qi Gong (Nei Gong – internally developed Qi) in a negative ion forest such as a pine forest, to assimilate cosmic Qi. They advise practicing the small sky microcosmic orbit that is described below.

Focus on CV 4 (Guanyuan). Bring this energy down to the GV channel and point by point, circulate the energy up the GV channel and down the CV channel. Don't pay much attention to breathing or there may be side effects.

Another exercise they suggest is:

Make small circles from GV 1 (Changqiang) to GV 4 (Mingmen) to CV 6 (Qihai) to CV 4 (Guanyuan). When you feel heat sensations in your palms you are ready to treat patients.

I have also included for the reader a formula that I obtained on a China study trip (Table 16.3). This was relayed as an excellent prescription for tonifying the Yuan Qi that the Chinese see as the root of our immunity. This theoretical position is consistent with the fundamental Chinese outlook on immunity outlined in Chapter 5.

The Chinese points used in the treatment of immune deficiency disease are CV 4 (Guanyuan), GV 4 (Mingmen), ST 36 (Zusanli), GV 14 (Dazhui) and BL 23 (Shenshu). It is important to point out that while Yuan (Source) points can be used to tonify the organs, they are not sufficient to tonify the Qi of the whole body. Remember Back Shu points are used for the Qi of the organs. This Qi can be transformed into Yuan Qi.

In my opinion the tonsillar formula and the Chinese immunity treatment constitute excellent approaches and in many ways are performing

Table 16.3 Analysis of point function in the Chinese treatment of immunity

Points	Functions
CV 4 (Guanyuan)	Tonifies the foundation Yin and Yang. Builds Yang and Blood, regulates Qi, restores Yang.
GV 4 (Mingmen)	Tonifies Kidney Yang, nourishes original Qi, warms the Gate of Vitality, expels Cold, benefits Essence, best point for Kidney Yang Xu with moxa. Primary point for allergies.
ST 36 (Zusanli)	Brings energy down. Tonifies Stomach and Kidney.
GV 14 (Dazhui)	Point of greatest Yang in the body – meeting of all Yang channels. Evil Wind reflex. Adrenal exhaustion reflex. Relieves the exterior, opens the Yang, clears the brain, calms the spirit. Increases white Blood cells. Strongly tonifies Wei Qi.
BL 23 (Shenshu)	Back Shu point of the Kidney for Kidney Qi Deficiency.

Table 16.4 Immunity treatment for cancer patients

Points	Functions
ST 36 (Zusanli)	Brings energy down, especially rebellious Stomach Qi that is a common sequel to chemotherapy or radiation. Prevents vomiting and loss of body fluids necessary to reestablish postnatal Qi. Tonifies Stomach and Kidney Yin Deficiency damaged by treatment.
PC 6 (Neiguan)	As master of Yin Wei channel, tonifies the Yin defensive energy. Brings energy down. Quiets the Heart. Helps the emotions. For the nausea that may accompany chemotherapy.
LI 4 (Hegu)	Stops pain, brings the energy down; for nausea due to chemotherapy.
SP 6 (Sanyinjiao)	Group Luo of the Three Leg Yin. Tonifies Yin of Liver, Spleen and Kidney, whose Yin is damaged by treatment.
CV 12 (Zhongwan)	As Front Mu point of the Stomach, tonifies Stomach Yin. Brings down rebellious Stomach Qi.
HT 7 (Shenmen)	Earth point, sedation point on the Heart meridian. Levels the Heart, calms the spirit, makes pain negligible because the spirit is addressed. A primary point for pain.

the same function. A comparison of Tables 16.2 and 16.3 shows that the energetic function of these approaches is more similar than not.

Yves Requena, French medical doctor and acupuncturist, reminds us that, 'A severe deficiency of Yuan Qi necessitates preventive treatment with moxa at CV 4, CV 6, and CV 8. These are the three basic points of the most severe organic states' (Requena 1986, p. 362). To these traditional points Shanghai physicians add BL 23 and GV 4, the point of origin of the Kidney meridian, and CV 17, Sea of Energy, all treated with moxibustion.

Guan An Men Hospital, a cancer specialty hospital in Beijing, proffers another formula on the treatment of immune problems with patients who have cancer. It consists of ST 36 (Zusanli), PC 6 (Neiguan), LI 4 (Hegu), SP 6 (Sanyinjiao), CV 12 (Zhongwan) and HT 7 (Shenmen). Their energetics can be found in Table 16.4. This formula can be modified based upon the patient's presentation. Points can be deleted or added according to signs and symptoms. The dual purpose of this prescription is to combat the side effects of chemotherapy or radiation and to support the antipathogenic Qi. More can be read about this in an article I have written on cancer (Gardner-Abbate 2000).

17

Japanese physical exam 5: differential diagnosis of back pain

Now we come to the treatment of a complicated healthcare problem – back pain. Patients complaining of this difficult disorder visit acupuncturists as well as almost every healthcare provider. While certain traditions specialize in back disorders, such as chiropractic and osteopathic doctors, a physician in any school of thought requires a treatment strategy for the back.

As many of us know, back problems are amongst the most challenging to treat. If they become chronic, their treatment generally becomes more elusive and more difficult to address. The purpose of this chapter is to explore an alternative treatment strategy for this complex area prone to tension, particularly from the Japanese perspective. Hence, it is included as the fifth and last component of the Japanese physical exam.

The back is a part of the body prone to tension because of its functions, physically and energetically. It is a large and powerful area protected by layers of muscles that make many movements possible and that encompass the posterior aspect of the organs. By nature it is Yang. It houses and protects the internal organs and is subject to movement and weight-bearing activities, especially the lower back. Within the back is the critical spinal column that makes motor movement and sensory awareness possible.

Acupuncturist David Legge (1990), in his book *Close to the bone*, provides an interesting evolutionary perspective on the tendency for the lower back to become subject to stress. He points out:

The low back forms the base of the spine. It bears the weight of the trunk, head and arms and transfers this weight to the hips. It must cope with more stress than

any other part of the spine. The vertebral column in four legged animals has much less significant weight-bearing role and is subjected to much less flexion and extension than is the human spine. As part of our development into two legged creatures there has been some adaptation in the low back to meet these additional requirements for strength and flexibility. This has involved incorporating larger vertebral bodies and intervertebral discs, stronger lumbar ligaments and a very strong L5. However this doesn't alter the fact that the low back occupies a position in the spine that it was not designed for. Furthermore, to accommodate the lumbar lordosis required by our upright posture, the superior faces of the sacrum and L5 have a marked anterior, as well as superior orientation. This tends to weaken the weight-bearing ability of this segment by:
1. Decreasing the component of the force of gravity that is transmitted through the discs and the vertebral bodies and 2. Increasing the anterior component of the transmitted forces that must be borne by the vertebral arch, the spinal ligaments, the intervertebral discs and the articular processes. Thus the low back, especially the L5/sacrum segment, is a weak link in the chain of support. The majority of low back complaints, as might be expected, are related in some way to this weak link. (p. 119)

ETIOLOGY AND EVALUATION

The most frequent back disorders come from postural, structural or occupational stress, although a sizable number come from trauma and injury to the area. Obviously, the more injured the back due to any reason, the more difficult and the longer it may take to treat. Keep this in mind when assisting these patients.

As we know in Oriental medicine, the important acupuncture points located on the back and relatively adjacent to the spinal column are the Back Shu points. The Back Shu points are infused with Qi and Blood and are diagnostic of Qi and Blood disharmonies of the internal organs. Hence, some back problems may be a reflection of the condition of the internal organs in the low back area, such as the Kidney and the Intestines.

Fundamentally in Chinese thought, the lower back belongs to the Kidney. As a result, all the factors that can make the Kidney weak can cause back problems. As we have seen throughout this book, one of the leading causes of Kidney problems is adrenal deficiency. Most adrenal defi-

ciency can be attributed to stress, followed by certain foods, medications and other lifestyle factors. Also weak immunity is ultimately viewed as a Kidney problem so some back problems may actually be a manifestation of weak immunity.

In order to determine the proper treatment of back pain, it first must be evaluated. Procedurally, back pain, like any major complaint, needs to be differentiated. As we have seen, differentiations in Japanese acupuncture may be phrased in different language so some new terminology is introduced here.

As with any major complaint, ask about the onset, duration, history of similar problems prior to this or within the family, what treatment was received and its effect. Obtain a thorough personal medical history and family medical history. Ask all the Ten Questions and obtain physical confirmation from the tongue, pulse and palpation.

Since the Japanese recognize several types of back pain, have the patient show you exactly where it is and mark it with a sterile marking pen or in some other way so you can go back and check your results after the treatment. The areas where back pain occurs include the following.

- On the midline of the back, that is, on the spine or the Governing Vessel channel
- At the end of the spine, specifically at the coccyx
- In the lumbar/sacral area
- At the sacrotuberous ligament
- Lateral to the spine, on the quadratus lumborum muscle or Bladder channel
- Along the border of the posterior superior iliac spine, the iliac crest
- At the mid-back
- In the upper back

Figure 17.1 depicts these areas.

TREATMENT
Chronic back pain

If the patient's back pain is of a chronic variety, determine where the pain is and then proceed with its treatment following the steps outlined below and summarized in Box 17.1.

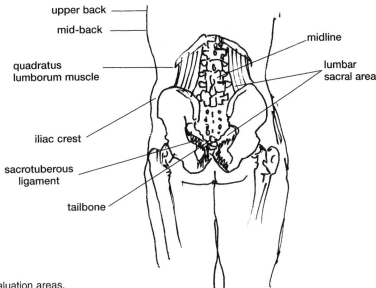

Figure 17.1 Back evaluation areas.

1. Conduct the healthy Hara examination to get the big picture on the condition of the Qi, Blood, Yin and Yang. Then inspect the portion of the back that is affected. Look for signs and symptoms of Excess, Deficiency or other signs of point pathology.
2. Next, using the modified abdominal examination, clear the abdomen and check the effect of this on the back. There should be some improvement in the condition of the back. Remember that the modified abdominal examination discloses the diagnosis of Qi, Blood, Yin and Yang and the abdominal clearing treats those entities. However, the abdominal clearing may not be specific enough to reduce the back pain.
3. Now, perform some of the other physical examinations discussed in this section of the book such as the inner thigh, checking scars, the sinuses, and the neck to see their potential relationship to the back problem.
4. Finally, specialized back procedures utilizing treatment-of-disease points may be employed to reinforce the clearance done by hand. These differentiations and their treatment points are listed in Figure 17.2 and will be discussed later in this chapter.

Case 17.1 offers a practical understanding of this procedure.

As part of the Japanese physical exam

If the back is not a major complaint but is either an inactive problem or a subpathology of the Ten Questions, still inspect it on the second or third visit since back problems, as part of the Japanese physical exam, are indicative of important energetic disharmonies. Follow the treatment protocol for the type of back pain the patient has.

For clinical convenience, Box 17.1 summarizes the basic treatment approach to backs.

Acute back pain

When a patient is suffering from acute back pain you may not be able to perform all the multiple exams that you might do for the patient who has chronic back pain. Because a general rule of thumb is to treat what you see, you need the person's presentation to guide you in treatment. However, there are some emergency points and some shortcuts that can be taken to assist in the remediation of their pain and they are presented below.

Box 17.1 Japanese back evaluations

When   Back evaluations may be performed:
1. if the back problem is the major complaint or one of the accompanying symptoms of a major complaint or
2. as an inactive problem (meaning part of the person's history) that is a subpathology of the Ten Questions or
3. as part of the Japanese physical exam when you are checking for significant physical pathologies that indicate a disharmony of the organism.

How   Have the patients show you where their back pain is. Possible locations are:
1. on the midline of the back, that is, on the spine or Governing Vessel channel
2. at the end of the spine, specifically at the coccyx
3. in the lumbar area
4. in the sacral area
5. lateral to the spine on the quadratus lumborum muscle or Bladder channel area
6. along the iliac crest
7. at the mid-back
8. in the upper back (in this case, treat as a neck problem).

These observations will help you differentiate the back problem.

Treatment

Chronic problem
1. Clear the abdomen and see if it releases the back.
2. Clear each of the following, one at a time, and see if they have a relationship to the back by rechecking it: the navel, inner thigh, scars, sinuses, and neck.
3. If required, treat the back according to its correct differentiation protocol, that is, use the treatment of-disease points. See Figure 17.2 for these specific protocols.

You do not necessarily need to perform all these examinations. Stop at the place where you obtain sufficient clearance of the back.

As part of the Japanese physical exam
1. Follow Figure 17.2.

Acute problem
1. Check the following clinically effective points one at a time and assess its relationship to the back: LR 4, KI 7, BL 62R and SI 3.
2. Consult Figure 17.2 and treat according to the corresponding differentiation.

Case 17.1 Back procedures

In a class in which I was teaching this material, I asked for a volunteer who had back pain in order to illustrate the procedural orientation to backs. The patient, who was in her 40s, had suffered from chronic back pain ever since she had her first period when she was in her teens.

First, I asked her to show me where the back pain was. I palpated the area and it was very tender and I marked it with a sterile marking pen since several other examinations needed to be done and I wanted to be able to check the tender area again with certainty and speed. Next, the healthy Hara examination was performed. Basically, Kidney Yang Deficiency, as seen through a puffy lower abdomen, and Blood Stagnation, as manifest through a tender ST 25L, were apparent. Then the abdominal clearing was performed. Her abdomen cleared 100%, which is not unusual once you become proficient with the process. I then rechecked the area of her back pain. Stunned, she reported that it had improved by 50%.

I then proceeded to clear her inner thigh by hand and when that was finished I rechecked her back. It had improved by another 25%. She was appreciably impressed. She had no problematic scars so they were not correlated with the back pain. The sinuses and the neck were then evaluated and cleared by hand. The sinuses totally alleviated it.

The patient, the entire class and myself were impressed by the ability of other body parts to remediate the back pain 100% and exclusively by hand. Certain significant clearance points for each of the specific exams could have been needled to reinforce what had been done by hand although I didn't do this due to time constraints. Those points were KI 1 (Yongquan) bilaterally (for the abdomen and the thigh), LR 4R (Zhongfeng) for the thigh, GB 41L (Zulinqi) for the neck portion of the sinus exam and a painful KI 16 (Huangshu) point for the sinuses. These five points were the most effective in clearance. We did not have to use any specific back protocols since the resolution was so effective.

The area where her specific back pain was located was on the quadratus lumborum muscle on the left side. Consulting Figure 17.2, under the quadratus lumborum protocol you will see that KI 1, LR 4 and SP 4 are primary points for that differentiation. KI 1 and SP 4 had already been palpated as part of abdominal clearing and LR 4 was for the clearance of the thigh so it is not surprising that they were effective for her variety of back pain because it was treated.

Note that in this treatment process, the rule is to proceed from the most general to the most specific and to accomplish as much as possible by hand. Needles, intradermals, moxa or palpation can be done for reinforcement.

Shortcuts/emergency treatment 1

1. First, always mark the area of pain with a sterile marking pen to allow you to go back and rapidly and accurately check the painful spot(s).
2. Positioning the patient on the table on their back, if this is possible, deeply press LR 4, one point at a time, for about 3–5 seconds. LR 4 is considered the best point for a strained back. It is typically very tender in cases of back pain. LR 4 is also the best treatment point for Blood Stagnation anywhere in the body, particularly in the Lower Jiao. To me, it is analogous to the role of PC 6 in the Upper Jiao. Check the patient's back and evaluate the improvement. It should have a significant effect in reducing the pain.
3. If the back pain is due to Kidney Deficiency, press KI 7 and then check the back. It is effective for this specific differentiation.
4. If the back pain also has concomitant cervical neck involvement, vigorously rub the base of the first metatarsal in the Spleen 3–4 area. This point is perhaps one of the most tender in the body so prepare the patient for the palpatory sensation. As usual, recheck the back and the neck.
5. Supplemental points for back pain along the spinal column accompanied by neck pain are BL 62R and SI 3L. Palpate each in the same method as described in Chapter 8 on abdominal clearing.
6. For added reinforcement the significant points can be needled according to the methods presented in this book.
7. Dependent upon the significance of their involvement, the patient can be taught to press them.

Shortcuts/emergency treatment 2

Another possible approach to the presentation of acute back pain is to test the treatment-of-disease points or the points that match the differentiation of the back pain. These back protocols presented here are quite efficacious and the reader is encouraged to try these procedures as well.

DIFFERENTIATION OF BACK PROBLEMS

In the Japanese system there are eight patterns of back differentiation. However, it is not uncommon that several types of back pain may coexist, thus making their treatment more confounding. Because back differentiations and their treatment are new and perhaps the most complex material presented in this book, all the relevant information about backs, including their differentiations, clinical manifestations and treatments, is summarized in Figure 17.2 and discussed below.

On the midline of the back, that is, on the spine or the Governing Vessel channel

This common form of back pain can be caused by several etiological factors including trauma to the area, invasion of exogenous pathogens which have a propensity to affect the Governing Vessel channel or other causative factors of illness in Oriental medicine. Specific clinical manifestations of this variety of back pain include disc problems, low back pain, midline back pain, neck, organ and shoulder problems, scoliosis, sciatica, hemorrhoids, prostatitis or urinary tract disorders.

The primary treatment point for this back pain as well as all the back pathologies presented in this chapter is Liver 4. LR 4 (Zhongfeng) is the Metal point on the Wood meridian. According to Five Element theory, Metal controls Wood. As such, this point facilitates the free flow of Qi and Blood, the lack of which causes pain. Remember that LR 4 is the primary point to move Stagnation in the Lower Burner so it is particularly effective for pain in the lower back. It benefits the ligaments that may be involved with back pain. In my opinion, LR 4 is similar in its effects on the Lower Burner as PC 6 (Neiguan) is on the Upper Burner.

Press LR 4 one side at a time with a strong rubbing motion. I have found that the right side is usually more clinically effective but doing both strengthens its effects. This point is generally tender. When needling this point, insert the needle obliquely upward 0.3–0.5 in. in the direction of the

Back differentiation	Etiology	Clinical manifestation	Treatment	Normal	Abnormal
1. On the midline of the back, specifically on the spine or GV channel	Trauma, exogenous pathogens, other causative factors	Back problems, disc problems, low back pain, midline back pain, neck problems, organ problems, shoulder problems, scoliosis, hemorrhoids, sciatica, prostatitis, urinary tract problems	1. LR 4 (Zhongfeng) with pressure or needle obliquely in the direction of the meridian 0.3–0.5 in. Tiger Thermie or massage. Best point for strained back. 2. SI 3L (Houxi – opens GV channel) obliquely 0.5–0.7 in. underneath the bone towards SI 1. With BL 62R (Shenmai – joins Bladder channel), 0.3–0.5 in. in the direction of the meridian towards the toe. Massage or intradermal. 3. Needle BL 20 (Pishu – strengthens muscles), perpendicularly 0.5–1.0 in. or implant intradermal inferiorly in the direction of the meridian. 4. GB 25 (Jingmen – Mu of KI), perpendicularly 0.5–1.0. MA. *Patient must be on their side.* 5. BL 25 (Dachangshu), perpendicularly 1.0–1.2 in. MA. 6. BL 1 (Jingming – moves meridian) perpendicularly 0.3–0.5 in. along the orbital wall. 7. Shiqizhui, (below L5) perpendicularly 0.5–1.0 in. MA.		
2. Pain at the end of the spine, specifically the coccyx	Trauma to the coccyx leads to adrenal cortex being affected which can produce hormonal problems	Back tension, spasm, chronic constipation, headache, herniated disc, hormone imbalances, low back pain, neck pain, sciatica, prostatitis, hypoglycemia, diabetes	1. Check for tailbone tenderness by palpating directly below the tailbone and to either side of it. The practitioner or the patient may do it. 2. If tender, the point can be needled (under the bone or into the tense area 0.5–1.0 in.) or the patient should be instructed to massage the point daily.		
3. In the lumbar/ sacral region	Same as #1. Area most structurally weak	Inspect for a flat lumbar area or a puffy sacrum	1. LR 4 (see method above). 2. GV 14 (Dazhui), perpendicularly 0.5–1.0 in., MA.		
4. Lateral to the spine on the quadratus lumborum muscle or Bladder channel	1. KI Deficiency; failure of the Kidney to dominate Water metabolism processes resulting in improper fat metabolism 2. Sinus problems 3. Feet not properly aligned 4. Sacrotuberous ligament may be involved	1. L4–5 subluxation 2. Tightness in the quadratus fasciae 3. Eating fat makes worse	1. With patient on side release thigh with KI 1 (Yongquan), LR 4 (Zhongfeng). 2. BL 20, GB 25, BL 25, Shiqizhui (same reasons as #1, see above). 3. SP 4 (Gongsun), perpendicularly 0.3–0.5 in. or Tiger Thermie 4. If sinus involvement BL 1 (see above) and BL 2 with Tiger Thermie or 0.3–0.5 in. subcutaneously towards the lateral aspect.		

Figure 17.2 Back evaluation and treatment form.

5. Sacrotuberous ligament	Sinus problems or ankle problems	Disc problems, cement back, frozen back, low back pain with occipital involvement	1. Check BL 62 (Shenmai) for any spinal problem. Could add SI 3. (See method above.) 2. Check GB 34 (Yanglingquan) to release muscles – the influential point which dominates the muscles, perpendicularly 0.8–1.2 in. MA. Rub with strong pressure or use an intradermal. Palpate, needle or use an intradermal. 3. If KI involvement add BL 23 (Shenshu), perpendicularly 1.0–1.5 in. MA. 4. TE 5R (Waiguan), perpendicularly 0.7–1.0 in. and GB 41L (Zulinqi), 0.3–0.5 in. in the direction of the meridian if there is neck involvement. 5. If ankle involvement (inverted or everted legs), needle or intradermal BL 62R (Shenmai), (see above) with KI 6 both (Zhaohai), transversely 0.1 in. towards the heel. In sitting position and have patient hold their leg straight.		
6. Pain along the iliac crest, posterior superior iliac spine	Weak lymphatic glands leading to secondary infections that create weak ligaments. This is then reinforced by other lifestyle variables	Back of knee problems, back problems, pubic bone pain	1. Check to see if TE 16 (Tianyou) and Naganos release pain. Tiger Thermie both or for TE 6 needle perpendicularly 0.3–0.5 in. For the Naganos perpendicularly 0.5–1.0 in. Puncture the most tender with a lift-and-thrust method. 2. ST 13 (Qihu) needle 0.3–0.5 in. transversely and bilaterally towards the lateral aspect or use the Tiger Thermie warmer.		
7. Upper back pain – see neck protocols			See sacrotuberous ligament with neck involvement or pain along the midline with neck involvement.		
8. Mid-back pain	Digestive imbalances	Mid-back pain spasm	1. Check BL 62R (see above). 2. Needle digestive points BL 17, 18, 19 (Geshu, Ganshu, and Danshu) in direction of meridian obliquely 0.5 in. 3. LR 2 (Xingjian), obliquely 0.3–0.5 in.		

R = right side
L = left side
B = bilateral
MA = Moxa is applicable

TE = standard abbreviation of the World Health Organization (1989) for the Triple Warmer.

Figure 17.2 *continued*

Summary – Basic back points:

LR 4 (Zhongfeng) – best point for strained back
KI 7 (Fuliu) – back pain due to KI Xu
SP 3, 4 (Taibai, Gongsun) – any spine problems involving the neck
BL 62 (Shenmai), SI 3 (Houxi) – spinal problems especially with neck involvement

Treatment:_____

_____
_____
_____
_____
_____
_____
_____
_____

Results:_____

_____
_____
_____
_____
_____

Figure 17.2 *continued.*

Liver meridian (upward). The Tiger Thermie warmer may also be applied to each point for about a minute and a half. This is an important point for patients to learn how to rub themselves or to have someone rub on them if it relieves the back pain.

Other primary treatment points include SI 3 (Houxi) and BL 62 (Shenmai). SI 3 is the Master of the Governing Vessel channel. It opens the channel, clearing it of obstruction. BL 62 is the Coupled point of the Governing Vessel channel and the Master of the Yangqiao channel. It works on midline back pain because it joins the Bladder channel, comforts the tendons, relaxes the muscle channels and straightens the legs.

Treat SI 3 on the left side. BL 62 is treated on the right side. Check whether the standard Chinese BL 62 or the Japanese BL 62 is the more tender. Note that Japanese BL 62, thereafter referred to as BL 62, has the same location as Chinese BL 61. Each point can be massaged, implanted with an intradermal needle or needled. Puncture SI 3 obliquely 0.5–0.7 in. underneath the bone towards SI 1. Puncture BL 62 0.3–0.5 in. in the direction of the meridian (towards the toe).

Supplemental points include BL 20, GB 25, BL 25, BL 1 and Shiqizhui. BL 20 (Pishu) is the Back Shu point of the Spleen. The Spleen has a connection with the muscles according to Five Element theory. Puncture perpendicularly 0.5–1.0 in. or implant an intradermal needle inferiorly in the direction of the meridian. GB 25 (Jingmen) is the Front Mu point of the Kidney and is a clinically effective point for back pain. Patients should recline on their side; this position is critical for maximum efficacy. Puncture perpendicularly as if needling towards the spine 0.5–1.0 in. Moxibustion is applicable. BL 25 (Dachangshu), Back Shu point of the Large Intestine, is effective for back pain due to Kidney Deficiency. Puncture perpendicularly 1.0–1.2 in.

BL 1 (Jingming) moves the meridian. It is a point of the Yangqiao channel. With your fingers, gently direct the eyeball to the side so that the needle can be inserted. Slowly puncture the point perpendicularly 0.3–0.5 in. along the orbital wall. It is not advisable to twist or lift or thrust the needle. Take the needle out slowly and apply a dry cotton ball for one minute to the area to the prevent bruising. The extra point, Shiqizhui, is located in the depression below the spinous process of the fifth lumbar vertebra. Puncture this point perpendicularly 0.5–1.0 in. Moxibustion is applicable. All needles can be retained 10–20 minutes with the exception of BL 1 which should be retained about 5 minutes.

Pain at the end of the spine, specifically at the coccyx

This is an interesting type of back pain that has its etiology due to trauma to the tailbone area. The patient may have other back manifestations such as back spasm, low back pain, herniated disc or sciatica and other clinical manifestations such as prostatitis, hypoglycemia, diabetes, chronic constipation, headache, hormonal imbalances and neck pain.

When trauma is experienced by the tailbone, it causes a reverberation throughout the spine. As that shock passes through the adrenal cortex of the Kidney it may release adrenal hormones, thereby precipitating a hormonal imbalance in the individual.

To treat the back pain or related clinical manifestations, follow the procedure outlined here.

1. Ask the patients if they have ever had a tailbone injury that they can remember. If it was a significant injury such as falling off a horse or roller-skates they will generally remember it.
2. Wearing protective gloves, palpate directly below the coccyx and to either side of it for residual tenderness. Either the practitioner or the patient may do this. If the area is tender it indicates that there is lack of free flow of Qi in the area.
3. Teach the patient how to massage this point for a few minutes every day. The point can also be needled by inserting a #1 needle 0.5–1.0 in. into the tense area. Apply a

lift-and-thrust method to break up the tension and retain for 5 minutes. I prefer to instruct patients on how to massage the point rather than needling it and I have obtained excellent results for low back pain, herniated disc and prostatitis using this method.

Pain in the lumbar/sacral region

This variety of pain may be due to some of the same etiologies described under midline pain; that is, trauma or the general causative factors of illness. It is found in the lumbar/sacral region. The lumbar region presents as flat and the sacral area as puffy. The normal lumbar spine should have a curvature to it and the sacrum should not be puffy or look edematous.

As always, have the patient point out the specific painful area in this region. It may be in the liaos (foramina) of the sacrum. LR 4 is the first point to check to see if it will release this as well as all varieties of back pain. (See previous method for LR 4 under midline back pain.) Additionally, GV 14 (Dazhui) may be an important treatment point. There are several reasons for this. First, when the lower spine is affected, there is usually a compensatory change in the neck area where GV 14 is located. Second, GV 14 is the point of greatest Yang of the body. When it is not performing its function of metabolizing Water, one of the clinical manifestations that may result is edema.

One place where that puffiness can accumulate is in the sacral area due to its connection with the Kidney. It can also present as a fat pad at GV 14, as we saw in Chapter 16. Commonly patients who have a puffy sacrum have a fat pad or a pre-clinical fat pad at GV 14. For this variety of back pain, GV 14 is a supplemental point. Puncture perpendicularly 0.5–1.0 in. or in the manner described in Chapter 16 if an actual fat pad exists. Moxibustion is applicable.

Lateral to the spine on the quadratus lumborum muscle or the Bladder channel

This is a common presentation of back pain that has several causative factors. One of the most common causes is Deficiency of the Kidney. Another clinical manifestation is subluxation of the vertebrae at the L4–L5 area. In this case, the patient feels tenseness in this part of the back.

When the Kidney is deficient, it fails to dominate the metabolism of Water. Unmetabolized Water can lead to the retention of Damp, Water, dilute Phlegm and Phlegm. Hence, the patient with this type of back pain may have difficulty digesting fats or the ingestion of fats may exacerbate the back pain because fat, as a type of Water, requires the energy of the Kidney to break it down. The patient is generally not aware that the fat may make the back worse so you need to establish this connection by asking the question so that the patient can become sensitized to it. The quadratus lumborum muscles may also evidence pain due to structural problems such as the ankles not being aligned properly.

But perhaps the most 'obscure' cause of this subset of back pain is due to sinus problems. Remember sinus problems are essentially Lung problems. When the Lungs are weak they fail to descend the Qi. The Kidney concomitantly can become weak because it does not grasp the Qi. The process for treating pain on the Bladder channel or the quadratus lumborum muscle is described below.

1. The first treatment strategy is to release the inner thigh using the two primary thigh treatment points, KI 1 (Yongquan) and LR 4 (Zhongfeng) (see Chapter 13).
2. BL 20 (Pishu), GB 25 (Jingmen), BL 25 (Dachangshu) and Shiqizhui can be useful, for the reasons listed above.
3. SP 4 (Gongsun) according to classical Chinese literature can be used for back problems. Puncture perpendicularly 0.3–0.5 in. Moxibustion in the form of the Tiger Thermie warmer is applicable.
4. If there is sinus involvement, BL 1 (Jingming) and BL 2 (Zanzhu) may need to be treated. Puncture BL 2 0.3–0.5 in. subcutaneously towards the lateral aspect. The Tiger Thermie warmer can be applied to this point in the eyebrow region for about one minute and is very effective and relaxing to the patient. This treatment can alleviate the back pain if it involves the sinuses. The patient should be taught how to Tiger Thermie the sinus area to expedite resolution of the back problem and to strengthen Lung and Kidney function.

Sacrotuberous ligament

The sacrotuberous ligament connects the sacrum to the ischial tuberosity. Sinus problems or misaligned ankles may cause this pathology. When the sacrotuberous ligament is involved, the patient experiences pain in the lower sacral area in the proximity of the ligament as well as symptoms such as disc problems, frozen back (cement back) or low back pain reflecting to the occipital region.

In the treatment of sacrotuberous ligament-induced back pain use the following procedure.

1. If there is also spinal involvement, use BL 62 (Shenmai) and SI 3 (Houxi) as described previously.
2. GB 34 (Yanglingquan) is a very useful point for this configuration. Remember that GB 34 is the Influential point which dominates muscles, tendons, nerves and ligaments. Use the Japanese location for GB 34, which is 1 cun posterior to the head of the fibula (about 1 cun posterior to the Chinese GB 34). GB 34 is a primary point for pain because pain usually has muscular involvement and this point influences the function of the muscles. Press the point deeply, implant an intradermal needle into the point or puncture perpendicularly 0.8–1.2 in. Moxibustion is applicable. This location is depicted in Figure 17.3.
3. If there is Kidney involvement add BL 23 (Shenshu), Back Shu point of the Kidney. Puncture perpendicularly 1.0–1.5 in. Moxibustion is applicable.
4. TE 5 (Waiguan) and GB 41 (Zulinqi) may be used if there is neck involvement. TE 5 facilities the circulation of Qi in the channels and relaxes the sinews and tendons. Puncture TE 5R perpendicularly 0.7–1.0 in. GB 41L is punctured 0.3–0.5 in. in the direction of the meridian (towards the toe) or rubbed with strong dispersive pressure. An intradermal needle can be inserted into

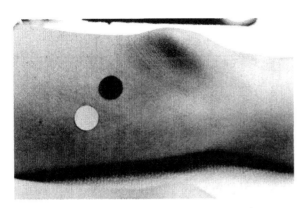

Figure 17.3 Two locations of GB 34 (Yanglingquan). Dark = Chinese, light = Japanese.

GB 41. Together, TE 5 and GB 41 loosen carotid compression of the neck that can affect the sinuses.

5. Finally, if the ankles are involved, BL 62 (Shenmai) and KI 6 (Zhaohai) are the treatment points to balance the Yangqiao and Yinqiao channels, respectively. Needle each point in the direction of the meridian. KI 6 is punctured subcutaneously towards the heel 0.1–0.2 in. and BL 62 is needled transversely 0.3–0.5 in. towards the toes. Have patients sit while you do this treatment and have them hold their leg upright to balance the meridians of the ankle.

Pain along the iliac crest, the posterior superior iliac spine

This is a very non-traditional and fascinating type of back differentiation, due to weak immunity. When immunity is impaired, various parts of the body are also weak, especially the lymphatic glands whose job it is to destroy pathogens so that disease does not develop. If those pathogens are not destroyed, secondary infection can attack other body parts such as the ligaments, weakening them. In this case of weak immunity, the patient may experience pain in the back of the knees, back pain, or pain in the pubic bone area.

Further immunological impairment can come from lifestyle factors which weaken immunity, such as excess alcoholic consumption, stress or not getting enough sleep. With this type of back presentation, the practitioner's treatment plan is to strengthen the immunity of the person. Note that the needles are not applied in the back but rather on the points aimed at fostering immunity.

Three sets of points comprise the basic treatment plan. They include TE 16 (Tianyou), the Naganos and ST 13 (Qihu). As we have seen in Chapter 16 TE 16 (four locations) is the diagnostic point on the neck for an overworked immune system. Check all four points. The one which is the most tender may be needled perpendicularly 0.3–0.5 in. or massaged. The most effective and non-invasive way of treating this area is to apply the Tiger Thermie warmer to the points since as a whole they tend to be very painful. In this way all four points can be addressed and the patient enjoys the soothing heat. The moxa in this implement is unsurpassed at loosening tense tissue.

The Naganos can be treated in the same manner. Puncture the most tender Nagano on each arm perpendicularly 0.5–1.0 in. Use the lift-and-thrust method to break up congestion in the points.

Finally, ST 13 is needled. This is a point of intersection of the ST, TE, SI and many divergent meridians. It is a treatment-of-disease point for weak immunity. Needle this point bilaterally in a transverse direction 0.3–0.5 in. towards the lateral aspect of the chest. Light moxibustion in the form of a rubbing motion with a Tiger Thermie warmer is applicable.

Upper back pain

See neck protocols or the treatment of the sacrotuberous ligament (with neck involvement) or the protocol for pain along the midline, if the pain is along the midline in the neck area.

Mid-back pain

The last variety of back pain can develop in the middle of the back which covers organs that primarily pertain to digestion. Hence, pain in this region is frequently due to digestive disorders including overconsumption of sugar. Dietary counseling should be provided as part of the treatment plan.

BL 17 (Geshu), BL 18 (Ganshu) and BL 19 (Danshu) can be needled. Puncture each bilaterally in an oblique direction 0.5 in. in the direction of the meridian, that is, downward. BL 62 can be used for any spinal problem so it can be used for midline back pain too. Liver 2 (Xingjian), the Fire point, may be added if the digestive problems are due to too much sugar consumption as this aggravates the Liver which has a role in sugar metabolism. Sugar creates 'Fire' in the Liver. That is why LR 2 is used. Puncture bilaterally in an oblique direction 0.3–0.5 in. in the direction of the meridian (proximally).

In conclusion, you are urged to try these approaches to back pain. Do not be discouraged by their apparent complexity. If you feel comfortable with the energetic explanations for the points, you should proceed. The more frequently these protocols are employed, the less foreign they will seem. Patient comfort and rate of improvement are expedited with these treatments because the entire process is aimed at treating the whole person and treating the root that is revealed in the various protocols.

NEW WORDS AND CONCEPTS

Quadratus lumborum muscle – the large muscle lateral to the spine in the area of the lumbar vertebrae.

Sacrotuberous ligament – the ligament which connects the sacrum to the ischial tuberosity.

QUESTIONS

1. What are the physical and energetic functions of the back?

2. What is the most common etiology of back pain?

3. How can the back be a reflection of the health of the internal organs?

4. What factors weaken the Kidney?

5. Why would GB 34 (Yanglingquan) be an effective point for back pain, specifically for a sacrotuberous ligament problem?

6. Why is GV 14 (Dazhui) an important point in the treatment of the lower spine?

7. What does pain in the quadratus lumborum muscle indicate?

8. Which pair of Confluent points helps to align the ankles to treat back problems?

9. Which pair of Confluent points may be used in the treatment of back pain when there is neck involvement?

10. Explain how sinus problems can cause back pain.

11. Explain how each aspect of treating the back (healthy Hara examination, abdominal clearing, inner thigh treatment, etc.) can affect the condition of the back.

12. What is the most important point in the treatment of back pain and why?

18

Treatment of pain

ORIENTAL MEDICAL APPROACHES TO PAIN

Oriental medicine is uniquely qualified to treat the ever-present condition of human pain because of its perception of pain. While we have seen that meridian-style acupuncture can be used to treat virtually every condition, in this supplementary chapter we will see why Japanese acupuncture is so adept at eliminating pain in the process of the physical examination presented in this book. I will begin with the theoretical differential diagnosis and treatment of pain from the perspective of both Chinese and Japanese medicine and then outline various point categories for pain. Many of these point categories are an integral part of the various physical examinations. They include Luo points, Xi (cleft) points, Influential points and Confluent points.

In this chapter I summarize:

- the criteria for assessing pain, including its subjective nature as perceived by the patient
- the differential diagnosis of pain according to pain characteristics
- a cross-reference of characteristics according to Chinese diagnostic category
- the clinical differentiation and energetics of the six categories of specialized acupoints including specific powerful points within each category
- the locations and needling parameters for the acupoints described.

Case studies illustrating the effectiveness of selected points are provided. The chapter concludes with a discussion of pain management and issues involving the loved ones of those with pain.

WHAT IS PAIN?

Pain is an inescapable experience of life for many people. Millions of people affected by pain either suffer in silence or seek a multitude of treatments, which yield varied outcomes. Some of their therapies, especially those involving Western medications, generally only mask the pain and indeed, these drugs often cause deleterious side effects. This is not to imply that there is no place for prescription or over-the-counter drugs in the management of pain, especially in the treatment of severe or acute pain. However, when prescription medications are taken on a continual basis or abused by patients they may become a serious health concern.

The functional role of pain in the body is that of signal, indicating that something is wrong. As such, it can act as a messenger of bodily imbalances if the message can be understood or 'read'. Western medicine defines pain as a complex subjective phenomenon comprising sensation, indicating real or potential tissue damage, and the affective response that it generates.

Oriental medicine, through its unique perspective of the body, maintains that pain is the lack of the 'free flow' of energy (Qi or Blood) or what I view as the physiological, psychological and emotional manifestations of Stagnation. This definition is not unlike the Western point of view; both recognize that pain involves more than a physical component. Whereas nerve involvement is considered to be a fundamental mechanism of pain in the Western paradigm, Stagnation is a fundamental mechanism in Oriental medicine.

Consequently, in Oriental medicine, a guideline in the root treatment for pain is not to conceal or anesthetize it but if possible, to eliminate it by resolving the underlying Stagnation and addressing those factors that may be responsible for its presence. Acupuncture, moxibustion and related Oriental modalities are effective tools for restoring the proper flow of Qi and Blood so that Stagnation can be addressed. However, this is not to imply that such redirection is an easy task or always possible. It must be recognized that some pain, such as that accompanying degenerative, chronic or terminal disease, may only be managed rather than fully corrected.

THE DIFFERENTIAL DIAGNOSIS OF PAIN

In any tradition, the key to the successful treatment of pain is the correct differentiation of that pain. As the Western definition acknowledges, pain is a complex phenomenon. Therefore, the differential diagnosis of any pain must be made by considering several criteria, summarized in Box 18.1.

As regards the character of pain, both Western and Oriental practitioners sometimes overlook the fact that, clinically, several types of pain may coexist, thus confounding its presentation. These types of pain do not present separately; rather, they are composites of the multiple types of pain that modify and influence the pain's appearance. In these cases, the nature of the pain may fail to reflect the classical characteristics from any one perspective. This confusing presentation should serve as a clue to the practitioner that several types of pain may be involved. The precise differentiation of this constellation of symptoms must be discerned to arrive at an exact diagnosis.

To the Oriental physician, the presence of multiple, coexisting types of pain should not be surprising. An understanding of Zang-Fu organ physiology, Five Element interrelationships, Qi and Blood physiology, Triple Warmer interactions and Yin/Yang philosophy posits that a change in one organ's proper functioning may lead to interrelated changes. Stagnation in one part of the body may influence the Qi and Blood flow in another part. I use this rule of thumb: the longer the duration of the body's current disharmonies, the more likely it is that multiple levels of pain may develop, which need to be diagnostically dismantled. For instance, Qi Stagnation may lead to Blood Stagnation, which in turn may lead to Blood Stasis with Heat.

As shown in Box 18.1, another significant factor that contributes to pain differentiation is

Box 18.1 Pain assessment criteria

1. Location	Pain can be anywhere. Location must be considered together with all the criteria found in this table.
2. Onset	Onset of pain includes any situations that lead up to the perception of pain. The patient's entire medical history, supplemented by the traditional Ten Questions of Chinese medicine, is necessary in determining the conditions under which the pain arose. By only concentrating on the pain, the practitioner may isolate the pain from the context of the whole person and thereby miss valuable clues about its possible etiology and proper diagnosis. This clinical faux pas is more likely to occur when the pain has taken a long time to manifest.
3. Character	The character or nature of pain includes variables such as temperature, intensity and the tension or pressure one may feel. Some pain is of a mixed nature that further complicates its differentiation. It refers both to what the patient reports and what the practitioner may feel.
4. Duration	Duration includes both generally how long the patient has been experiencing the pain as well as the specific duration of the current pain.
5. What makes the pain better or worse?	This is an extremely significant consideration for determining the fundamental diagnosis of the pain. Patients tend to naturally seek these solutions – it is their body's way of attempting to achieve homeostasis, of trying to rectify the imbalance. Probing questions by the practitioner can attune the patient to these bodily clues.
6. How does the pain impact the person?	This insightful question, often overlooked, serves to inform the practitioner regarding how the patient is coping with the pain, how it affects their life and the lives of those who live and/or work with them. Pay attention to the words the patient uses to describe the pain. Language is an expression of the spirit. Listen to the tone of the voice, the Five Element sounds, expressions and emotions conveyed in the language, volume of the voice, and so on. It signifies their experience of pain, the way in which it affects their spirit. According to traditional Chinese medicine, the way in which the spirit is affected will influence the flow of Qi and Blood and accordingly, Qi and Blood flow affects the spirit. Hence, pain has enormous implications for the emotional, spiritual and physical well-being of the patient.

how the patient perceives and articulates it. This is a highly complex response that involves cultural, social and individual perceptions of the threshold of pain: what is or is not proper to report; one's ability to verbalize the sensations associated with the pain; fatigue, stress levels and many other factors.

Not only is there a language of pain in Oriental and Western medicine but, perhaps more importantly, there is the personal language of pain. While clinicians may prefer the terms used in Table 18.1, such as 'fixed, stabbing or boring', to help arrive at a diagnosis, patients may not perceive their pain in the language of the clinician. The report of their pain can range anywhere from imprecise to intensely hyperbolic. It is the task of the practitioner to listen to the specific language of the patient, which in all cases is the body's

attempt to describe its subjective experience. This emotional description of pain should not be denied or discounted simply because the practitioner may not know how to translate it. The person's emotional verbiage about their pain is indeed an image of how the energy in the body is somatizing itself and affecting the viscera, the psyche (Shen) and ultimately the Qi and the Blood. It provides important clues as to the nature and etiology of the pain.

Table 18.1 provides a fairly comprehensive guide for the differential diagnosis of pain from the Oriental perspective. While this chapter does not address the etiology of each of the diagnoses found here, a strong foundation in the etiology and pathogenesis of disease will enable the practitioner to understand the mechanism by which these states come about.

Table 18.1 Characteristics of pain and their corresponding diagnoses according to classical Chinese medicine

Pain characteristics	Diagnosis
A. Onset	
1. Sudden onset	Excess or Deficiency
2. Acute onset (the transitory nature of the pain experience)	Excess, sudden, sharp, severe
3. Gradual onset	Deficiency
4. Intermittent and irregular pain	Diseases of the biliary tract, stomach, intestine and parasites
B. Nature of the pain	
1. Distending, feelings of oppression, non-specific location, fluctuating intensity with bloating or fullness	Qi Stagnation
2. Dull, mild, bothersome, nagging, discomfort	Irregular flow of Qi and Blood
3. Slight and accompanied by fatigue	Dampness or Qi Deficiency
4. Numb	Qi and/or Blood Deficiency or Phlegm
5. Tingling	Blood Deficiency
6. Pricking	Localized Blood Stasis
7. Sharp, cutting, penetrating, intense	Blood Stagnation
8. Moderate	Qi and Blood Stagnation
9. Localized with distended or stifling sensation, may be localized swelling or mass, fixed hard pain or painful upon pressure, resists dispersion under pressure	Stasis of Qi followed by stasis of Blood, Phlegm
10. Stabbing, boring, piercing	Severe Blood Stagnation
11. Gaseous	Excess pathogenic factor which has led to an obstruction in the flow of Qi and Blood
12. Swelling and bone deformities	Phlegm (turned to bone) obstruction
13. After childbirth	Blood or Yin Deficiency (Xu) or Blood Stagnation
14. Sensation of heaviness	Dampness
15. Moves from place to place	Qi Stagnation, internal or exogenous Wind
16. Continuous, no respite, equal intensity	Symptoms of Yang diseases in their last stage
17. Mild prolonged pain	Beginning of Yin diseases
C. Temperature	
1. Heat, fever locally or systemic, red and swollen	Heat
2. Burning, searing, scalding	Pathogenic Fire or preponderance of Yang due to Yin Deficiency
3. Cool, cold, freezing	Cold
D. Pressure or tension	
1. Gnawing	Blood Stasis
2. Severe pain	Obstruction of the channels by pathogenic Cold or Blood Stagnation
3. Sharp	Excess
4. Cramping, wrenching	Cold, Yang Xu
5. Colicky	Intestinal blockage due to Qi or Blood Stagnation
6. Tugging, pulling, taut	Qi Stagnation
7. Tight, pinching, pressing	Qi Stagnation, sinking Qi
8. Heavy, squeezing, crushing, suffocating	Severe Blood Stagnation
9. Slight and accompanied by fatigue	Qi Deficiency and/or Dampness
10. Lancinating pain around the navel	Blood repletion
11. Swollen	Qi Stagnation
12. Feels full with no pain	Obstruction
13. Feels full with pain	Full condition
E. Duration	
1. Dull/lingering	Deficiency
2. Intermittent scurrying in the umbilical region, paroxysmal with drilling sensation	Stagnation due to parasites (Chong ji)
3. Constant, steady, enduring	Blood Stagnation
4. Periodic, intermittent, brief	Qi Stagnation
5. Pulsing, throbbing, pounding	Cold Stagnation
F. Location	
1. In many areas of the body accompanied by pathogenic soreness and heaviness	Pathogenic factors invading the channels and collaterals

Table 18.1 *continued*

Pain characteristics	Diagnosis
2. Wandering, migrating	Wind (draft)
3. Focal, fixed, heavy	Dampness
4. Generalized, diffuse	Qi Deficiency
5. Deep	Interior problems
6. Superficial	Exterior problems
7. Spreading, radiating	Heat
8. Jumping, shooting	Internal Wind
9. Actual location (e.g. chest, abdomen, etc.)	
G. What makes it better or worse?	
1. Relieved by pressure, palpation	Deficiency, usually of Qi, Blood or Yin, Cold
2. Exacerbated by pressure	Excess, mainly from exogenous pathogenic factors, obstruction of the channels, Qi and Blood Stagnation, food or Phlegm retention, intestinal parasites
3. Soothed by heat	Cold
4. Better with cold	Heat
5. Aggravated by food	Excess
6. Alleviated by food	Deficiency
7. Better with rest	Deficiency
8. Better with movement	Excess or Cold or Yang Deficiency
9. Worse with movement	Heat
10. Better with lying down	Deficiency
11. Better with sitting	Excess
12. Increases in humid weather	Dampness
13. Increases in cold weather	Yang Deficiency and/or Cold
14. Relieved by passing flatus or belching	Qi Stagnation
H. How does the pain impact the person? Nauseating, sickening, killing, unbearable, frightful, agonizing, distressing: 'It's going to give me a stroke'; 'It's a challenge, an opportunity or lesson to learn something about my life', etc.	Interpret each according to your insight and Chinese medical theory

Table 18.2 cross-references the various presentations of pain according to the diagnosis of pain. Additionally, common clinical manifestations are provided to illustrate each type of pain.

TREATMENT

The proper treatment of pain disorders in traditional Chinese medicine is based upon an understanding of how that pain developed. In the *Classic of internal medicine (Neijing)*, Chapter 1 of *Simple questions (Suwen)* points out that, 'Injured Qi is pain'. Hence, pain arises from a problem in the flow of Qi and Blood through the channels, organs and tissues. Additionally, Chapter 74 of *Simple questions* instructs that, 'When the Heart is serene, all pain is negligible'. This statement implies that the perception of pain is through the spirit. Thus, acupuncture can relieve pain utilizing two therapeutic mechanisms:

1. by restoring the flow of Qi and the Blood, such that blockages or obstructions to the flow of Qi and Blood are regulated
2. by changing the patient's perception of pain by treating the spirit.

With these guidelines in mind, acupoints can be selected to treat the multiple manifestations of pain, such that Stagnation may be set in motion and/or the spirit may be changed.

Many practitioners address pain with various electrical stimulation devices such as TENS machines. Painful areas can be anesthetized and Stagnation dispersed with this method of stimulation. However, electrical stimulation is most effective when treating the Stagnations that are

Table 18.2 Diagnostic categories of pain

Pain category	Pain characteristics	Clinical manifestations
Qi Stagnation	a. Distension, feeling of oppression, non-specific location, fluctuating intensity with bloating or fullness b. Slight and accompanied by fatigue c. Periodic, intermittent, brief d. Generalized, diffuse e. Numb f. Tugging, pulling, taut, occasional twitching g. Tight, pinching, pressing h. Moves from place to place i. Exacerbated by pressure j. Colicky k. Moderate l. Dull, mild, bothersome, nagging, discomforting m. Moves slowly	Dull headaches, stomachache, backache, abdominal distension, pain in the chest and abdomen due to emotional disturbances, fullness in the hypochondrium
Blood Stagnation	a. Moderate b. Stabbing, boring, piercing c. After childbirth d. Gnawing e. Severe f. Colicky g. Heavy, squeezing, crushing, suffocating h. Constant, steady, enduring i. Exacerbated by pressure j. Pricking k. Localized with distended or stifling sensation; may be/localized swelling or mass, fixed hard pain or painful upon pressure	Severe headache, stomachache, appendicitis, hard lumps, lancinating pain around the navel and abdomen, tumors, local fixed palpable masses worse at night
Wind (draft)	a. Internal or exogenous Wind b. Jumping, shooting c. Wandering, migrating, shifting around fast	Joint pain, rheumatic arthritis, headache
Damp	a. Slight and accompanied by fatigue b. Sensation of heaviness c. Focal, fixed, and heavy d. Increases in humid weather	Heavy, swollen joints, headache or sinusitis
Phlegm Stagnation	a. Numb b. Swelling and bone deformities c. Exacerbated by pressure d. A mix of Qi and Blood Stagnation feelings	Chest and substernal pain, headache with nausea, bronchitis
Fluid Stagnation	a. Similar to Phlegm but more watery	Gurgling, swelling
Food Stagnation	a. Exacerbated by pressure b. Feelings of fullness	Stomachache, intestinal fullness, frontal headache, nausea, belching with foul odor, indigestion
Cold Stagnation	a. Cool, cold, freezing b. Cramping, wrenching c. Severe pain d. Pulsing, throbbing, pounding e. Soothed by heat f. Better with movement g. Increases in cold weather h. Relieved by pressure, aching pain	Cold sensations accompanying the pain, such as limb or abdominal pain
Heat Stagnation (Fire)	a. Heat, febrile locally or systemic fever, red and swollen b. Burning, searing, scalding c. Spreading, radiating	Heat and swelling sensations, abscesses, hard lumps

Table 18.2 *continued*

Pain category	Pain characteristics	Clinical manifestations
	d. Better with cold e. Worse with movement	
Worm Stagnation	a. Intermittent 'scurrying' or paroxysmal drilling sensation in the umbilical region b. Exacerbated by pressure c. Similar to Qi and Blood Stagnation	Vague feelings of uneasiness in the liver, intestines and umbilical region, generalized abdominal pain, rebound pain, some abdominal distension, slight abdominal tenderness on deep pressure
Deficiency	a. Sudden onset (although has been developing) b. Gradual onset c. Dull, lingering d. Relieved by pressure, may feel hollow e. Better with rest f. Alleviated by food g. Better with movement (Yang Xu) h. Better with lying down i. After childbirth (Yin or Blood Xu) j. Tingling (Blood Xu) k. Numb (Blood Xu) l. Tight, pinching, pressing (sinking Qi) m. Increase in cold weather (Yang Xu) n. Usually manifests as Yin, Yang, Qi or Blood Deficiency	Feelings of emptiness, hunger, fatigue
Excess	a. Sudden onset b. Acute onset c. Sharp d. Pathogenic factor, which has lead to an obstruction of the flow of Qi and Blood, leading to gaseous pain e. Pathogenic factors invading the channels and collaterals in many areas of the body accompanied by soreness and heaviness f. Aggravated by food g. Better with sitting h. Better with movement i. Exacerbated by pressure (exogenous pathogens or obstruction of the channels)	Pain which lasts a long time, difficult to relieve, migraines, gallstones

true Excesses, as opposed to Stagnations due to underlying Deficiencies. Not having a penchant for electricity or machines, I have observed that a strong needle technique or vigorous palpation style can accomplish the same result in most cases.

As we know, the spirit resides in the Heart. The classical paradigm of the Three Treasures (Jing, Shen and Qi) reminds us that when the spirit (Shen) is affected, it must be treated first. Treating the spirit first 'roots it in the body' so that the Qi can then be manipulated. Failing to initially treat the spirit often leads to an improper treatment.

Treatment strategies for each type of pain with classical categories of Chinese acupoints

The Chinese knowledge of acupoint functions is summarized in their repertoire of point energetics. Some classical categories of acupoints that practitioners should consider as part of their arsenal in the treatment of pain come to mind. These include Luo points, Xi (cleft) points, Influential points, Confluent points, Five Seas and auricular points. As we have seen in this text, Luo points, Xi (cleft) points, Influential points and Confluent points constitute a large portion of the clearance points (Table 8.2).

Table 18.3 summarizes the clinical differentiation of these six categories, including specific powerful points within each category. Cases illustrating the effectiveness of certain points are provided at the end of this chapter. Table 18.3 lists locations and needling parameters for these selected acupoints. With the exception of Gall Bladder 34, all of these locations have been previously depicted in Figures 8.8, 8.9, 8.11, 8.12, 8.13, 8.14, 8.16 and 8.17. Figure 17.3 illustrates the Chinese and Japanese locations of GB 34.

My training in both the Chinese and Japanese acupuncture systems and my preference for palpating points as part of the diagnostic process have revealed that certain locations are more clinically significant in relieving pain. This finding has been verified through repeated practice. Knowledge of diverse locations offers the practitioner varied options for the multiple ways in which pathology can manifest. The Japanese locations presented in Table 18.4 are recommended by Kiiko Matsumoto and the Chinese locations are the standardized locations taught in China (Beijing College 1980). I frequently check both of them for tenderness.

As you may have noted, Cases 18.2, 18.3 and 18.4 did not utilize abdominal clearing, although they could have. What I am trying to stress here is the efficacy of certain types of points for the immediate treatment of pain.

PAIN MANAGEMENT PLAN

For people living with pain, a coping strategy is essential. For example, a patient who experiences daily headaches due to vascular constriction in the neck may need to have regular chiropractic treatments, do exercises to relax the musculature of the neck and shoulders, receive acupuncture to regulate the Liver or examine the occupational hazards or stress in his life. A plan that acknowledges the existence of the pain and then leads to a course of action not only empowers patients to take care of themselves but may reduce or relieve the pain. Different approaches to pain management are effective with different types of pain.

Table 18.3 Six classical acupuncture point categories and the treatment of pain

Point category	Functional purpose	Examples
1. Connecting (Luo xue)	'Drainage ditches' to divert Excess from an organ–meridian complex or its coupled organ–meridian complex	Particularly useful Luo points include: LR 5 (Ligou), PC 6 (Neiguan), LU 7 (Lieque), SP 4 (Gongsun)
2. Xi (cleft) (Xi xue)	Points of accumulation or blockage (reflex points) in the organ–meridian complex	ST 34 (Liangqui), Xi (cleft) point of the Stomach channel, is a clinically effective point in the treatment of pain
3. Influential (Ba hui xue)	Points that exert a specific effect over certain functions and associated entities of the body	GB 34 (Yanglingquan) dominates the 'muscles' and CV 12 (Zhongwan) dominates the Yang organs: two powerful Influential points
4. Confluent (Ba mai jiao hui xue)	'Rain barrels' or reservoirs for collecting Excess or supplementing Deficiency. Also known as the Master points of the Eight Extraordinary Meridians. They activate the physiology pertaining to those vessels	LU 7 (Ren mai), KI 6 (Yinqiao mai), SP 4 (Chong mai), PC 6 (Yinwei mai), SI 3 (Du mai), BL 62 (Yangqiao mai), TE 5 (Yangwei mai), GB 41 (Dai mai)
5. Five seas	Pertains to energetic zones of the body, powerful foci of essential substances	SP 10 (Xuehai) in particular is a potent Sea acupoint – a Sea of Blood
6. Auricular	Vortices of energy which work rapidly due to the amount of Qi and Blood with which they are infused, their proximity to the brain and the number of meridians that pass through and around the ear	Shenmen, Prostate, Liver, Sympathetic, etc.

TE = standard abbreviation of the World Health Organization (1989) for Triple Warmer.

Table 18.4 Locations and corresponding needling parameters for selected acupoints from Table 18.3

Point	Locations	Needling parameters
LR 5 (Ligou)	Three locations: see Fig. 8.14 Chinese: 1. On the medial aspect and near the medial border of the tibia (in a small vertical depression on the bone) 2. On the medial aspect and near the medial border of the tibia (right off the bone) Japanese: 3. Midway between SP 9 (Yinlingquan) and the tip of the medial malleolus (off the bone)	Posteriorly, horizontally, 0.3–0.5 in. Same as above Horizontally upward in the direction of the meridian; depth: 0.1–0.2 in.
ST 34 (Liangqiu)	Japanese location: see Fig. 8.9 Two cun above the laterosuperior border of the patella. (Cup your palm over the patella. The point is located where the thumb rests on the lateral aspect of the leg.) This point is more lateral than the Chinese equivalent	Insert using standard direction angles and depths
SP 10 (Xuehai)	Japanese location: see Fig. 8.12 Two cun above the mediosuperior border of the patella. Similar to Chinese SP 10 but much more medial. Use same technique as for finding ST 34 (Liangqiu) described above but on the inside of the leg	Insert using standard direction angles and depths
GB 34 (Yanglingquan)	Japanese location: see Fig. 17.3 One cun posterior to Chinese GB 34, i.e. behind the head of the fibula	Insert using standard direction angles and depths
KI 6 (Zhaohai)	Japanese location: see Fig. 8.8 One cun directly below the medial malleolus at the junction of the red and the white skin	Insert the needle 0.1–0.2 cun transversely towards the heel
GB 41 (Zulinqi)	Japanese location: see Fig. 8.13 Anterior to the cuboid bone	Insert the needle 0.3–0.5 in. towards the toes
BL 62 (Shenmai)	Japanese location: see Fig. 8.17 The same location as Chinese BL 61	Insert the needle 0.3–0.5 in. towards the toes

---

Case 18.1 Prostatitis treated with Luo and auricular points

The patient was a 42-year-old medical doctor diagnosed with multiple sclerosis. He manifested a complex of problems that were part of his syndrome pattern. His major complaint centered on extreme, intermittent fatigue for the previous 7 years. It was accompanied by the following symptoms: 1) leg spasticity and burning pain, 2) lack of bladder control with fluctuations between urgency and a weak stream and/or painful urinary retention, 3) blurred vision and spots before his eyes, 4) loss of balance, and 5) painful constipation and bowel cramps.

His tongue was red, thin, trembling and slightly deviated. The sides and tip of the tongue were redder and rough. There were cracks in the Stomach and chest areas. The tongue coating was thick, white, dry and unrooted. On the Kidney and Liver areas, where there was no coating, the tongue had a glossy or mirror appearance.

His voice was quivery and weak; his lips were pale and sometimes slightly purple in color. He looked pale and tired and usually felt hot on palpation. The pulse was slightly fast, deep, thin and wiry with an irregular missed beat. The Lung, Kidney and Liver positions were particularly deficient.

Because of the overall Deficiency of his condition and the chronic nature of the complaint, I treated him for a period of 2 years, usually on a weekly basis. However, when acute, painful obstructions developed due to underlying Deficiencies, immediate relief was required which entailed treatment several times per week. During such acute episodes, Luo points and auricular points were selected because of their unique attributes.

Case 18.1 Prostatitis treated with Luo and auricular points (*continued*)

From time to time, the excess energy manifested as prostatitis, a sequela of his urinary disturbance. His prostate gland would become enlarged and produced symptoms of referred burning pain to the penis with perineal and suprapubic aching, urinary frequency, urgency, discomfort during urination, difficulty initiating the stream, night-time urination and an inability to ejaculate.

When these symptoms developed, I tried several different approaches including Chinese herbs, plum blossom needling therapy and acupuncture, all of which worked. However, the most immediate and most lasting results arose from the use of two points used alone or in combination, depending upon his condition. They are presented here.

1. Auricular point – prostate. Upon needle insertion and a strong dispersion technique, the patient would report that he could feel the burning, achiness and referred pain diminish in less than 10 seconds. Tremendously relieved from the pain, he would become relaxed, even sleepy. To maintain the results, I would treat him daily for 3 days, which appeared successful in bringing about the reversal of his symptoms.
2. Liver 5 (Ligou), the Luo point of the Liver channel, worked very well for draining off or dispersing excess, stuck or perverse energy. Initially, to confirm that Liver 5 was appropriately selected, as I do with every point that I consider needling, I palpated the three locations of the points (see Fig. 8.14). A strong Ah shi reaction at this point indicated that the Liver channel was in Excess. The Liver meridian encircles the external genitalia which is one of the reasons why it was chosen.

The point was needled in the direction of the meridian (upward), using it as a longitudinal Luo to stimulate the channel but with a strong dispersion technique to relieve the Excess. Often, simply the strong palpation of the point provided relief but I always inserted a needle to reinforce the dispersion brought about by the palpation. In this way, the Luo point was one of the best points to use for draining the Excess from the organ–meridian complex.

Case 18.2 Xi (cleft) points: an energetic, philosophical model for pain and blockage

The patient was a 39-year-old male with acute lumbago following vigorous exercise. He hadn't exercised strenuously in a long time and had a history of minor episodes of back strain usually brought on by lifting heavy objects, a common cause of acute lumbago.

Mindful of the self-care considerations for this familiar type of injury, he proceeded to rest, take hot baths using bath salts, applied Chinese liniments and bruise plasters, all of which provided some relief but only for a limited time. In this instance, the back strain was quite severe and 6 weeks later, despite his efforts, he had not recovered. He sought relief via acupuncture.

In this case, I chose distal points because of their effectiveness. The Six Division model* (Liu jing bian zheng) was implemented. I chose SI 6 (Yanglao) and BL 63 (Jinmen), the Taiyang Xi (cleft) points that specifically treat acute lumbago.

SI 6 (Yanglao), in the upper part of the body, was needled first on the left side. The acupoint was needled with a coarse (#28 gauge) Chinese needle and strong stimulation; that is, a dispersive technique but in the direction of the flow of the meridian. The patient described strong energy going up his arm. At the same time he was instructed to stand and to mobilize his back by swaying to activate the affected area. His back immediately felt better, even though he had endured 6 weeks of pain that had ranged from residual discomfort to immobilization.

To consolidate the effect, BL 63 (Jinmen), the corresponding Xi (cleft) point, was also needled on the left side against the flow of energy in the meridian. However, the effect was not as great as with SI 6 (Yanglao) because SI 6 had worked so effectively. The needles were retained only for the time required to achieve the desired needle sensation and to note improvement. After this treatment the patient reported that his back was fine! Application of the Six Division model of coupled Xi (cleft) points can be an elegant, understated treatment strategy that yields dramatic and effective results when appropriately selected.

---

* The Six Division energetic model is used here as a treatment strategy in which the Xi (cleft) points of the meridians are paired together. This treatment strategy reflects the Chinese cosmological view of 'as above, so below'. This expression means that both the organ–meridian complex which is impaired 'above' (upper part of the body) and the corresponding complex 'below' (lower part of the body) will tend to be affected in acute conditions because of their Six Divisions coupling (see Gardner-Abbate 1996, pp. 75–79).

A fundamental rule of treatment in Chinese medicine is to treat what you see; hence, an understanding of the etiology and pathogenesis permits insight into the root of a problem so that the causative factors can be addressed. When causative factors can be ascertained, a pain management plan can be formulated that directly addresses these factors. One's preferred health-

---

Case 18.3 Blockage in the Heart treated with a Xi (cleft) point

The patient was a 28-year-old woman with an unusual complaint of profuse but odorless daytime sweating of the hands and feet. This complaint was a source of great consternation to the patient. I was called in to see her in a fast-paced clinical setting.

The patient craved large glasses of cold drinks and her face was red. From observation I detected two emotions fluctuating between grief and excess joy. The other practitioners had diagnosed her with 'Excess Dampness'. I did not agree based upon the clinical data mentioned above.

According to Chinese medicine, sweat is the body fluid that pertains to the Heart. It is a derivative of the Blood. The loss of too much body fluid can lead to both Blood and Yin Deficiency, so this is not a superficial problem. Profuse daytime sweat can be diagnosed as Heat Stagnation in the Heart leading to Heart and Lung Qi Deficiency.

To the amazement of the other practitioners, my point of choice was Heart 6 (Yinxi), the Xi (cleft) point of the Heart. It relieves Stagnation; in this case, the Excess Heat or Fire which causes (1) the fluid to be driven out of the blood, and (2) sweating to occur through the pores, which are regulated by the Lungs. When the Fire element is excessive it overacts on Metal and makes the Lungs weak, hence the sweating.

Upon the arrival of Qi, the patient began to cry with much emotion. The observers thought it was because of a painful needle technique. As we pursued the significance, she revealed feelings that she had harbored for many years – that her mother had never said that she loved her, even though she knew this was not the case. The other practitioners had not expected this development. Following this treatment session, the sweating subsided.

This is an interesting case of the use of a Xi (cleft) point to treat emotional pain that had turned to Heat Stagnation and caused the physical symptom of excess daytime sweat.

Case 18.4 Trauma from an automobile accident treated with auricular and Confluent points

The patient was a 44-year-old man who had been in an automobile accident on the previous day; he had been seen in a hospital emergency room and released following the accident. When I met him in the waiting room he was clearly disturbed. His eyes were wandering uncontrollably, his pupils were dilated and he couldn't seem to maintain normal eye contact. His speech was affected and, although coherent, he spoke excessively and rambled; he complained of multiple aches and pains as a result of the impact. (He had also made an appointment to see a chiropractor later in the week to have his spine and neck evaluated.)

It was apparent that this patient was suffering from post-traumatic disorientation and did not need any more trauma or invasion in the form of too many needles. Before attending to secondary aches and pains, the first thing that needed to be done was to treat him as a 'whole person'; this included integrating his spirit, which clearly needed to be 'rooted' and secured in his body.

I chose two points: ear Shenmen (Spirit Gate) to quiet the Heart, calm the spirit and reduce pain* and Kidney 6 (Zhaohai), the Confluent point of the Yin heel vessel to root the spirit. The Kidney channel has a branch that intersects with the Heart and needling Kidney 6 (Zhaohai) in combination with Shenmen has the synergistic effect of calming the Heart, nourishing the Yin, relieving trauma and anxiety.

Upon needle insertion at ear Shenmen, the patient immediately became quiet, calm and tranquil. He reported that when the needle was inserted at Kidney 6 (Zhaohai) he saw a 'restful sea'. Interestingly, translations of this point name include Reflection on the Sea, Shining Sea and Luminous Sea. During treatment I verbally tried to reinforce this important image for him.

Upon completion of the treatment, the patient appeared extremely rested and peaceful, in contrast to his previous state. Much of the emotional trauma had subsided; he was now re-rooted in the world.

---

* HT 7 (Shenmen) could have been used instead of auricular Shenmen; however, ear points work remarkably fast, as discussed here.

care provider should be consulted to formulate a plan with which the patient can comply. However, particularly in cases of progressive, degenerative, terminal disease with pain, pain management may be just that – a way to cope with the pain.

At this juncture, pain experts are better than I at providing strategies to relieve this type of suffering. Their therapies include, but are not limited to, pain support groups, metered medication, physical therapy intervention, hospice care and multidisciplinary team care. Of the cases that I have treated (that have not involved degenerative illness), most of the pain has been associated with daily occurrences like accidents, emotional problems and organ dysfunction. The modalities and the acupoints described above have yielded profound clinical results.

Just as coping mechanisms vary for patients who live with pain, so too does the response of partners or those who live with them. In my experience, both as a patient and a practitioner, I have observed varying reactions to pain. Frequently, the family and friends of pain patients do not know how to help them. As a result, feelings of helplessness on both sides are not uncommon and such helplessness may often lead to avoidance of the problem. While there is no shortage of books by pain specialists on how family members can learn to cope with the pain that affects their loved ones, my assessment of this topic focuses on three factors – acknowledgment, awareness and articulation.

Acknowledgment means recognizing that pain is part of the patient's experience. It is their reality. Not to reckon with it is, in effect, to deny it and this attitude will not help the sufferer. It tends to cause further Stagnation which in turn causes pain because the problem is in essence ignored.

Awareness is a further step on the continuum of acknowledgment. It means being attentive to the person, 'tuning in' to how they are feeling, being sensitive and compassionate. 'Touching base' with them daily simply by asking how the person is doing and being truly available to listen to the response has a tremendous healing capacity.

Articulation allows talking about the experience, letting people describe their pain and how it is affecting them. I believe that not giving patients an outlet to express their pain, whether in the form of talking, sighing, crying or any other reaction, only serves to cause more 'injured Qi' and Stagnation and indeed may exacerbate their pain. The simplest human responses, such as saying 'It must be awful to have that pain' and allowing the person to say, 'Yes, it is', may have more therapeutic effect than any chemical medication, herb, acupuncture point or device.

In conclusion, while doctors, psychologists, pain specialists and other healthcare providers certainly have an important role in assisting people with their suffering, when confronted with those in pain we can all be, genuinely and simply, a human being 'reaching out' to another with great healing effect. Sometimes that reaching out includes professional and simple human touch.

NEW WORDS AND CONCEPTS

Five Seas – classical literature refers to the Si Hai (Four Seas). However, various sources designate these seas differently. Universally recognized are the Sea of Qi, Sea of Blood and Sea of Marrow. Some sources refer to a Sea of Nourishment and others have added the Sea of Internal Pollution. I have taken the liberty of combining them, thus I refer to the Five Seas (Liu & Liu 1989, pp. 40–44).

Shang Han Lun – *Discussion of Cold-induced disorders* by Zhong Zhong-Jing, written around 220 CE.

Three Treasures – the classical diagnostic framework utilizing Qi, Jing and Shen as essential substances.

TENS machines – transcutaneous electrical nerve stimulation devices, used to inhibit the physiological pain response.

QUESTIONS

1. Extrapolating from the Chinese medical definition of pain, the author views pain as different manifestations of Stagnation. What are the three general types of manifestation proposed by the author?

2. What is the functional role of pain in the body?

3. Why and how might multiple levels of pain develop within the body?

4. Discuss the importance of the patient's personal description of their pain.

5. What are the two therapeutic mechanisms by which acupuncture can relieve pain?

6. Which point is the primary pain point? What energetics give it this distinction?

7. Pick one of the acute abdominal syndromes from Table 11.1 Then try to diagnose and categorize the symptoms of pain for that illness. Use the classical Chinese tables on pain given in this chapter to help you.

19

The modalities

In this final chapter the use of the various treatment modalities in this system is recapitulated. Each of these methods was listed throughout this book in relevant chapters. Now as a summary they will all be brought together to remind the practitioner of their broad range of use as well as their specific clinical applications.

The primary modalities discussed in this work are the basic tools of Oriental medicine. The modalities center around the use of palpation, needles, moxa in its various forms, particularly with the Tiger Thermie warmer or insulations like ginger or salt, intradermal needles, liniments and the rolling pin. What makes them different is the specificity of use and how the Chinese and Japanese use of the modalities differs, as was pointed out in Table 2.1.

PALPATION

Palpation is the primary modality for both diagnosis and treatment by the practitioner and self-treatment by the patient. It can be used on its own to maintain health, as the leading diagnostic and treatment style, or as an adjunct for practitioners who have established their own method of treatment but seek information derived through touch. It is involved in the three major physical exams in this book and all the subsets of evaluations that make up the Japanese physical exam.

The palpation modality frees up the surface, contacts the Qi of the meridians, including the secondary vessels, and allows the Jing or core level to be reached. It provides an immediate and verifiable index to the patient and the practitioner of the degree of bodily disharmony and its remediation. In addition, it confers the subtle therapeutic benefits of human touch.

NEEDLES

The use of needles is the second major modality for regulating Qi and Blood, especially to re-inforce any of the palpation exams that are first cleared by hand but also as treatment-of-disease points for certain conditions. As we have seen, the aim within this system is to reduce the number of needles in treatment, so that the points finally selected for needling rectify the root pathology. The needling method tends to be superficial, gentle, obtains little or no Qi and is frequently a tonification method because most root pathologies are Deficiencies. The tonification is usually achieved by a shallow insertion and especially by needling in the direction of the meridian flow.

MOXIBUSTION

Moxibustion is an unsurpassed modality for regulating the Qi and Blood due to its unique therapeutic properties. It can be administered in many forms. The following list comprises the most common methods of delivery.

Tiger Thermie warmer

The Tiger Thermie warmer is an extremely effective method of moxa application for several reasons.

1. It allows the application of the moxa virtually onto the skin so that the heat is more precisely targeted. It can be used like direct moxa by holding the implement on the surface of the skin until it feels hot. Each time the patient says it is hot it is the equivalent of a direct moxibustion method.
2. It has the unrivaled benefit of simultaneously conferring the therapeutic benefits of moxa while applying the pressure of palpation in order to break up obstruction or loosen tissue.

3. The tool and the moxa are inexpensive.
4. It is easy to learn how to use it and patients can use it to treat themselves at home on a frequent basis, thus expediting the healing process.
5. Patients love the soothing heat of the Tiger Thermie. They find it relaxing and comply well with using it.

Belly bowl

The belly bowl is a relatively small metal stand that keeps the moxa over a point or area (Fig. 19.1). This is actually a Korean tool that can be adapted to Japanese or Chinese treatments. I use it exclusively over the navel when performing navel treatments. The belly bowl moxa is crude, thick and coarse and so burns quickly. Therefore it is important to lift it frequently to make sure that the patient's skin is not burned. Use cautiously with patients who have sensitive skin or who have diminished pain perception such as the elderly, diabetics or those with neurological disorders. The moxa produces a rich resin on the skin that can be covered and affixed with a gauze pad for a few hours so that the moxa oil can be absorbed.

Rice grain or mini-thread size moxa

Rice grain or mini-thread size moxa is directly applied to the point and burned down until the patient says 'hot'. It is a direct, non-scarring method of directing heat precisely into the point.

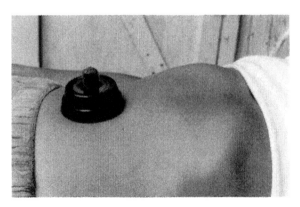

Figure 19.1 The belly bowl.

Only pure-grade moxa should be burned directly onto the skin to avoid introducing impurities into the burn that might cause infection. The rice grain size can be rolled prior to application. The thread size can be purchased from most suppliers. To avoid burning the patients, ignite these very small moxa with an incense stick instead of a match or other tool. The amount of smoke created is very small and less noxious to the patients or the practitioner if they have an aversion to large amounts of smoke.

Moxa insulations (such as on ginger and salt)

Used with ginger, moxa is unsurpassed in tonifying the Yang, especially of the Lung, Spleen and Kidney. Ginger is a hot herb. When the moxa is burned on top of the ginger, the Yang of the moxa and the ginger is conveyed to the area and the physiological functions that the point controls. When salt is put in the navel it acts as both an insulator from burns but also a conductor of the moxa specifically to the point CV 8.

INTRADERMALS

Intradermals are small subcutaneous needles used to implant an acupoint to promote the same effects as needling but on a sustained basis. They reinforce the action of the point because they are retained. Guard against infection by retaining the intradermals for approximately 3–5 days depending upon humidity levels or exposure to water. Provide patients with written instructions on how to remove them or ask them to return to your office for removal so that infection does not develop.

LINIMENTS

Each liniment has its own therapeutic properties. The ones I am most inclined to use are those which are warm or hot in nature such as Zheng Gu Shui (hot), Tieh Da Yao Gin (warm) or Possum On (Warm). They are unsurpassed at moving Qi and Blood and dispersing Stagnation. While they can be used on their own, generally the combination of a liniment with a modality

such as the Tiger Thermie warmer has added clinical effect.

ROLLING PIN

The simple device of a rolling pin can be used to regulate the Yin and the Yang energies of the meridians of the legs. It is useful in breaking down fat, Phlegm and Damp, resolving inner thigh compression and regulating the Blood and Blood pressure.

CONCLUSION

Upon completion of this book, I hope you now feel that Japanese acupuncture is a valuable system. One of its greatest strengths is that it is based on the *Nanjing*, with its sensitivity to the natural laws of life. This Taoist view posits that energy is infused in the universe and in man, specifically in the meridians of the body. Through palpation, the energy of the meridian can be contacted and adjusted in order to bring the person back into balance and health.

Do not look at this material as the best way to do things; it is simply part and parcel of the most ancient Chinese material. The techniques that are best for you are based upon your skill and your ability to reach out and to touch another human being with compassion. The diagnostic paradigm or treatment modality with which you have success is the proper one for you to use.

As D H Lawrence maintained, touch is more than epidermal, it is a profound penetration into the core of one's being (Ackerman 1990, p. 71). And the *Neijing* likewise asserts that the purpose of treatment is to establish contact with another person's spirit. Palpation, with the accompanying sensations evoked through it, such as laughter and curiosity, heightened awareness of bodily processes and their remediation, achieves this.

On the physical level, even the simplest touch – a hand on the shoulder, an arm around the waist – has been shown to reduce heart rate, lower Blood pressure and decrease levels of the stress hormones cortisol and norepinephrine. Such studies have sometimes shown this touch to be a matter of life or death. Surely palpation is that magic hand which, by touching the person, the organs, the meridians, and the spirit, can penetrate to the core of our vital Essence, our life force, the Spring that is within us all and bestows renewed life upon us.

NEW WORDS AND CONCEPTS

Direct moxa – a method of moxibustion in which moxa is burned directly on the skin. It can be of a scarring or non-scarring variety.

Indirect moxa – a method of moxibustion in which moxa is applied to the body but not directly on the skin. For instance, it may be administered in an implement such as a Tiger or Lion Thermie warmer, moxa box, moxa stick, belly bowl or other moxa instrument.

QUESTIONS

1. According to the system presented in this book, what will almost always be the core strategy for any illness and what will be the primary modality used to achieve this?

2. For each modality presented in this chapter, give the clinical indications for which it would be most effective.

Forms

SECTION CONTENTS

FORM 1 ABDOMINAL DIAGNOSIS: THE HEALTHY HARA EXAMINATION

Patient's name: _____ Date: _____

Major complaint: _____

Check (✓) in the Normal column if the patient has this healthy characteristic, check (✓) in the Abnormal column if the finding is abnormal.

Characteristics (The Healthy Hara)	Significance/Comments Keep hands there a short amount of time	Normal	Abnormal	Diagnosis
1. Temperature: a) fairly uniform	As warm-blooded mammals, the human body is more Yang than Yin.			
b) cooler above umbilicus	Why should there be a cool Stomach and *not* a warm Stomach? Warmth consumes Yin which leads to ST Yin Xu and Heat which leads to KI Yin Xu.			
c) warmer in the lower right quadrant (LRQ), the Mingmen area	LRQ = Yin, Yin, Yin. Needs Mingmen Fire to balance it. Therefore should feel warm.			
2. Moisture: a) slightly moist	Not dried up, withered, scaly or fatty deposits.			
3. Resilient: a perpendicular assessment. Check: CV 12, ST 25L, ST 25R, CV 6, CV 4 a) bouncy, elastic, not hard or mushy (If abnormal note quality found in Abnormal column.)	1. Hard, Excess, replete, aggravated by pressure = tense, unhealthy tissue. 2. Mushy = Deficiency, vacant, soft or full but not aggravated by pressure; pain may be relieved. 3. Hardness on top often has Deficiency below or the reverse. Patient says doesn't feel anything.			
CV 12				
ST 25L				
ST 25R				
CV 6				
CV 4				
4. Strength: a surface assessment done at CV 12 and ST 25L a) looser above umbilicus especially at CV 12	1. Substernal tension is the cause of many problems; seen in TCM as KI Yin Xu (because tight = ST Yin Xu). ST Yin Xu leads to KI Yin Xu. Mental degeneration begins with a tight stomach.			
b) stronger on left side ST 25 (Tianshu) (If abnormal, comment on quality found.)	2. Strong ST 25 (Tianshu) = sufficient Blood.			
5. Shape: a) even, symmetrical, including umbilicus, rib cage and size of the sternocostal angle (SCA). Not sunken, fat, thin, puffy, etc. (see Fig. 6.1B)	1. Sunken, thin = Deficiency 2. Puffy, fat = Yang Deficiency 3. Narrow SCA = ST Yin Xu → KI Yin Xu			
6. Pulsation at CV 6: a) palpable in the middle to deep position	Upon palpation should feel pulse at CV 6 (Qihai) = energy of the Kidneys communicating with each other. More important than radial pulse.			

7. Depression along Ren channel and slight depression at CV 12 and above umbilicus	Ren Channel, primordial channel, formed after the first cell division from 1 to 2 cells. Structural meridian. Controls all the Yin meridians. Good constitution, good genetic inheritance.			
8. Breathing: a) noticeable rise and fall of abdomen below umbilicus	To bring LU Qi to KI area. The Kidney grasps the Qi.			
9. Point inspection (for pathology)	See Table 6.2			
10. Other (specify)				

General diagnosis: _____

Treatment plan: _____

FORM 2   THE MODIFIED ABDOMINAL EXAM

Patient's name:_____ Date:_____

Major complaint and accompanying symptoms: _____
_____

Palpate these points	Palpation sensation, degree of tenderness or vacancy	Signs of point pathology	Clinical significance of point pathology or palpation sensation	Clearance points used and degree of clearance obtained
CV 15/14 (Jiuwei/Juque)				
CV 12 (Zhongwan)				
ST 25 (Tianshu) Left and Right				
CV 6 (Qihai)				
CV 4 (Guanyuan)				

General abdominal map: circle points which were tender:

Results of clearance:_____
_____
_____
_____
_____
_____

FORM 3   NAVEL DIAGNOSIS FORM

Patient's name:_____ Date:_____

Major complaint and accompanying symptoms: _____

_____

Record the results of observation and palpation of the navel in the appropriate column

Healthy navel description	Healthy	Unhealthy
1. The navel is well shaped with strong surrounding tissue, a slight depression above it. No interruptions, indentations. Not 'looking up or down'		
2. It has a firm navel border		
3. There is no puffiness around it		
4. There is a full pulsation around it		
5. It is tucked in		
6. It is not too wide		
7. It is not too tiny, too narrow, too deep or too long (specify)		
8. It is not small, flat or shallow		
9. It is centrally located on abdomen		
10. It is loose above and resilient below		
11. The area surrounding the navel is not hard		
12. The area surrounding the navel is without pain or reactivity		
13. There is a slight depression above navel in the area around CV 9 (Shuifen) and no tenderness upon palpation		

Other:_____

Drawing:

Tenderness – where? Describe:_____
_____

Ability to clear navel. What points had the most clearance value?:_____
_____

Treatment with what modalities:_____
_____

Effect on major complaint if any and/or reaction to treatment:_____
_____
_____
_____

FORM 4   THIGH CLEARANCE FORM

Patient's name:_____   Date:_____

Major complaint and accompanying Symptoms: _____

_____

1. After abdominal clearing, what was the most significant pathology remaining that you were unable to obtain sufficient clearance on?_____

_____

_____

_____

_____

2. Circle the leg, meridian and point which was the most tender.

        Right SP 1 2 3 4
               LR 1 2 3 4
               KI 1 2 3 4
         Left SP 1 2 3 4
               LR 1 2 3 4
               KI 1 2 3 4

3. Record points used to clear the most painful thigh points.

Points	Degree it contributed to clearance
KI 1	
LR 4	
SP 6	
KI 6	
KI 3	
KI 7	

4. Describe the patient's reaction to thigh palpation, what you felt if anything upon palpation, presentation of patient's thighs. Then record the results of the thigh clearance/patient's reaction to thigh clearance.

_____

_____

_____

_____

_____

_____

_____

5. After the thigh clearance go back and check the points on the abdomen on which you did not obtain 100% clearance. Was there any change in abdominal presentation? Describe.

_____

_____

_____

_____

FORM 5   SCAR TREATMENT FORM

Patient's name:_____ Date:_____

Major complaint and accompanying symptoms: _____

_____

The Scar – Inspection

1. Description (shape, size, color, texture, height, or any other sensations associated with it): _____

_____

_____

_____

_____

_____

2. Location:_____

_____

_____

_____

Palpation

3. Sensation upon palpation:_____

_____

_____

_____

Treatment

4. Treatment (which modalities used and why):_____

_____

_____

_____

_____

5. Result of treatment of scar (changes in color, size, shape, texture, height, accompanying sensations, other):

_____

_____

_____

_____

_____

6. Effect on major complaint if any:_____

_____

_____

_____

_____

7. Other comments:_____

_____

_____

_____

FORM 6 SINUS EVALUATION FORM

Patient's name:_____ Date:_____

Major complaint and accompanying symptoms: _____

_____

Check off any of the signs and symptoms the patient may have under the appropriate column.

Signs/symptoms	Etiology and diagnosis	Needle techniques	Observations	Abnormal	Normal
1. Sinus problems or history of same.	Weak Lung function, broken nose, birth trauma, etc.	Consult specific manifestation described below and treat			
2. Deviated septum	1. Same as #1 plus lack of free flow of Qi and Blood in the local area leads to insufficient oxygenation. 2. Local infection 3. Trauma – birth, broken nose 4. Drugs	Palpate between nose and facial bones; needle at 45° angle transversely towards the lateral aspect of the face or apply Tiger Thermie to the area. Retain 10–20 minutes.			
3. Floating facial capillaries (engorgement of nasal Blood vessels) on orbital ridge of nose or below eye and/or puffy cheek	1. Focal infection, Heat in the Blood or Heat and Blood Stasis. Can be due to inverted postures, hot water, LR Heat, coffee, alcohol, weather, pollution	Needle transversely towards lateral aspect of face or bleed locally. Relieves hemostasis, invigorates Qi and Blood. Can add LI 4 and LU 7 for facial edema			
4. Tenderness in sinus areas (ST 2, GB 1, Yuyao, BL 2)	Preclinical or clinical sinus problems	Needle perpendicularly or transversely toward the lateral aspect or apply Tiger Thermie moxa around the orbital area for about 3 minutes			
5. Red coloration in the glabella (Yintang) region	1. Pituitary gland reflex can lead to thyroid problems, insomnia, infertility or memory problems 2. Heat in Blood, HT or SP 3. Serious, chronic sinus infection in cavity	Needle or bleed or intradermal Yintang. Can add SI 3			
6. Tight sternocleidomastoid muscle	Particularly posterior SCM = weak immunity or autonomic nervous system problems	See neck protocols ST 9R, use KI 6; ST 9L, use KI 7 then TE 5R, GB 41L for both Needle ST 9 for 1 min. Massage works just as well 1. To treat muscle as a whole: KI 6, KI 7, TE 5, GB 41 2. TE 16 Check – turn head a. ST 25R may clear neck. Why? Neck could = pathogen and ST 25R treats LU and immunity b. Naganos 3. ST 9 – TE 3 releases carotid compression			
7. Pathology at the KI 16 area (or ST 25R)	1. Kidney disorders, Front Mu of the Kidney (according to Dr Manaka) – Kidney is the root of the Qi 2. KI 16 = SP is mother of LU and grandmother of KI	See navel protocols in Chapter 10			

Treatment with additional points:
GV 4 = Tonifies Source Qi – needle 45° upward or Tiger Thermie.
ST 44 = Water point of ST – needle perpendicularly or Tiger Thermie or massage deeply.
TE 3 – Loosens carotid compression to release SCM/compressed carotid. Needle obliquely or proximally.

FORM 7   NECK EVALUATION FORM

Patient's name:_____   Date:_____

Major complaint and accompanying symptoms:_____

_____

Check yes if the neck area is normal, no if it is not.

Area of the neck to examine	Clinical significance	Yes	No	Treatment
1. Evaluation of the sternocleidomastoid muscle (SCM):				With palpation, needles, intradermals, or moxa
a. muscle itself	Right side = sympathetic nervous system disharmony; Left side = parasympathetic nervous system disharmony			For R use KI 6; for L use KI 7; for both use TE 5R, GB 41L Can also use TE 3R or bilateral
b. ST 9 area	Same as above plus possible thyroid problems – see #4			Same as above or needle or massage ST 9
c. posterior border (TE 16 area)	Immune system response (overworked or active battle)			Moxa Naganos or moxa local TE 16 area with Tiger Thermie
2. Scalene muscle evaluation:				
a. height of muscle (GB 21 area) (scalene compression of underlying Blood vessels and nerves)	a. Tight, hard, rock-like = scalene compression b. One side hard/thick, one side soft/thin = scoliosis			Needle LU 7, massage, intradermal Needle LU 7, massage, intradermal
3. Supraclavicular fossa evaluation:	This can lead to Blood Stasis pattern in the occipital region			
a. brachial plexus involvement	Sends Qi and Blood to the musculature of the upper limbs			Tiger Thermie or needle ST 12* or massage
b. vertebral artery	Sends Blood to the brain, head			Tiger Thermie or needle ST 12* or massage
c. subclavian artery	Source of Blood flow to the upper limbs			Tiger Thermie or needle ST 12* or massage
d. left ST 12	Heart Qi Xu			Tiger Thermie or needle ST 12* or massage
e. right ST 12	Spleen Qi Xu with Damp, right lymphatic duct congestion			Tiger Thermie or needle ST 12* or massage
4. Thyroid evaluation	KI Qi, Essence, Yin Xu, with Fire. Hypothyroid = KI Qi or Yang Xu; Hyperthyroid = KI Yin Xu with Fire			Check ST 9, LI 18 and height (top) of SCM muscle, KI 3
5. Fat pad at GV 14	Adrenal exhaustion (severe KI Yang Xu)			Needle GV 14 or moxa Can add GV 4, KI 6, KI 16 or KI 27
6. Blood Stasis patterns in the occipital region	Blood Stagnation			Bloodletting techniques, see Table 16.1

*Remember, when needling ST 12, position patient in the lateral recumbent position. Do not obtain Qi.

FORM 8   TONSILLAR TREATMENT FORM

Patient's name:_____   Date:_____

Major complaint and accompanying symptoms: _____

_____

1. How did you use this treatment?

    On its own ☐

    As the skeletal outline to treatment ☐   List other points_____

    Preventively ☐

    For immunodeficient symptoms ☐

2. How do you feel this prescription might benefit the patient; that is, what is the rationale for the treatment?

_____

_____

_____

_____

3. After abdominal clearing what was the most significant pathology on which you obtained less than satisfactory clearance?

_____

_____

_____

_____

4. Describe the tenderness of the tonsillar points upon palpation.

    TE 16R   _____

    TE 16L   _____

    KI 6R   _____

    KI 6L   _____

    LI 10R   _____

    LI 10L   _____

    GV 14   _____

5. Describe fully the method administered (moxa, needles, including depths of insertion, retention time, etc.).

_____

_____

_____

_____

_____

_____

6. Describe the results of treatment (changes on the difficult point(s) to clear on the abdomen (recorded in #3), how patient felt, problems you had, assessment of treatment, changes in major complaint, accompanying symptoms, etc.).

_____

_____

_____

FORM 9   HOW TO PERFORM BACK EVALUATIONS AND TREATMENT

Back differentiation	Etiology	Clinical manifestation	Treatment	Nor-mal	Abnor-mal
1. On the midline of the back, specifically on the spine or GV channel	Trauma, exogenous pathogens, other causative factors	Back problems, disc problems, low back pain, midline back pain, neck problems, organ problems, shoulder problems, scoliosis, hemorrhoids, sciatica, prostatitis, urinary tract problems	1. LR 4 (Zhongfeng) with pressure or needle obliquely in the direction of the meridian 0.3–0.5 in. Tiger Thermie or massage. Best point for strained back. 2. SI 3L (Houxi – opens GV channel) obliquely 0.5–0.7 in. underneath the bone towards SI 1. With BL 62R (Shenmai – joins Bladder channel), 0.3–0.5 in. in the direction of the meridian towards the toe. Massage or intradermal. 3. Needle BL 20 (Pishu – strengthens muscles), perpendicularly 0.5–1.0 in. or implant intradermal inferiorly in the direction of the meridian. 4. GB 25 (Jingmen – Mu of KI), perpendicularly 0.5–1.0. MA. *Patient must be on their side.* 5. BL 25 (Dachangshu), perpendicularly 1.0–1.2 in. MA. 6. BL 1 (Jingming – moves meridian) perpendicularly 0.3–0.5 in. along the orbital wall. 7. Shiqizhui (below L5), perpendicularly 0.5–1.0 in. MA.		
2. Pain at the end of the spine, specifically the coccyx	Trauma to the coccyx leads to adrenal cortex being affected which can produce hormonal problems	Back tension, spasm, chronic constipation, headache, herniated disc, hormone imbalances, low back pain, neck pain, sciatica, prostatitis, hypoglycemia, diabetes	1. Check for tailbone tenderness by palpating directly below the tailbone and to either side of it. The practitioner or the patient may do it. 2. If tender, the point can be needled (under the bone or into the tense area 0.5–1.0 in.) or the patient should be instructed to massage the point daily.		
3. In the lumbar/ sacral region	Same as #1. Area most structurally weak	Inspect for a flat lumbar area or a puffy sacrum	1. LR 4 (see method above). 2. GV 14 (Dazhui), perpendicularly 0.5–1.0 in., MA.		
4. Lateral to the spine on the quadratus lumborum muscle or Bladder channel	1. KI Deficiency; failure of the Kidney to dominate Water metabolism processes, resulting in improper fat metabolism 2. Sinus problems 3. Feet not properly aligned 4. Sacrotuberous ligament may be involved	1. L4–5 subluxation 2. Tightness in the quadratus fasciae 3. Eating fat makes worse	1. With patient on side release thigh with KI 1 (Yongquan), LR 4 (Zhongfeng). 2. BL 20, GB 25, BL 25, Shiqizhui (same reasons as #1, see above). 3. SP 4 (Gongsun), perpendicularly 0.3–0.5 in. or Tiger Thermie 4. If sinus involvement BL 1 (see above) and BL 2 with Tiger Thermie or 0.3–0.5 in. subcutaneously towards the lateral aspect.		

5. Sacrotuberous ligament	Sinus problems or ankle problems	Disc problems, cement back, frozen back, low back pain with occipital involvement	1. Check BL 62 (Shenmai) for any spinal problem. Could add SI 3 (see method above). 2. Check GB 34 (Yanglingquan) to release muscles – the influential point which dominates the muscles, perpendicularly 0.8–1.2 in. MA. Rub with strong pressure or use an intradermal. 3. If KI involvement add BL 23 (Shenshu), perpendicularly 1.0–1.5 in. MA. 4. TE 5R (Waiguan), perpendicularly 0.7–1.0 in. and GB 41L (Zulinqi), 0.3–0.5 in. in the direction of the meridian if there is neck involvement. 5. If ankle involvement (inverted or everted legs), needle or intradermal BL 62R (Shenmai), (see above) with KI 6 both (Zhaohai), transversely 0.1 in. towards the heel. In sitting position and have patient hold their leg straight.		
6. Pain along the iliac crest, posterior superior iliac spine	Weak lymphatic glands leading to secondary infections that create weak ligaments. This is then reinforced by other lifestyle variables	Back of knee problems, back problems, pubic bone pain	1. Check to see if TE 16 (Tianyou) and Naganos release pain. Tiger Thermie both or for TE 6 needle perpendicularly 0.3–0.5 in. For the Naganos perpendicularly 0.5–1.0 in. Puncture the most tender with a lift-and-thrust method. 2. ST 13 (Qihu) needle 0.3–0.5 in. transversely and bilaterally towards the lateral aspect or use the Tiger Thermie warmer.		
7. Upper back pain – see neck protocols			See sacrotuberous ligament with neck involvement or pain along the midline with neck involvement.		
8. Mid-back pain	Digestive imbalances	Mid-back pain spasm	1. Check BL 62R (see above). 2. Needle digestive points BL 17, 18, 19 (Geshu, Ganshu and Danshu) in direction of meridian obliquely 0.5 in. 3. LR 2 (Xingjian), obliquely 0.3–0.5 in.		

R = right side
L = left side
B = bilateral
MA = Moxa is applicable

Summary – Basic back points:

LR 4 (Zhongfeng) – best point for strained back
KI 7 (Fuliu), – back pain due to KI Xu
SP 3, 4 (Taibai, Gongsun) – any spine problems involving the neck
BL 62 (Shenmai), SI 3 (Houxi) – spinal problems especially with neck involvement

Treatment:_____
_____
_____
_____
_____
_____
_____
_____
_____

Results:_____
_____
_____
_____
_____
_____
_____

Integrated Japanese point location, energetics and needle technique

---

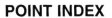

POINT INDEX

Lung

Large Intestine

Stomach

Spleen

2 and 3	Dadu and Taibai
4	Gongsun
6	Sanyinjiao
8	Diji
9	Yinlingquan
10	Xuehai

Heart

7	Shenmen

Small Intestine

3	Houxi
11	Tianzong

Bladder

1	Jingming
2	Zanzhu
17	Geshu
18	Ganshu
20	Pishu
23	Shenshu
57	Chengshan
62	Shenmai
66	Zutonggu

Kidney

1	Yongquan
2	Rangu
3	Taixi
6	Zhaohai
7	Fuliu
9	Zhubin
13	Qixue
16	Huangshu
23, 24, 25	Shenfeng, Lingxu, Shencang
27	Shufu

Pericardium

4	Ximen
6	Neiguan
8	Laogong

Triple Warmer

3	Zhongdu
5	Waiguan
6	Zhigou

16	Tianyou
17	Yifeng

Gall Bladder

1	Tongziliao
15	Toulinqi
25	Jingmen
31	Fengshi
34	Yanglingquan
40	Qiuxu
41	Zulinqi

Liver

2	Xingjian
3	Taichong
4	Zhongfeng
5	Ligou
8	Ququan
12	Jimai
14	Qimen

Governing Vessel

1	Changqiang
2	Yaoshu
3	Yaoyangguan
4	Mingmen
5	Xuanshu
6	Jizhong
11	Shendao
12	Shenzhu
13	Taodao
14	Dazhui
15	Yamen

Conception Vessel

1–2 area	Huiyin-Qugu
3	Zhongji
4	Guanyuan
5	Shimen
6	Qihai
7	Yinjiao
8	Shenque
9	Shuifen
12	Zhongwan
14–15 area	Juque and Jiuwei
17	Tanzhong

THE TREATMENT-OF-DISEASE POINTS

The points listed in this section are what I refer to as the treatment-of-disease points which are simply the acupuncture points of the 14 channels. Here I list the unique energetics of these points and how they fit into the acupuncture system I have described in this book. Many of these points have already been discussed as diagnosis points, clearance points or treatment-of-disease points for the specific illnesses which I have referred to. Additional treatment-of-disease points for illnesses not discussed in the body of the book are provided for the practitioner. These can be used when the treatment approaches described here are not specific enough for the particular illness that your patient has. Practitioners are urged to consult this section in the following way.

- As a reference and a reminder of what you have already learned.
- To learn more Japanese point energetics for additional diseases.

The points which are included here may be somewhat different from their Chinese counterpart in some respect.

- **Location** – there may be a difference of location. If the point has the standard Chinese location this will be noted by the key 'SCL'. That location will be described for clinical convenience. If the location is different it will say Japanese location (JL) and the location will be both described and, in most cases, illustrated.
- **Energetics** – the point may be used in a slightly different way, that is, its energetics may be articulated somewhat differently. The energetics listed here are by no means meant to be an exhaustive list; I have only listed those energetics which reinforce the reader's understanding of the primary role which each point plays in this system. To differentiate them, these energetics are italicized.
- **Modalities** – the needle technique and moxibustion methods may likewise be different. This includes some angles and depths of insertion.

In summary, remember, as I pointed out in Chapter 2, that Japanese needling depths are generally more shallow, hence they are more likely to have a subcutaneous insertion. Moxa use is more liberal than the Chinese in the sense that some points which the Chinese would not moxa the Japanese do but in small, precise places, usually with the Tiger Thermie warmer or mini-thread moxa. Contraindications or cautions for needling or moxa are in bold.

Codes used in this section:

- JL = Japanese location
- MA = moxibustion is applicable
- PO = puncture obliquely
- PP = puncture perpendicularly
- PT = puncture transversely
- SCL = standard Chinese location
- TD = treatment-of-disease point
- TE = standard nomenclature of the World Health Organization (1989) for Triple Warmer
- Italics = unique energetics
- Bold = contraindications or notes

Two indices are provided for the practitioner following this chapter. The first is an alphabetical index by disease of point energetics in the Japanese acupuncture system, that is, which diagnosis, clearance point or treatment-of-disease point is used for a particular illness. The second is a cross-reference by meridian of the same energetics. These are provided to assist the practitioner in recalling what points are used for certain diseases.

THE LUNG MERIDIAN

Point: LU 1 (Zhongfu) – LU 2 (Yunmen)
Location: SCL: LU 1 – 1 cun directly below LU 2.
LU 2 – directly below the acromial extremity of the clavicle, 6 cun lateral to the Ren channel.
Think of both points as similar in function.
Palpate both.

Energetics:
1. Front Mu point of Lungs: it adjusts and tonifies LU Qi (Yin and Yang).
2. Point of entry of energy into the body: increases energy of the entire body.

3. *First clearance point for ST 25 (Tianshu) R in abdominal clearing.*
4. Expands and relaxes the chest, disperses fullness from the chest and stops pain, stops cough, stimulates the descending of Lung Qi, clears the Upper Burner as well as Heat from the Lungs and the Upper Jiao.
5. Opens relevant emotional blockages.
6. Meeting of Taiyin (Lung/Spleen).

Needle technique: PO 0.3–0.5 in. towards the lateral aspect of the chest. Exercise caution with needling depth and angle to avoid puncturing the Lungs. As a clearance point, rub both points horizontally and bilaterally, first on the right and then on the left. MA.

Point: LU 4 (Xiabai)
Location: JL: Raise the arm to the nose. Point is where nose rests on radial side of m. biceps brachii (4 cun below the end of axillary fold).
Energetics:
1. Increases oxygenation to the body. *TD for chest pain.*
Needle technique: PP 0.3–0.5 in. MA.

Point: LU 5 (Chize)
Location: Three locations:
- SCL: on the cubital crease, on the radial side of the tendon of m. biceps brachii. This point is located with the elbow slightly flexed.
- JL: 1 cun above Chinese LU 5 or
- JL: 1 cun below Chinese LU 5.

Locate with elbow slightly flexed.
Energetics:
1. He (sea) point: He (sea) points have a special effect upon the organs. In this case it regulates and tonifies the Lungs,

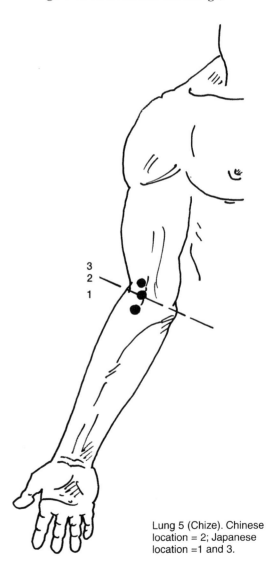

Lung 5 (Chize). Chinese location = 2; Japanese location =1 and 3.

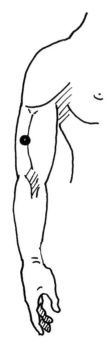

Lung 4 (Xiabai). Japanese location.

especially Yin and Qi, alleviates exterior (Excess) conditions.

2. As the Water point, LU 5 clears Heat from Lungs, expels Phlegm from Lungs, moistens dryness of the Lungs.
3. Being the Water point on the Metal meridian makes it the sedation point. As such, it helps Lung Qi descend and brings down rebellious Lung Qi. Has a strong effect on the throat (tonsillitis) and Lungs (bronchitis). *TD for asthma and bronchitis.* Also for tonsillitis with muscular pain.
4. Tonsil reflex.

Needle technique: PP 0.3–0.5 in. or apply firm pressure. **No moxa. Direct moxa may permanently bend the elbow by shortening the tendon of the m. biceps brachii.**

Point: LU 6 (Kongzui)
Location: JL: 3 cun below (distal to) Lung 5 (Chize).
Energetics:
1. As the Xi (cleft) point (point of accumulation or blockage), it breaks up stuckness and congestion of the meridian. It adjusts Lung Qi and cools Heat in the Lungs.
2. *TD for hemorrhoids and rectal vein congestion.*

Needle technique: PP 0.5–0.7 in. MA.

Point: LU 7 (Lieque)
Location: SCL: superior to the styloid process of the radius, 1.5 cun above the transverse crease of the wrist. When the index fingers and the thumbs of both hands are crossed with the index finger of one hand placed on the styloid process of the radius of the other, the point is in the depression under the tip of the index finger.

Energetics:
1. Master of Ren channel: opens the Ren channel: allows its energy to flow upward. The Ren channel is one of the best meridians for controlling Qi in the chest and the Lungs. *Second clearance point for CV 14.*
2. Luo point: stimulates the descending and dispersing function of the Lungs. General body tonification point. Regulates the Water of the entire body; benefits the Bladder and opens Water passages. Point of exit: circulates defensive Qi and releases exterior. Expels exterior Wind.
3. As a longitudinal Luo, it moves the Lung meridian because the meridian passes through the shoulder area. *Opens compression of the scalene muscles. TD for carpal tunnel and thoracic outlet syndrome.* Also tonifies the Qi of the Lungs as well as that of the whole body.
4. As a general Luo point, promotes the free flow of Qi in the body. One of the best controlling points for rebellious Qi in the chest.
5. As a transverse Luo, assists the Large Intestine in removing the dregs from the body.
6. Sends the Qi downward to be grasped by the Kidney.
7. In the Extra Meridian system it is coupled with KI 6 (Zhaohai). The two points

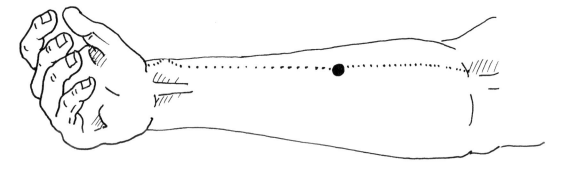

Lung 6 (Kongzui). Japanese location.

together, like a wheel, put Stagnation in motion.

8. Regulates Water passageways and Water metabolism.
9. With LI 4 (Hegu), circulates energy to the face.

Needle technique: PO 0.3–0.5 in. MA. As the clearance point, rub on the right side only. Needle direction dependent upon how the point is used.

Point: LU 8 (Jingqu)
Location: SCL: 1 cun above the transverse crease of the wrist, in the depression on the radial side of the radial artery.
Energetics:
1. Jing (river) point, Metal point, horary point: it has the same elemental energy as the Lungs. As such it treats 'Metal' problems – throat and Lungs problems.
2. *TD along with LU 7 (Lieque) for opening scalene compression.*

Needle technique: PP 0.1–0.2 in. **Avoid the radial artery. No moxa.**

Point: LU 10 (Yuji)
Location: SCL (with a slight variation): on the radial aspect of the midpoint of the first metacarpal bone, at the junction of the red and the white skin (but a big area on the hypothenar eminence).
Energetics:
1. The Fire point: this point can add or take away Fire from the Lungs.
2. *TD for fecal stagnation.* Inspect the color of the hypothenar area that may be green or grayish if there is fecal Stagnation.

Needle technique: Massage works best. Can needle, PP 0.5–0.7 in. Needle as close to the first metacarpal bone as possible, not on the palm of the hand. Pull the skin down to locate the place to needle. MA although not used that much clinically.

THE LARGE INTESTINE MERIDIAN

Point: LI 1 (Shangyang)
Location: SCL: on the radial side of the index finger, about 0.1 cun posterior to the corner of the nail.

Energetics:
1. Metal point, horary point: can add or take away 'Metal' energy.
2. *TD for toothache in the lower quadrant* since the branch from the supraclavicular fossa goes to the gums.

Needle technique: Prick with a three-edge needle to cause bleeding to reduce Heat/Fire or pick up the Qi of the Intestine on a superficial level. Or PP or PO 0.1 in. **Clinically moxa is not used**.

Point: LI 4 (Hegu)
Location: SCL: between the first and second metacarpal bones, approximately in the middle of the second metacarpal bone on the radial side.
Energetics:
1. Source point: tonifies the Lungs and the Qi of the entire body. It contains the Yuan Qi that reflects the condition of the organ.
2. *TD for toothache in the upper quadrant.*
3. *Second clearance point for ST 25R.*
4. Brings energy down, clears the Large Intestine channel, clears Heat from the orifices of the head and face, expels Wind, relieves the surface, elevates the clear and descends the turbid. Removes obstructions from the channels, disperses Cold, regulates the Qi of the Large Intestine, regulates the bowels, causes sweating, suppresses pain, stimulates the descending and dispersing function.
5. Calming and antispasmodic, stops pain, soothes the mind, promotes labor, strengthens Qi Deficiency, subdues Stomach Qi.
6. Spreads Lung Qi. Point of entry of the Lungs to the Large Intestine. Tonifies Taiyin (LU/SP).
7. Brings energy down for nausea due to chemotherapy.
8. With LU 7 (Lieque), it circulates energy to the face.

Needle technique: PP 0.5–0.8 in. MA. Press vigorously and bilaterally as the clearance point on both sides. **Contraindicated in pregnancy to needle, moxa or press (massage)**.

Point: Between LI 6 (Pianli) and LI 7 (Wenliu)
Location: Place the two hands together as you do when you locate LU 7 (Lieque) on the styloid process. The point is on the anterior aspect of the arm between where the index and middle finger rest.
Energetics:
1. Located between the Luo, LI 6 (Pianli) and LI 7 (Wenliu), the Xi (cleft), it has energetics similar to those points. Essentially it moves energy in the meridian and drains stuckness. It affects the mouth because of these features and its internal pathway.
2. *TD for mouth problems such as periodontitis, gingivitis, stomatitis, thrush and oral herpes.*
Needle technique: PO and proximally 0.5–0.7 in. MA although not commonly used.

Points: LI 10 (Shousanli) and LI 11 (Quchi) area: the Naganos

Location: These points run lateral and parallel to the LI 11 and LI 10 area. There are four of them. They are about one fingerbreadth apart as you proceed distally from the elbow crease.
Energetics:
1. Their functions are similar to the points on the Large Intestine meridian. LI 10 (Shousanli) is the upper He (sea) of ST; ST is where the manufacture of postnatal Qi begins. It is a powerful Qi and Blood tonic. LI 11 (Quchi), He (Sea) and Earth point, builds nutritive Qi and Blood, clears Heat and Fire, dispels Wind and Damp (which are all evil Qi). Cools and disperses, for fever in general, Heat in Intestines, cools Blood, good for hives, lowers Blood pressure, has a general tonification effect as well. Helps induce sweating. Benefits the sinews and joints.
2. *TD for immunity*: these points boost the immune system (Zheng or True Qi). Used

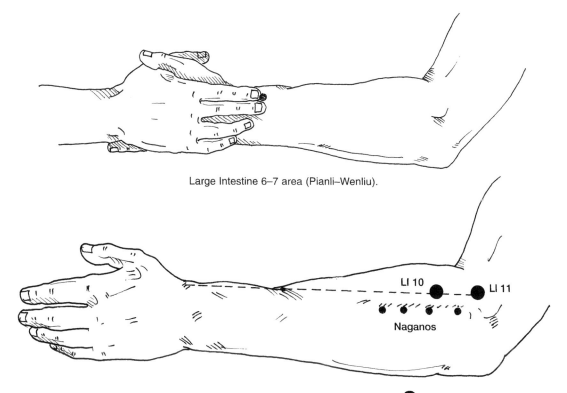

Large Intestine 6–7 area (Pianli–Wenliu).

Large Intestine 10 and 11 (Shousanli and Quchi). Chinese location = ●, Naganos = ●.

for immunity treatments. With TE 16 (Tianyou), boosts immunity and fights off evil Qi.

Needle technique: PP 0.5–1.0 in. Look for a gummy, sticky area as you lift and thrust thought it. Once you get through the gummy area, raise the needle and slowly look for a crunchy area above the gummy spot that you have pierced. Don't get Qi or twist. The needle is used mechanically to break down free ionized calcium (crunchiness). MA highly recommended, especially with the Tiger Thermie warmer. These are extremely tender points to palpate. Needling produces a heavy sensation during and after needling.

Point: LI 14 (Binao)
Location: SCL: on radial side of humerus, at the lower end of the m. deltoideus, on the line connecting LI 11 (Quchi) and LI 15 (Jianyu).
Energetics:
  1. *TD: resolves Phlegm and disperses masses anywhere in the body, particularly in the Upper Jiao and head.*
Needle technique: PP or PO proximally 0.5–0.7 in. MA.

Point: LI 18 (Futu)
Location: SCL: on the lateral side of the neck, level with the tip of the Adam's apple, between the sternal and clavicular heads of the SCM.
Energetics:
  1. *TD for thyroid problems.*
  2. Diagnostic point in neck evaluation for thyroid problems.
Needle technique: PP 0.3–0.5 in. MA.

THE STOMACH MERIDIAN

Point: ST 2 (Sibai)
Location: SCL: below ST 1 (Chengqi), in the depression at the infraorbital foramen. Directly below the mid-eye at the junction of the infraorbital ridge and the zygomatic arch in the foramen.
Energetics:
  1. *TD for sinus problems and sinus infections.*
  2. Diagnostic point for sinus problems.

Needle technique: PP or PO 0.2–0.3 in. **Deep puncture not advisable because the point is precisely on the course of the infraorbital nerve. Use a fine needle. While it is not forbidden to moxa this point, it is generally not used due to its proximity to the eye. Tiger Thermie moxa may be used as in the sinus treatments since the amount of smoke is negligible and you do not linger long on the point.**

Point: ST 9 (Renying)
Location: SCL: level with the tip of the Adam's apple, just on the course of the common carotid artery, on the anterior border of the SCM.
Energetics:
  1. As the Sea of Qi, regulates energy in the head and sends Qi down. Regulates Qi, especially of the Stomach, by subduing rebellious Stomach Qi, resulting in hiccups, belching, nausea and asthma that is related to the Stomach channel.
  2. Affects the thyroid. It is a local point for the thyroid because it is located at the superior thyroid artery on the bifurcation of the internal and external carotid artery.
  3. *TD for high Blood pressure and thyroid problems.*
  4. *ST 9L is diagnostic of a parasympathetic nervous system problem and ST 9R is diagnostic of a sympathetic nervous system disorder.*
Needle technique: Pressure is sufficient. PP 0.3–0.5 in. **Avoid the carotid artery. No moxa because the point is on the course of the common carotid.**

Point: ST 12 (Quepen) area
Location: SCL: in the midpoint of the supraclavicular fossa, 4 cun lateral to the CV channel.
Energetics:
  1. *TD for nervous system disharmonies, thyroid problems, immune problems, Heart Qi Deficiency (on the left), right lymphatic duct congestion (on the right) and vascular disturbances.*
  2. All Yang meridians meet here with the exception of the GV and BL channels.

3. *Most important point for carpal tunnel syndrome because the brachial plexus and the subclavian artery run beneath it.*
Needle technique: PP 0.3–0.5 in. **Avoid the transverse cervical artery. Deep puncture is not advisable. Needle with caution because the point is on the apex of the Lungs. The Japanese technique is, with patients lying on their side, puncture perpendicularly towards the spine, not downward. Treat with Tiger Thermie with gentle pressure or loosen by palpation. With the Tiger Thermie, moxa downward (perpendicularly) into the point.**

Point: ST 13 (Qihu)
Location: SCL: at the lower border of the middle of the clavicle on the mammillary line, 4 cun lateral to the Ren channel.
Energetics:
  1. Connects with ST, LI, TE, SI and many divergent meridians.
  2. *TD for prolapses such as hernias, etc. Pulls things up. Much prolapse due to weak immunity. Use in immunity treatments.*
Needle technique: PT 0.3–0.5 in. towards the lateral aspect. MA.

Point: ST 18 (Rugen)
Location: SCL: in the fifth intercostal space, one rib below the nipple.
Energetics:
  1. *TD for Heart problems.* Below the left nipple. Is the source of all Blood vessels. It is the point where the heart is closest to the surface. It corresponds to the apical pulse in Western medicine. Too strong or too weak a pulsation indicates insufficiency of Heart Qi (downward draining of ancestral Qi).
Needle technique: PO towards lateral aspect 0.3–0.5 in. MA.

Point: ST 21 (Liangmen)
Location: SCL: 4 cun above the umbilicus, 2 cun lateral to CV 12 (Zhongwan).
Energetics:
  1. *TD for stomach problems such as ulcers.* Reinforces the effects of CV 12.

Needle technique: PP 0.5–0.8 in. Puncture the right side very carefully due to possible Liver enlargement. MA.

Point: ST 25 (Tianshu)–27 (Daju) area
Location: SCL: ST 25 (Tianshu) – 2 cun lateral to the center of the umbilicus.
ST 26 (Wailing) – 1 cun below the umbilicus, 2 cun lateral to CV 7 (Yinjiao).
ST 27 (Daju) – 2 cun below the umbilicus, 2 cun lateral to CV 5 (Shimen).
Energetics:
  Diagnostic point of the modified abdominal map.
  Right side:
  1. Front Mu of LI – *Neijing*: can add Yin to the organ. Can adjust the Large Intestine in any condition be it a problem of (Yin/Yang), or stagnant Qi and Blood.
  2. Front Mu of LU – *Nanjing*: moves Stagnant Qi and Blood in the intestines and elsewhere and indicates the condition of the Qi of the body.
  3. Front Mu of TE (Manaka): *used in the treatment of immunity.*
  4. *Reflex of lymphatic glandular exhaustion (Dr Nagano): for weak immunity.*
  5. Appendix reflex.

  Left side:
  1. *Blood Stagnation anywhere in the body.*

  Both:
  1. Meeting point of the Yangming energetic layer of the Stomach and Large Intestine. Can be used to regulate them.
  2. Regulates menstrual flow and reinforces the Qi of the Stomach and Spleen.
  3. Can be used for chronic Deficiency of the Spleen and Kidney.
  4. Reflex point for problems of the nose and throat.
Needle technique: PP 0.7–1.2 in. MA.

Point: ST 28 (Shuidao)
Location: SCL: 3 cun below the umbilicus, 2 cun lateral to CV 4 (Guanyuan).

Energetics:
1. Ovary reflex for gynecological problems.
2. Name of point is Water Passage. Water Stagnation reflex. Stimulates urination. Strengthens Kidney's ability to separate the pure from impure. *TD for Damp-Heat in the Lower Jiao.* Treats bladder infection.

Needle technique: PP 0.7–1.2 in. MA.

Point: ST 30 (Qichong)
Location: SCL: 5 cun below the umbilicus, 2 cun lateral to CV 2 (Qugu), superior to the inguinal groove, on the medial side of the femoral artery.
Energetics:
1. Local point: regulates Qi and Blood in the lower abdomen.
2. Point of the Penetrating Vessel (Chong mai): enhances the therapeutic effect to the lower abdomen. Sea of Blood point.
3. Point of departure of the ST meridian: connects with Spleen. Sends energy up.
4. *TD for prolapse. Use with ST 13 (Qihu).*

Needle technique: PP 0.3–0.5 in. MA but be careful with heat in the pubic hair area.

Point: ST 31 (Biguan)
Location: SCL: directly below the anterior superior iliac spine, in the depression on the lateral side of m. sartorius when the thigh is flexed. Level with the pubic symphysis, when the thigh is flexed.
Energetics:
1. *TD for pain in the thigh, muscular atrophy, motor impairment, numbness and pain of the lower extremities, atrophy or blockage of the muscles of the thigh and buttocks, inhibited movement of the leg muscles due to sinew tension, low back pain and cold knees.*

Needle technique: PP 1.0–1.5 in. MA.

Point: ST 32 (Futu)
Location: SCL: 6 cun above the laterosuperior border of the patella, on the line connecting the anterior superior iliac spine and lateral border of the patella in line with the outside of the leg. Flex the thigh to locate.
Energetics:
1. Union of veins and arteries: useful for circulatory problems.

2. *TD for cold knees, edema, numbness of the lower limbs.*

Needle technique: PP 1.0–1.5 in. MA. **Classically forbidden to moxa; could impair function of raising the leg.**

Point: ST 33 (Yinshi)
Location: SCL: 3 cun above the laterosuperior border of the patella.
Energetics:
1. *TD for aching and prolapse of the knee, numbness, soreness and motor impairment of lower extremities, painful knee joints.*

Needle technique: PP 0.7–1.0 in. MA.

Point: ST 34 (Liangqiu)
Location: JL: slightly more lateral and superior to the SCL, which is 2 cun above the laterosuperior border of the patella.

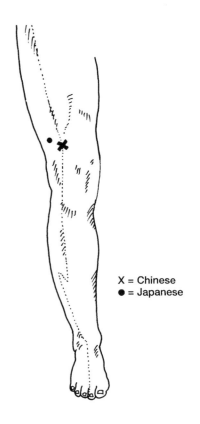

X = Chinese
● = Japanese

Stomach 34 (Liangqiu).

Energetics:

1. Xi (cleft) point.
2. *Clearance point for CV 12 in the abdominal clearance protocol.*
3. *TD for acute stomachache, food poisoning, allergies, bleeding gums, bad breath, migraines, Yangming headache.*
4. Clears Heat from the Stomach, harmonizes and pacifies the Stomach and rebellious Qi, opens the flow to the meridian. Reflex point of the meridian.
5. It dispels Stagnation and accumulation of the Yangming, clears the channels, removes obstructions and quickens the collaterals.
6. Expels Dampness and Wind.
7. Relieves spasm and stops pain.
8. Benefits the knees.

Needle technique: PP 0.5–1.0 in. MA but not used much clinically. Rub vigorously on the right side only in the clearance protocol.

Point: ST 35 (Dubi)
Location: SCL: ask the patient to flex the knee. The point is in the depression below the patella and lateral to the patellar ligament.
Energetics:

1. *TD for heavy knee, fluid in knee.*

Needle technique: PO 0.7–1.0 in. towards the medial side. MA.

Point: ST 36 (Zusanli)
Location: SCL: 3 cun below ST 35 (Dubi), one fingerbreadth lateral from the anterior crest of the tibia.
Energetics:

1. Regulates hydrochloric acid. Moxa for insufficiency. Needle for Excess.
2. *TD for immunity treatments* and cancer patients.
3. Brings energy down, especially rebellious Stomach Qi that is a common sequela to chemotherapy or radiation, such as vomiting and loss of body fluids.
4. Tonifies Stomach and Kidney Yin Deficiency damaged by chemotherapy or radiation.

Needle technique: PP 0.5–1.2 in. MA.

Point: ST 44 (Inner Neiting)
Location: JL: alternative location of ST 44. On the sole of the foot at the junction of the margin of the web between the second and third toes.
Energetics:

1. Water point and Ying (spring) point: cools and drains Heat from the Stomach and the other end of the channel. Regulates Qi and suppresses pain of the channel in relation to Stomach Fire so good for toothache. Also cools Heat of the Yangming so helpful for epistaxis.
2. *TD for Stomach Fire manifestations such as allergic reactions, toothache, migraines, eczema, hydrochloric acid excess, acute stomachache, periodontal gum disease.*
3. Promotes bowel movements.
4. Regulates rebellious Qi.
5. Stops abdominal pain with fever, eliminates Wind from the face.
6. Cools Stomach Heat that may develop from Liver Heat.

Needle technique: PP 0.3–0.5 in. Use strong pressure or Tiger Thermie with dredging method. MA. This is a good example of the application of Tiger Thermie for Hot conditions.

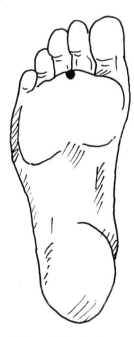

Stomach 44 (Inner Neiting). Japanese location.

THE SPLEEN MERIDIAN

Point: SP 2 (Dadu)–SP 3 (Taibai) area
Location: SCL: area between SP 2 (Dadu) and 3 (Taibai). SP 2 (Dadu) – on the medial side of the big toe, distal and inferior to the first metatarso-digital joint, at the junction of the red and white skin. SP 3 (Taibai) – proximal and inferior to the head of the first metatarsal bone, at the junction of the red and white skin.
Energetics:
1. SP 2 (Dadu) – tonification point, Fire point: adds Fire to the Spleen for SP Qi Xu or takes Fire away, in this case arthritic bone deformities. *Bunions (bone deformities) in this area are due to sugar improperly metabolized (Phlegm) due to SP Qi Xu.*
2. SP 3 (Taibai) – Shu (stream) point, Yuan (source) point, Earth point, horary point: adds or takes away Earth energy. Adds for SP Qi Xu, removes to take away Dampness.

Needle technique: PP 0.1–0.2 in. MA. Tiger Thermie this area following the generous application of Zheng Gu Shui to break down bunions.

Point: SP 4 (Gongsun) area
Location: JL: the area beneath the base of the first metatarsal.
Energetics:
1. Luo point: (a) drains Excesses, (b) stimulates the affected meridian and (c) communicates with the Coupled channel. Regulates circulation of the Middle Burner, regulates Spleen/Stomach disharmonies, pacifies the Stomach, dispels fullness and obstruction.
2. *The third clearance point for CV 12 (Zhongwan).* Tonifies SP Qi Xu. Removes Damp, resolves Excess.
3. Opens and regulates the Chong mai. Most effective meridian for cold feet. Dispels Cold from the Heart and abdomen. Affects adrenals, stops bleeding, regulates menstruation.
4. Tonifies Spleen Qi and Yang, creates Blood.

Needle technique: PP 0.3–0.5 in. MA. Tiger Thermie. Rub both vigorously as the clearance point.

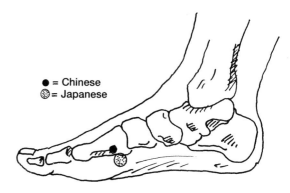

● = Chinese
◉ = Japanese

Spleen 4 (Gongsun).

Point: SP 6 (Sanyinjiao)
Location: SCL: 3 cun directly above the tip of the medial malleolus, on the posterior border of the tibia, on the line drawn from the medial malleolus to SP 9 (Yinlingquan).
Energetics:
1. Group Luo of the Three Leg Yin: powerful effect on circulation of the three Yin meridians of the leg. Tonifies Yin of the Spleen, Liver and Kidney. Improves circulation, especially of the lower limbs.
2. *TD for inner thigh congestion. Clears SP line on upper thigh when Blood Stagnation in abdomen is due to poor venous circulation or Spleen meridian obstruction.*

Needle technique: PP 0.5–1.0 in. MA but **no moxa or needling in pregnancy**.

Point: SP 8 (Diji)
Location: SCL: 3 cun below the medial condyle of the tibia, on the line connecting SP 9 (Yinlingquan) and the medial malleolus. Posterior to the bone.
Energetics:
1. Xi (cleft) point.
2. *TD for dysmenorrhea.*

Needle technique: PP 0.5–0.8 in. MA. Palpation is effective.

Point: SP 9 (Yinlingquan)
Location: SCL: on the lower border of the medial condyle of the tibia, in the depression between the posterior border of the tibia and m. gastrocnemius.

Energetics:
1. He (sea) point: for digestive problems. Indicates the presence of gas or toxins.
2. Water point: it resolves and drains Dampness and Damp-Heat and promotes urination.
3. *TD for gas or constipation due to nervous colon.*

Needle technique: PP 0.5–1.0 in. Palpate for a knotty lump (Damp or Phlegm). This indicates a chronic problem. Needle with the same lift-and-thrust method as used on the Naganos. Obtain no Qi. Work through the gummy area until crunchy. MA.

Point: SP 10 (Xuehai)
Location: JL: cup your right palm to the patient's left knee, with the thumb on its medial side and the other four fingers directed proximally. The point is where the tip of your thumb rests. It is a big area, more medial than Chinese SP 10.

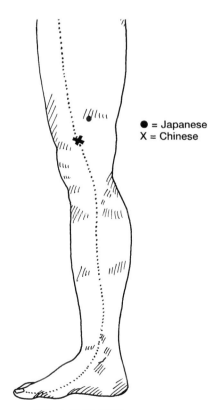

● = Japanese
X = Chinese

Spleen 10 (Xuehai).

Energetics:
1. Sea of Blood: intersects with the Chong mai which regulates Blood, especially menses. SP 10 (Xuehai) has a strong energetic effect upon Blood so it is consistently used for Blood problems in Chinese and Japanese systems.
2. *The point for Blood Stagnation anywhere in the body, but particularly in the lower abdomen. Diagnostic point and primary clearance point for ST 25 (Tianshu) L to move stagnant Blood.*
3. Cools Heat in Blood.
4. Eliminates Damp, perfuses the lower abdomen, tonifies and strengthens the Blood.

Needle technique: PP 0.7–1.2 in. but usually palpated strongly since it is a clearance point. As a clearance point, rub on the left side with firm pressure. Generally extremely tender. MA.

THE SMALL INTESTINE MERIDIAN

Point: SI 3 (Houxi)
Location: SCL: when a loose fist is made, the point is proximal to the head of the fifth metacarpal bone on the ulnar side, in the depression at the junction of the red and white skin.
Energetics:
1. Master of the Du channel, affects pituitary gland, pituitary gland reflex, opens the Du channel to allow Yang energy to circulate properly. Eliminates interior Wind from the GV channel, expels exterior Wind, disperses Heat from the exterior, benefits sinews, comforts tendons, muscles, moves and controls GV, disperses Excess Yang of the GV channel, resolves Dampness affecting the chest and Gall Bladder, relaxes the muscle channels, clears the spirit, consolidates the surface. Regulates the Yang energy of the head. Because the channel passes through the head and the brain, it has an effect on hormonal problems.
2. *Major clearance point for ST 25R (Tianshu). Tender when the person has hormonal problems such as those induced by the birth control pill,*

diet pills or other hormonal problems regulated by the pituitary gland.

3. Shu (stream) point, Wood point, tonification point.
4. Removes obstruction from the channel, expels Wind-Heat, meridian reflex area, promotes lactation.

Needle technique: PO distally under the bone 0.5–0.7 in. MA. Press firmly and bilaterally as the clearance point.

Point: SI 11 (Tianzong) area
Location: the Chinese location is in the infrascapular fossa, at the junction of the upper and middle third of the distance between the lower border of the scapular spine and the inferior angle of the scapula. The Japanese location is slightly more lateral to this location. Feel for the tendinous cord.
Energetics:

1. *A knotty lump may be found on the left side, which indicates the condition of the Qi of the Heart. Only check left side.* I have found it clinically effective for headaches due to stress, neck misalignment and circulatory problems.

Needle technique: Palpate for a tendinous cord in this area on left side only. May treat with needle going into it in three directions. Pick three tender areas. Break up like SP 9 (Yinlingquan) and the Naganos. MA.

THE HEART MERIDIAN

Point: HT 7 (Shenmen)
Location: JL: on the transverse crease of the wrist, in the articular region of the pisiform and the ulna, in the depression on the ulnar side of the tendon of the m. flexor carpi ulnaris (Chinese is on radial side of the tendon).
Energetics:

1. Shu (stream) point, Source point, Earth point, sedation point: quiets the Heart, calms the spirit, makes pain negligible because the spirit is addressed. A primary point for pain and for emotional problems.
2. *TD for constipation due to anxiety.*

Needle technique: PP 0.3–0.5 in. MA but not used clinically.

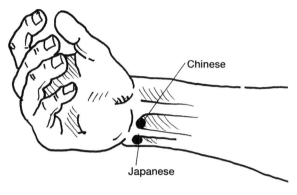

Heart 7 (Shenmen).

THE BLADDER MERIDIAN

Point: BL 1 (Jingming)
Location: SCL: 0.1 cun superior to the inner canthus. Ask the patient to close the eyes when locating the point.
Energetics:

1. *TD for sinus problems – expels Wind, clears vision, brightens eyes, cools Heat and nourishes Water.*
2. *Reflex point of the pituitary gland.*

Needle technique: PP 0.3–0.7 in. along the lateral wall. **When inserting, push the eyeball to the lateral side. A lift or thrust technique is not advisable. Puncture slowly and perpendicularly. Apply cotton ball and press after withdrawal to avoid bruising. No moxa.**

Point: BL 2 (Zanzhu)
Location: SCL: on the medial extremity of the eyebrow, in the supraorbital notch.
Energetics:

1. Removes channel obstructions.
2. *TD for sinus problems.*
3. Reflex point of the pituitary gland.
4. Diagnosis point for sinus problems.

Needle technique: Prick to bleed or puncture 0.3–0.5 in. transversely towards the lateral aspect. Traditionally no moxa but Tiger Thermie is effective.

Points: BL 17 (Geshu), 18 (Ganshu), 20 (Pishu)
Location: SCL: BL 17 (Geshu) – 1.5 cun lateral to the lower border of the spinous

process of the seventh thoracic vertebra.

BL 18 (Genshu) – 1.5 cun lateral to the lower border of the spinous process of the ninth thoracic vertebra.

BL 20 (Pishu) – 1.5 cun lateral to the lower border of the spinous process of the 11th thoracic vertebra.

Energetics:

1. *TD for sugar cravings, diabetes, mid-back spasm and digestive problems.*
2. BL 17 (Geshu) – Back Shu point of diaphragm; Influential point that dominates Blood. Moves and produces Blood.
3. BL 18 (Ganshu) – Back Shu point of Liver. Regulates Qi and Blood of Liver.
4. BL 20 (Pishu) – Back Shu point of the Spleen. Regulates Qi of Spleen, builds Blood.

Needle technique: PP 0.5–0.7 in. MA.

Point: BL 23 (Shenshu)
Location: SCL: 1.5 cun lateral to the lower border of the spinous process of the second lumbar vertebra.
Energetics:

1. Back Shu point of the Kidney: used for Kidney Qi Deficiency.

Needle technique: PP 1.0–1.2 in. MA.

Point: BL 57 (Chengshan)
Location: SCL: directly below the belly of m gastrocnemius, on the line connecting BL 40 (Weizhong) and tendo calcaneus, about 8 cun below BL 40 (Weizhong).
Energetics:

1. Regulates the Qi of the Yang channels. Opens circulation. For low back pain, spasm of the gastrocnemius, lumbago, leg pain, relieves cramping of the back of the legs, twisted muscles of the calf.

Needle technique: PP 0.8–1.2 in. MA.

Point: BL 62 (Shenmai)
Location: JL: equivalent to Chinese BL 61 (Pucan)

location, posterior and inferior to the external malleolus, directly below BL 60 (Kunlun), in the depression at the junction of the red and the white skin.

Energetics:

1. Master of Yangqiao mai. Joins BL channel with Yang head channels, opens heel channels, comforts tendons, relaxes muscle channels, straightens the spine and legs. Brings energy down. With BL 1 (Jingming) and KI 6 (Zhaohai) reduces hot flashes, a Yinqiao/Yangqiao disharmony.

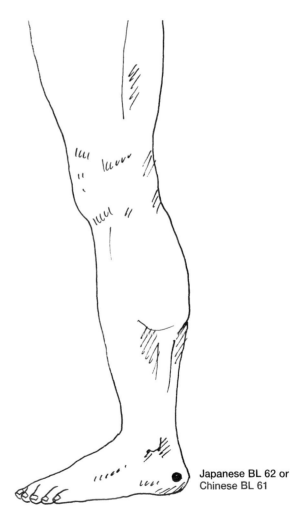

Japanese BL 62 or Chinese BL 61

Bladder 62 (Shenmai).
Note: Japanese BL 62 = Chinese BL 61.

2. *Abdominal clearance point for CV 4 (Guanyuan) and CV 6 (Qihai).*
3. *TD point for back pathology.*

Needle technique: PP 0.3–0.5 in. MA. Apply intradermal needle in direction of meridian, i.e. towards toe. Rub firmly on right side as the clearance point.

Point: BL 66 (Zutonggu)
Location: SCL: in the depression anterior and inferior to the fifth metatarsophalangeal joint.
Energetics:
1. Ying (spring), Water point, horary point.
2. *TD for edema of the foot and leg.*

Needle technique: PP 0.2–0.3 in. or implant with intradermal transversely towards toe. MA.

THE KIDNEY MERIDIAN

Point: KI 1 (Yongquan)
Location: SCL: in the depression appearing on the sole when the foot is in plantar flexion, approximately at the junction of the anterior and middle third of the sole.
Energetics:
1. Jing (well) point, Wood point, sedation point. Opens orifices.
2. *KI 1 (Yongquan) is one of the primary clearance points in the Japanese system.* It tonifies Yin, clears Heat, subdues Wind and empty Heat, calms the mind, restores consciousness and clears the brain. Nourishes Kidney to suppress Liver Fire.
3. Sedation point: *its primary use relates to adjusting blood pressure or vascular disturbance. As a result it helps release inner thighs. Promotes circulation of blood due to vascular disturbance of the lower limbs.* If there is inner thigh congestion, there is poor circulation. When this point is tender it must be cleared for, as the classics remind us, where there is a Blood problem there may be severe vascular disturbances. *TD for Blood problems.*
4. *The primary clearance point for CV 4 (Guanyuan) and CV 6 (Qihai) and the inner thigh.*

Needle technique: This point is extremely tender in many patients. Patients should be taught to clear this point by hand. Push with firm, deep, dispersive pressure on a daily basis for several minutes. Continue until the point is no longer tender. May be needled to consolidate the effect. PP 0.3–0.5 in. Many health problems will resolve as a result of this. MA especially with the Tiger Thermie warmer.

Point: KI 2 (Rangu)
Location: SCL: anterior and inferior to the medial malleolus, in the depression on the lower border of the tuberosity of the navicular bone.
Energetics:
1. Ying (spring) point/Fire point: reduces Heat. Calms the mind.

Needle technique: PP 0.3 in. MA.

Point: KI 3 (Taixi)
Location: JL: equivalent to Chinese KI 5 (Shuiquan), in the depression anterior and superior to the medial side of the tuberosity of the calcaneum.
Energetics:
1. Shu (stream) point, Source point, Earth point: has four major functions in Chinese medicine relating to KI Qi, Essence, Fire and Yin/Yang. Benefits Essence, bones and marrow (brain). Regulates the uterus (Essence nourishes the uterus and the fetus). Clears Deficiency Heat by nourishing Yin. Tonifies Kidney Yin or Yang. Strengthens the lower back and knees.
2. *Major clearance point for CV 4 (Guanyuan) and CV 6 (Qihai) in abdominal clearance.*
3. *Thyroid gland reflex. TD for thyroid problems.* Thyroid hormones stimulate the metabolism of every cell. The Kidney similarly can be seen as the basis for all the functions in the body. When the thyroid function is low, the thinking abilities can be dulled, much like when Kidney Essence is low and not nourishing the brain.
4. Increases Water of the whole body, moistens the Heart, subdues Fire.

Needle technique: PP 0.3–0.5 in. With the needle directed upward (up the leg). As the clearance

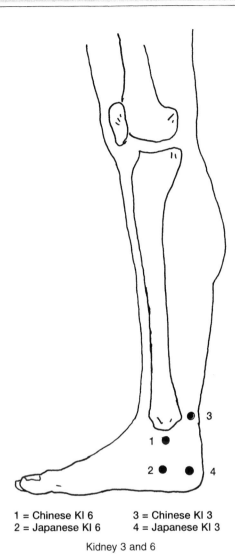

1 = Chinese KI 6   3 = Chinese KI 3
2 = Japanese KI 6   4 = Japanese KI 3

Kidney 3 and 6

the Yinqiao mai. Cools the Blood. Benefits the throat.
2. *Abdominal clearance point for CV 14, CV 6 and CV 4.*
3. *Reflects the condition of the adrenal glands. Strengthens the adrenals (adrenals become weak from emotional shock, speed, steroids, birth control pills, chronic illness, stress and trauma because they consume Yin).*
4. *With LR 5 (Ligou), reduces inflammation. For any 'itis'.*
5. *Primary point for bronchitis with LU 5 (Chize). Opens the chest.*
6. *TD for neck tension and sympathetic nervous system weakness related to KI Yin Xu with GB 41 (Zulinqi).*

Needle technique: PT 0.1 in. towards the heel. Extremely tender on most patients. Patients should rub it. As a clearance point, rub firmly on both sides. MA.

Point: KI 7 (Fuliu)
Location: SCL: 2 cun directly above KI 3 (Taixi), on the anterior border of tendo calcaneus.
Energetics:
1. Jing (river) point, Metal point, tonification point, especially of Kidney Yang. Regulates the Qi of the Kidney, clears Heat, eliminates Damp, strengthens Wei Qi, regulates pores, dispels dryness, disperses Stagnation, moves Water, organ reflex point of the Kidney, regulates Bladder, menses, Water pathways, stimulates or restrains sweating, strengthens back, unblocks pulses, restores collapsed Yin.
2. *Clearance point of CV 4 (Guanyuan) and CV 6 (Qihai) in abdominal protocol.*
3. *TD for adrenal and thyroid problems.*
4. *Clearance point for neck tension on left SCM muscle (parasympathetic nervous system weakness). Restores balance or redresses Deficiency of parasympathetic nervous system.*

Needle technique: Perpendicular 0.3–0.5 in. Rub firmly on both sides. MA.

Point: KI 9 (Zhubin)
Location: SCL: on the line drawn from KI 3 (Taixi) to KI 10 (Yingu), at the lower end of the

point, press firmly against the bone bilaterally. MA.

Point: KI 6 (Zhaohai)
Location: JL: equivalent to one of the Chinese locations, 1 cun directly below the tip of the malleolus at the junction of the red and the white skin.
Energetics:
1. KI 6 (Zhaohai) is to Japanese acupuncture what ST 36 (Zusanli) is to Chinese medicine. *Its primary function relates to the Yin.* Nourishes the Yin. Calms the mind. Invigorates the Yin heel vessel as Master of

belly of gastrocnemius in the medial aspect, about 5 cun above KI 3 (Taixi).

Energetics:
1. Xi (cleft) of Yinwei mai (which connects all the Yin channels). Tonifies KI Yin that benefits the Blood and the Heart. Helps replenish the Yin channels from depletion due to toxicity.
2. *TD for drug detox.*

Needle technique: PP 0.5–0.7 in. MA.

Point: KI 13 (Qixue)
Location: SCL: 3 cun below the umbilicus, 0.5 cun lateral to CV 4 (Guanyuan).
Energetics:
1. Tonifies Kidney and Essence.
2. Point on the Chong mai (Penetrating Vessel): responsible for the circulation of Qi and Blood in the abdomen. Removes masses and obstructions in the abdomen and chest from channel.
3. *TD that has a strong effect on the uterus because it is on the Penetrating Vessel. Uterus reflex.*

Needle technique: PP 0.5–1.0 in. MA.

Point: KI 16 (Huangshu)
Location: JL: 0.5 cun lateral to the center of the umbilicus all around the navel (see Fig. 10.18).
Energetics:
1. According to Yoshio Manaka and the *Nanjing* it is the Front Mu of the Kidney.
2. According to the *Nanjing* it corresponds to the Spleen. Can tonify the Lungs and the Kidney since Spleen is the mother of Lungs and the grandmother of Kidney.
3. *Missing Organ Shu point (the placenta):* the 'storehouse of energy' – prenatal Qi. Strengthens the root Qi of the body.
4. Associated point of the Intestines.
5. Point of the Penetrating Vessel; tonifies the Kidneys; Kidney energy goes through this point to connect with the Heart.

Needle technique: PO 0.5–1.0 in. towards the navel. MA especially with the Tiger Thermie warmer or the belly bowl.

Points: KI 23 (Shenfeng), 24 (Lingxu), 25 (Shencang)

Location: SCL: KI 23 (Shenfeng) – in the fourth intercostal space, 2 cun lateral to the CV channel.
KI 24 (Lingxu) – in the third intercostal space, 2 cun lateral to the CV channel.
KI 25 (Shencang) – in the second intercostal space, 2 cun lateral to the CV channel.
Energetics:
1. Reflex area of the Heart: these points all relate to the 'spirit' or the 'mind'. Named Mind Storage (Heart Pertaining), Spirit Burial-Ground (Heart Mound) and Mind Seal (Heart Housing), respectively. These points are close to the Heart and they can all calm the mind. They reduce anxiety and mental restlessness deriving from KI Xu.
2. Bring down rebellious Qi and aid the Lung Qi to descend and disperse.
3. KI 25 – good for chest pain. Invigorates local Qi Stagnation. Used for chest pain, cough, asthma due to KI Deficiency. Strengthens the Kidney's ability to grasp the Qi.

Needle technique: PO towards the lateral aspect 0.3–0.5 in. MA but generally not used.

Point: KI 27 (Shufu)
Location: SCL: in the depression on the lower border of the clavicle, 2 cun lateral to the CV channel.
Energetics:
1. The Shu of Shus: activates all the Bladder Back Shu points. Extra associated point for all the Yin points on the back.
2. Diagnostic point for the Lungs: regulates LU for cough, asthma, difficult breathing, stimulates the KI function of reception of Qi, resolves Phlegm. For abdominal distension – harmonizes ST/SP. Adrenal imbalance: tonifies KI Yang.
3. *Bone Mu, parathyroid Shu – adjusts calcium levels.* In Western thought the parathyroid gland releases a hormone (parathormone) which controls the level of calcium in the blood. The level of calcium in the body is

regulated by the kidney physiology of filtration and reabsorption. Parathyroid hormone increases the movement of calcium from the bone into the extracellular fluid.

4. *Stress reflex.*

Needle technique: PP 0.3 in. or PO towards lateral aspect. MA.

THE PERICARDIUM MERIDIAN

Point: PC 4 (Ximen)
Location: SCL: 5 cun above the transverse crease of the wrist, on the line connecting PC 3 (Quze) and PC 7 (Daling) between the tendons of the palmaris longus and flexus carpi radialis muscles.
Energetics:

1. Xi (cleft) point: opens the chest, expands the diaphragm, assists the Qing Qi from the air to enter the Lungs. Sends oxygen to all areas.
2. Pacifies and regulates the Heart, calms the spirit, moves Blood Stasis.

Needle technique: PP 0.5–0.8 in. MA.

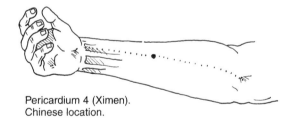

Pericardium 4 (Ximen).
Chinese location.

Point: PC 6 (Neiguan)
Location: SCL: 2 cun above the transverse crease of the wrist, between the tendons of the palmaris longus and flexor carpi radialis muscles.
Energetics:

1. *Primary clearance point for the abdominal map as well as the first clearance point for CV 14.*
2. Removes Stagnation anywhere in the body with a special effect on the upper part of the body.
3. As a longitudinal Luo point, regulates the Qi and Blood of the Heart, opens the Heart orifice, calms the spirit and the mind and

Heart. Expands the diaphragm, decongests the chest and diaphragm, broadens the chest and controls the chest above the Stomach. It can drain off excessive stuck energy of the Upper Jiao, the Heart and chest in particular, including stuck emotional energy which can cause stagnant Qi and Blood.

4. As a transverse Luo point, it connects to the Triple Warmer. Calms and harmonizes the Stomach, promotes and regulates the functional Qi of the Middle Burner and regulates the function of the Triple Warmer.
5. Master of the Yinwei mai: opens the Yinwei mai to distribute Qi to the Stomach, chest and Heart. It links all of the Yin channels together. Coupled to the Chong mai; thus it has a connection to the Kidney.
6. Suppresses rebellious Qi and disperses stagnant Liver Qi. Suppresses pain, stops vomiting and regulates the Jueyin meeting of the Three Arm Yin (PC, LR, HT).
7. All of the extra meridians meet here.
8. Good for miscommunication between the Upper and Lower Jiao, particularly the uterus because there is a special vessel from the Pericardium that goes to the uterus.
9. Benefits the Heart, brain, the emotions and the mental state.
10. Stimulates the production of the essential substances.

Needle technique: PP 0.5–1.0 in. or apply deep dispersive pressure on the left side only. MA but not generally used.

Point: PC 8 (Laogong)
Location: SCL: when the hand is placed with the palm upward, the point is between the second and third metacarpal bones, proximal to the metacarpophalangeal joint, on the radial side of the third metacarpal bone. When making a soft fist, the point is where the tip of the middle finger touches the palm.
Energetics:

1. PC 8 (Laogong) as a distal point of the channel will pull down any Heat or Heat

in the Blood creating pain or obstruction in the axilla area, Heart and breast. The Pericardium channel emerges from the costal region below the anterior axillary fold and ascends to the axilla and further runs downward from the medial aspect of the upper arm. Additionally it has an effect on Heat because it is the Ying (spring)/Fire point. As the horary point, its nature is also Fire related.

2. *TD for the treatment and prevention of Heart disease and fibrocystic breasts.*

Needle technique: PP 0.3–0.5 in. or press firmly with deep dispersive pressure for the desired therapeutic effect. Use preventively. MA but generally not used since it is a Fire point.

THE TRIPLE WARMER MERIDIAN

Point: TE 3 (Zhongdu)
Location: JL: when the hand is placed with the palm facing downward the point is on the dorsum of the hand between the fourth and fifth metacarpal bones, in the depression distal to the metacarpophalangeal joint.
Energetics:
1. Shu (stream) point, Wood point, tonification point. Moves the meridian.
2. *TD which promotes salivation which aids digestion and Yin Deficiency.*
3. *Third abdominal clearance point for ST 25R (Tianshu).*

Needle technique: PP 0.3–0.5 in. or PO towards elbow. Implant intradermal needle. MA. Rub vigorously and bilaterally as a clearance point.

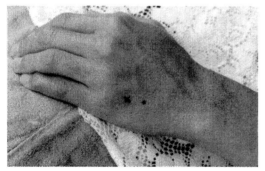

X = Chinese; ● = Japanese. Triple Warmer 3.

Point: TE 5 (Waiguan)
Location: SCL: 2 cun above TE 4 (Yangchi), between the radius and ulna.
Energetics:
1. The primary point of the Triple Warmer. Luo point.
2. Main point for treating any kind of ear disease.
3. *Second clearance point for ST 25L (Tianshu).*
4. Master of the Yangwei mai (increases Yang defensive energy).
5. Works with GB 41 (Zulinqi), Master of the Dai channel, to open the Dai and thereby circulate Yang defensive energy over the whole body like a spiral (see Fig. 5.2).
6. *Clearance point for both sides of the SCM. In the neck protocol the Triple Warmer meridian passes through the neck, running along the posterior border of the ear. It maintains the health of the neck, improves Blood flow, lymphatic drainage and nervous conduction.*

Needle technique: PP 0.5–1.0. in. Press deeply on the right side as a clearance point for ST 25 and on the right as the clearance for the neck. MA.

Point: TE 6 (Zhigou)
Location: SCL: 3 cun above TE 4 (Yangchi), between the ulna and radius.
Energetics:
1. Jing (river) point, horary point, Fire point: regulates Qi therefore has an effect on constipation. Primary point for constipation.
2. *TD for LR Qi Stagnation of chest and Intestines.*

Needle technique: PP 0.7–1.0 in. MA.

Point: TE 16 (Tianyou) area
Location: JL: an area of four points on the posterior border of the SCM.
Energetics:
1. *Infection reflex, adenoid reflex, evil Wind reflex.* Clears Heat, drains Fire. Dispels Wind and eliminates Damp. Reduces swelling, stops pain, softens and relaxes the neck.
2. *TD for immunity, lymphatic glandular exhaustion and neck disorders. Frees the channels and quickens the connecting vessels.*

The diagnosis point for an overworked immune system.

3. Window of the Sky point: brings energy to or takes it away from head.

Needle technique: Apply pressure or massage to this area which tends to be achy to painful. Check both sides of the neck. Choose the most tender point to treat if needling is done. PP 0.3–0.5 in. MA especially the Tiger Thermie warmer to the affected area.

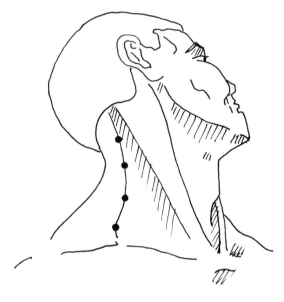

Triple Warmer 16 (Tianyou). Japanese location.

Point: TE 17 (Yifeng)
Location: SCL: posterior to the lobe of the ear, in the depression between the mandible and mastoid process.
Energetics:
1. *TD for lack of salivation: increases salivation with TE 3 (Zhongdu) for digestive and Yin Xu problems.*
2. Expels wind.
3. Benefits the ear.

Needle technique: PP 0.5–1.0 in. towards the mandible. MA.

THE GALL BLADDER MERIDIAN

Point: GB 1 (Tongziliao)

Location: SCL: lateral to the outer canthus, in the depression on the lateral side of the orbit.
Energetics:
1. *TD for hip joint pain* (internal meridian runs down hypochondriac region to lateral side of abdomen and reaches GB 30 (Huantiao)).
2. Dispels Wind, clears Fire and Heat.

Needle technique: PT 0.3–0.5 in. towards lateral aspect. Traditionally no moxa but Tiger Thermie is OK.

Point: GB 15 (Toulinqi)
Location: SCL: directly above GB 14 (Yangbai), 0.5 cun within the hairline, midway between GV 24 (Shenting) and ST 8 (Touwei).
Energetics:
1. *TD for sinus problems.*

Needle technique: PT 0.3–0.5 in. towards the lateral aspect. MA.

Point: GB 25 (Jingmen)
Location: SCL: on the lateral side of the abdomen, on the lower border of the free end of the 12th rib.
Energetics:
1. Back Shu point of the Kidney.
2. *TD for specific differentiation of back pain, namely puffy sacrum, flat lumbar area, pain on the center line.*

Needle technique: With patient in lateral recumbent position, needle towards spine, PP 0.5–1.0 in. MA.

Point: GB 31 (Fengshi)
Location: SCL: on the midline of the lateral aspect of the thigh, 7 cun above the transverse popliteal crease. When the patient is standing erect with the hands close to the sides, the point is where the tip of the middle finger touches.
Energetics:
1. Wind reflex. Expels Wind. For Gall Bladder type sciatica.

Needle technique: PP 0.7–1.2 in. MA.

Point: GB 34 (Yanglingquan)
Location: JL: the Chinese location is anterior and inferior to the head of the fibula. Use the Japanese location which is 1 cun posterior to

Chinese GB 34 (Yanglingquan), that is, behind the head of the fibula.

Energetics:
1. He (Sea) point, Earth point: resolves Damp-Heat.
2. Primary treatment point for pain as the Influential point that dominates the tendons and the muscles.

Needle technique: PP 0.8–1.2 in., implant intradermal or apply deep dispersive pressure. MA.

Point: GB 40 (Qiuxu)
Location: SCL: anterior and inferior to the external malleolus, in the depression on the lateral side of the tendon of m. extensor digitorum longus.
Energetics:
1. Source point: strengthens the Gall Bladder.
Needle technique: PP 0.5–0.8 in. MA.

Point: GB 41 (Zulinqi)
Location: SCL: in the depression lateral to the tendon of the extensor digiti minimi muscle. JL: anterior to the cuboid bone.
Energetics:
1. Shu (stream) point, Wood point, horary point. Resolves Damp-Heat, particularly in the genital region, promotes the smooth flow of Liver Qi, spreads and drains the Liver and Gall Bladder. Clears Fire and extinguishes Wind, brightens eyes and sharpens hearing, transforms obstructing Phlegm-Heat, removes coagulation and Stagnation of Blood and Phlegm from the Jueyin (LR/PC), for women's problems due to Liver imbalance.
2. Opens the Dai channel: used with TE 5R (Waiguan), Master of the Yangwei mai, to circulate Yang defensive energy.
3. *Abdominal clearance point for ST 25L (Tianshu) or ST 25R to open Dai channel.*

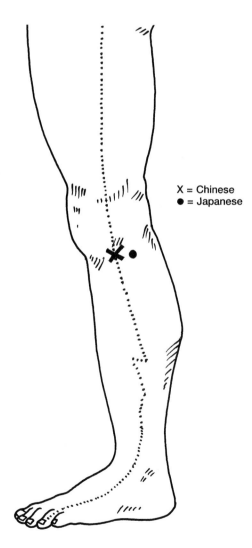

X = Chinese
● = Japanese

Gall Bladder 34 (Yanglingquan).

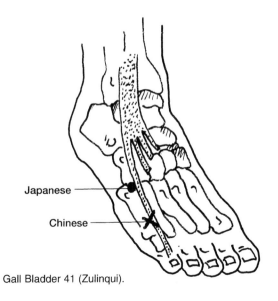

Japanese ——

Chinese ——

Gall Bladder 41 (Zulinqui).

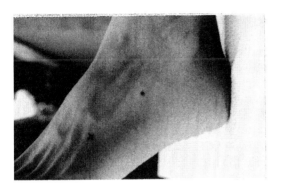

X = Chinese; ● = Japanese. Gall Bladder 41.

4. *TD for Liver Yang rising out of Yin Deficiency, i.e. migraines.*
5. *TD for tight SCM with TE 5R.*

Needle technique: Very tender point when palpated. PT 0.3–0.5 in. Apply strong, deep, dispersive pressure to the left side or implant intradermal needle. MA.

THE LIVER MERIDIAN

Point: LR 2 (Xingjian)
Location: SCL: between the first and second metatarsal bones, proximal to the margin of the web.
Energetics:
1. Ying (spring) point, Fire point, sedation point: clears Liver Fire.
2. Affects pancreas' regulation of sugar.

Needle technique: PO 0.3–0.5 in. in direction of the meridian. MA.

Point: LR 3 (Taichong)
Location: SCL: in the depression distal to the junction of the first and second metatarsal bones.
Energetics:
1. Shu (stream) point, Earth point, Source point: balances Liver function.
2. *Clearance point for ST 25L (Tianshu) when due to portal vein congestion or Liver Blood Deficiency.*

Needle technique: PP 0.3–0.5 in. or thread LR 2 (Xingjian) to LR 3 (Taichong). Implant intradermal needle. Rub vigorously and bilaterally. MA.

Point: LR 4 (Zhongfeng)

Location: SCL: 1 cun anterior to the medial malleolus, midway between SP 5 (Shangqiu) and ST 41 (Jiexi), in the depression on the medial side of the tendon of m. tibialis anterior.
Energetics:
1. Metal point on the Wood meridian: promotes the smooth flow of LR Qi in the Lower Burner because Metal controls Wood. Benefits the ligaments, opens pelvic blockage (structural).
2. *Primary TD for any type of back pain or Qi Stagnation without much Fire.*
3. Effective point for Blood Stagnation because Blood follows Qi.
4. *Primary clearance point for inner thigh congestion.*

Needle technique: PP 0.3–0.5 in. or PO in direction of meridian. Intradermals may be implanted. As a clearance point, rub firmly. MA.

Point: LR 5 (Ligou)
Location: Three locations:
1. Chinese – 5 cun above the tip of the medial malleolus on the medial aspect and near the medial border of the tibia.
2. Chinese – 5 cun above the tip of the medial malleolus posterior to the medial border of the tibia.
3. Japanese – midway between the tip of the medial malleolus and SP 9 (Yinlingquan) on the posterior border of the tibia.

Energetics:
1. Luo connecting point of the Liver channel: promotes smooth flow of LR Qi, pulls Excess out of Liver, also for Liver toxicity. Has specific affinity for genital and urinary area. Resolves Damp-Heat. Primary point for prostatitis. As the longitudinal Luo, it can be used to stimulate its own organ–meridian complex to drain Excess from the meridian such as Damp-Heat, stagnant Qi and toxicity. As the transverse Luo, connects to the source point of its Coupled meridian, the Gall Bladder, thus harmonizing Wood energy.
2. *TD for inflammation. Antiinflammatory point; can be used for any kind of inflammation, that is, any 'itis'. Works well with KI 6*

(Zhaohai) for inflammation and with KI 9 (Zhubin) for strengthening elimination and detoxification.

3. *Clearance point for ST 25L.*

Needle technique: PO upward 0.3–0.5 in. Rub vigorously on left side. MA.

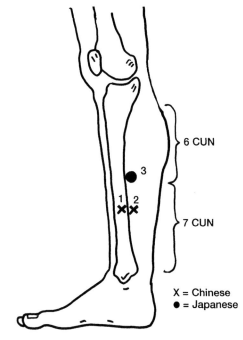

Liver 5 (Ligou).

Point: LR 8 (Ququan)
Location: SCL: on the medial side of the knee joint. When the knee is flexed, the point is above the medial end of the transverse popliteal crease, posterior to the medial condyle of the tibia, on the anterior border of the insertion of m. semi-membranosus and m. semitendinosus.
Energetics:

1. He (Sea) point, Water point, tonification point: cools and disperses Damp-Heat. Brings down Liver Yang; builds Liver Yin.

Needle technique: PP 0.5–0.8 in. MA.

Point: LR 12 (Jimai)
Location: SCL: inferior and lateral to pubic spine, 2.5 cun lateral to the CV channel, at the inguinal groove lateral and inferior to ST 30 (Qichong).

Energetics:

1. *Local clearance point for inner thigh.*

Needle technique: No needling due to pudendal artery and vein, femoral vein and external pubic branch of inferior epigastric artery. MA. Intradermal needle may be implanted.

Point: LR 14 (Qimen)
Location: SCL: on the mammillary line, two ribs below the nipple, in the sixth intercostal space.
Energetics:

1. *Clearance point for ST 25L (Tianshu) due to portal vein congestion. Clearance point for ST 25L (Tianshu) if due to Liver Deficiency (as the Front Mu point of the Liver regulates Liver Yin and Yang).*

Needle technique: PO 0.3–0.5 in. towards the lateral aspect. MA.

THE GOVERNING VESSEL MERIDIAN

Point: GV 1 (Changqiang)
Location: SCL: midway between the tip of the coccyx and the anus.
Energetics:

1. Luo point of the GV channel: it sends energy all through the spine and moves the meridian.
2. Adjusts the intestines.
3. *TD for rectal vein congestion.*

Needle technique: PP 0.5–1.0 in. MA.

Point: GV 2 (Yaoshu)
Location: SCL: in the hiatus of the sacrum.
Energetics:

1. Associated point of the renal region. Affects renal and sacral region. Strengthens low back. Dispels Wind-Cold.
2. *TD for back pain and hormonal problems due to an injured tailbone.*

Needle technique: PO upward 0.5–1.0 in. or massage upward. MA.

Point: GV 3 (Yaoyangguan)
Location: SCL: below the spinous process of the fourth lumbar vertebra. On the level with BL 25 (Dachangshu), the Back Shu point of the Large Intestine.

Energetics:
1. Adjusts the Kidney. Tonifies Yang of KI and weak adrenal glands. Benefits the back and knees. Adrenal reflex.
2. *TD for deficient KI Yang, a parasympathetic nervous system problem. Could also see cold feet, low body temperature, low Blood pressure, tendency to develop ovarian or breast cysts. Might have puffy sacrum (fluid retention due to deficient KI Yang).*

Needle technique: PP 0.5–1.0 in. MA.

Point: GV 4 (Mingmen)
Location: SCL: below the spinous process of the second lumbar vertebra, on the level with BL 23 (Shenshu), Back Shu of the Kidney.
Energetics:
1. The Gate of Life: supports and guards ancestral Qi. Tonifies KI Yang. Nourishes original Qi. Warms the Gate of Vitality, especially with moxa. Expels Cold. Strengthens lower back, benefits lumbars. Benefits Essence. Benefits SP Yang. Best point for KI Yang Xu. Strengthens immunity by tonifying source Qi.
2. *A primary TD point for allergies. Good for sinus problems.*
3. *TD for spinal back pain.*

Needle technique: PP 0.5–1.0 in. MA.

Point: GV 5 (Xuanshu)
Location: SCL: below the spinous process of the first lumbar vertebra between the Back Shu points of the Triple Warmer, BL 22 (Sanjiaoshu).
Energetics:
1. Regulates and tonifies SP, regulates the ST and benefits the lower back.
2. *TD for diabetes.*

Needle technique: PP 0.5–1.0 in. MA.

Point: GV 6 (Jizhong)
Location: SCL: below the spinous process of the 11th thoracic vertebra between BL 20 (Pishu), Back Shu point of the Spleen.
Energetics:
1. *TD for digestion and sugar metabolism problems.*

Needle technique: PP 0.5–1.0 in. **No moxa –** moxa will displace the spinous process of the 11th thoracic vertebra.

Point: GV 11 (Shendao)
Location: SCL: below the spinous process of the fifth thoracic vertebra below T5, between BL 15 (Xinshu), Back Shu point of the Heart.
Energetics:
1. Clears Heart Fire. Calms the mind. For Excess Heart patterns.

Needle technique: PP 0.5–1.0 in. **Classically forbidden to needle as it affects the Heart.**

Point: GV 12 (Shenzhu) areas
Location: SCL: below the spinous process of the third thoracic vertebra, between BL 13 (Feishu), Back Shu point of the Lungs.
Energetics:
1. Located at the same level as the Back Shus of the Lungs, it tonifies Lung Qi and generally strengthens the body. It readjusts the Qi of all the Yang organs and helps to fight off any attack of Wind. It can strengthen the body after a debilitating chronic illness.

Needle technique: PP 0.5–1.0 in. MA.

Point: GV 13 (Taodao)
Location: SCL: below the spinous process of the first thoracic vertebra between BL 11 (Dazhu), Back Shu point of the Bones.
Energetics:
1. Union of BL and GV channels: cools Heat, releases exterior, eliminates Wind-Cold, Wind-Heat, affects Lungs; calms the spirit, clears the mind.
2. Affects bones: for any bone condition.
3. Like GV 14 (Dazhui), can also treat all Yang channels.

Needle technique: PP 0.5–1.0 in. MA.

Point: GV 14 (Dazhui)
Location: SCL: between the spinous processes of the seventh cervical and the first thoracic vertebrae (approximately at the level of the shoulder).
Energetics:
1. Meeting of all Yang channels: point of greatest Yang in body. For febrile diseases,

disperses Excess Yang. Also can tonify Yang, especially HT Yang with moxa. Strongly tonifies Wei Qi. Increases white blood cells. Relieves the exterior, opens the Yang, clears the brain and calms the spirit.

2. *Evil Wind reflex. Adrenal exhaustion reflex if there is a fat pad.*
3. *TD for immunity.*

Needle technique: PP 0.5–1.0 in. MA. Frequent moxibustion is advisable to tonify Yang.

Point: GV 15 (Yamen)
Location: at the midpoint of the nape, 0.5 cun below GV 16 (Fengfu), in the depression 0.5 cun within the hairline.
Energetics:

1. *TD for lack of salivation with TE 3.*
2. Expels Wind. Benefits the ear. Removes channel obstruction.
3. Window to the Sky point: regulates Qi.
4. Sea of Marrow: lifts the mind.

Needle technique: Deep puncture not advisable. PP 0.5–0.8 in. CAN KILL! Do not needle obliquely upward due to proximity to medulla. MOXA FORBIDDEN.

THE CONCEPTION VESSEL MERIDIAN

Point: CV 1 (Huiyin)–2 (Qugu) area
Location: JL: on the midline of the abdomen in the depression on the pubic bone.
Energetics:

1. *TD for dripping urine.*
2. Urogenital problems.

Needle technique: PP 0.3–1.0 in. or obliquely upward. MA. Caution with moxa around the pubic hair.

Point: CV 3 (Zhongji)
Location: SCL: on the anterior midline, 1 cun above the upper border of the symphysis pubis.
Energetics:

1. Front Mu of Bladder: resolves Damp-Heat. Promotes the Bladder function of Qi transformation. Clears Heat.
2. Union of CV, SP, KI, LR channels.
3. Warms the Essence Palace.

Needle technique: PP 0.5–1.0 in. MA.

Point: CV 4 (Guanyuan)
Location: SCL: on the midline of the abdomen, 3 cun below the center of the umbilicus.
Energetics:

1. Kidney reflex area: tonifies foundation Yin, Yang and Blood. Regulates Qi; restores Yang.
2. Front Mu of SI, energetically equivalent to Spleen Yang.
3. Connects to Chong mai.
4. *Abdominal diagnosis point for Kidney dysfunction.*

Needle technique: PP 0.8–1.2 in. Frequent moxibustion is indicated.

Point: CV 5 (Shimen)
Location: SCL: on the midline of the abdomen, 2 cun below the center of the umbilicus.
Energetics:

1. Front Mu of the Triple Warmer: activates the Yuan Qi.

Needle technique: PP 0.5–1.0 in. MA.

Point: CV 6 (Qihai)
Location: SCL: 1.5 cun below the center of the umbilicus on the midline of the abdomen.
Energetics:

1. The center of the energy in the body. Strengthens KI Qi, Yin and Yuan Qi.
2. Connects to the Chong channel. Regulates Blood and hemorrhage.
3. *Abdominal diagnosis point for KI.*

Needle technique: PP 0.8–1.2 in. MA.

Point: CV 7 (Yinjiao)
Location: SCL: on the midline of the abdomen, 1 cun below the umbilicus.
Energetics:

1. Abdominal reflection of SP 6 (Sanyinjiao) – Three Yin Crossing.
2. Lower controlling point of Triple Warmer.

Needle technique: PP 0.8–1.2 in. MA.

Point: CV 8 (Shenque)
Location: SCL: the center of the umbilicus.

Energetics:

1. *Spleen reflex area according to the* Nanjing – *strengthens the Spleen.*
2. Gate of Shen: tonifies original Qi, increases will to live, strengthens the spirit.
3. Birth Trauma Mu point.

Needle technique: No needling directly but can needle around it in the KI 16 radius area (See KI 16). Moxa is applicable in any form and highly recommended.

Point: CV 9 (Shuifen)
Location: SCL: on the midline of the abdomen, 1 cun above the umbilicus.
Energetics:

1. Water metabolism reflex: tonifies SP Qi.
2. Heart reflex area.

Needle technique: PP 0.5–1.0 in. MA.

Point: CV 12 (Zhongwan)
Location: SCL: on the midline of the abdomen, 4 cun above the center of the umbilicus.
Energetics:

1. Front Mu of ST: indicates the condition of the Stomach, tonifies ST Yin. The point reflects stress.
2. Controlling point of the Middle Burner: adjusts the Stomach, tonifies the Spleen and Stomach, regulates the Qi and transforms Damp.
3. The Influential point that dominates the Fu organs.
4. It is the source of all Yin, hence its ability to diagnose the Yin of the body.
5. Brings down rebellious ST Qi.
4. *Abdominal diagnosis point for Stomach problems.*

Needle technique: PP 0.3–0.8 in. MA.

Point: CV 14 (Juque)–CV 15 (Jiuwei)
Location: SCL: on the midline of the abdomen, 6 cun above the center of the umbilicus.
Energetics:

1. Front Mu of HT: indicates the physical and energetic condition of the Heart. Pacifies the spirit, adjusts the Qi, harmonizes the Stomach and benefits the diaphragm.
2. Luo point: spreads energy through chest. Signifies Stagnation in the Upper Jiao and the lack of free flow of Liver Qi.
3. Good emotional release point.
4. *Abdominal diagnosis point for Heart pathology, LR Qi Stagnation and chest function.*

Needle technique: PO 0.4–0.6 in. with arms uplifted. **No moxa. Caution in case of elongated xiphoid process.** When palpated as an abdominal diagnosis point, locate CV 14 but slide down from CV 14 to the first available point that you feel you can go into and palpate obliquely upward.

Point: CV 17 (Tanzhong)
Location: SCL: in the midline of the sternum, between the nipples, level with the fourth intercostal space.
Energetics:

1. Front Mu of Pericardium. Influential point that dominates the Qi: tonifies energy of the chest. Chest reflex – all energy of channels concentrates at this point. Regulates and suppresses rebellious Qi. Major asthma point. Expands diaphragm. Grief point.
2. Upper controlling point of Triple Warmer.
3. *Thymus Mu point.*

Needle technique: PT upward 0.3–0.5 in. MA.

Answers

Chapter 4

3.   A = South
      B = East
      C = North
      D = West
      E = Center

4.   A = Heart
      B = Stomach and Spleen
      C = Spleen
      D = Liver
      E = Kidney
      F = Lung

5.   A = Fire
      B = Wood
      C = Water
      D = Metal
      E = Earth

6.   A = Spring
      B = Summer
      C = Winter
      D = Fall
      E = Late Summer

Chapter 6

1. a
2. c
3. b
4. a
5. d
6. b

1. d
2. d
3. a
4. e
5. a
6. b
7. c
8. f

1. d
2. b
3. f
4. c
5. g
6. a
7. e

Chapter 8

6.
      a = CV 4
      b = ST 25
      c = CV 12
      d = CV 14
      e = CV 6

14. b

Chapter 9

14. b

Chapter 10

1. c
2. d
3. a
4. e
5. f
6. c
7. b

Chapter 11

1.
    1. b
    2. a
    3. e
    4. c
    5. d

Chapter 12

1. l
2. f
3. a
4. c
5. i
6. h
7. m
8. k
9. d
10. e
11. g
12. b
13. j

Chapter 15

1. b
2. c
3. a
4. d, e
5. e, h
6. g
7. f

Chapter 16

1. d
2. c
3. f
4. a
5. b
6. e
7. g
8. h

Chapter 18

8a. KI 1, 6, 3, 7 or LU 7
8b. SP 10, TE 5, GB 41
8c. KI 1, 6, 3 or 7

References

Ackerman D 1990 A natural history of the senses. Vintage Books, New York

Alphen J van, Aris A 1995 Oriental medicine: an illustrated guide to the Asian arts of healing. Shambala Publications, Boston, MA

Balch J, Balch P 1990 Prescriptions for nutritional healing. Avery, New York

Baldt M 1996 Deep venous thrombosis of the lower extremity: efficacy of spiral CT venography compared with conventional venography in diagnosis. Journal of the American Medical Association 276(16): 1284

Beijing College of Traditional Medicine 1980 Essentials of Chinese acupuncture. Foreign Language Press, Beijing

Bell WR, Simon TL 1982 Current status of pulmonary thromboembolic disease. American Heart Journal 103: 239–262

Catlett R, Welch M 1996 Deep venous thrombosis: guide to tailoring the prophylactic regimen. Consultant 36(7): 1489

Center for Positive Living 1990 Positive living and health. Rodale Press, Emmaus, PA

Chaitow L 1991 Palpatory literacy. Thorson's, London

Challem J 1996 Probiotics: these 'friendly' bacteria improve digestion and boost immunity. Natural Health 26(5): 21–24

Cheung CS 1996 Phlegm. Abstract and Review of Clinical Traditional Chinese Medicine, 3: entire issue

Clayman C (med ed) 1994 The American Medical Association family medical guide, 3rd edn. Random House, New York

Cleary T (trans/ed) 1993 The spirit of the Tao. Shambala Publications, Boston, MA

Denmei S 1990 Japanese classical acupuncture: introduction to meridian therapy. Eastland Press, Seattle

DeVito PL 1994 The immune system vs. stress. USA Today 123(2590): 27

Doner K 1996 Heal your angry heart. American Health 15(7): 74

Dzung TV 1989 The curious meridians. American Journal of Acupuncture 17(1): 45–46

Epstein D 1994 The 12 stages of healing. Amber-Allen Publishing, California

Flaws B 1988 Allergic rhinitis. Blue Poppy Press research report # 97. Blue Poppy Press, Boulder, CO

Frager R 1980 Touch. Working with the body. In: Complete guide to holistic medicine. Westview Press, Boulder, CO

Fratkin J 1986 Chinese herbal patent formulas: a practical guide. Institute of Traditional Medicine, Portland, OR

Fratkin J 1995 Sushi versus Stir-fry. My move from TCM acupuncture to Japanese acupuncture. North American Journal of Oriental Medicine July: 28–29

Fratkin J 1996a Denmei Shudo workshop at the Pacific Symposium. North American Journal of Oriental Medicine 3(8): 21

Fratkin J 1996b Root and branch: clinical applications of Japanese meridian therapy. North American Journal of Oriental Medicine 3(7): 9–13

Gagne D 1994 The effects of therapeutic touch and relaxation therapy in reducing anxiety. Archives of Psychiatric Nursing 8(3): 184

Gardner-Abbate S 1995a New insight on the eitology and treatment of cellulite according to Chinese medicine: more than skin deep. American Journal of Acupuncture 23(4): 336–339

Gardner-Abbate S 1995b Assessing and treating pericardium 6 (Neiguan): gate to internal well-being. American Journal of Acupuncture 23(2): 231–239

Gardner-Abbate S 1995c The treatment of periodontal gum disease: a protocol for prevention, maintenance and reversal within the paradigm of traditional Chinese medicine. American Journal of Acupuncture 23(3): 238

Gardner-Abbate S 1996 Holding the tiger's tail: an acupuncture techniques manual in the treatment of disease. Southwest Acupuncture College Press, Santa Fe, NM

Gardner-Abbate S 2000 Immune enhancement for oncology patients through auricular acupuncture. Acupuncture Today 1(3): 18–19

Hammer L 1988 Dragon rises, red bird flies. Station Hill Press, Barrytown, New York

Hirshowitz B, Ullmann Y, Har-Shai Y, Vilenski A, Peled IJ 1993 Silicone occlusive sheeting in the management of hypertrophic and keloid scarring, including the possible mode of action of silicon by static electricity. European Journal of Plastic Surgery 16: 5–9

Howard S 1995 The paradox of paradigms and points. Acupuncture Society of Massachusetts Newsletter, May: 6

Johns R 1997 Pericardium 6 Neiguan: the wild card. American Acupuncturist 17: 3–4

Kagoshima M 1996 Immunity studies get down to gut issues: widening research on the role of the intestinal tract in body's defense is yielding medical applications. Nikkei Weekly (Japan) 3334(753): 10

Keller E, Bzdek VM 1986 Effects of therapeutic touch on tension headache. Nursing Research 35(2): 101

Kischer CW, Bunce H, Sheltar MR 1978 Mast cell analyses in hypertrophic scars treated with pressure and mature scars. Journal of Investigative Dermatology 70: 355–357

Larree C 1995 Rooted in spirit. Station Hill Press, New York

Larree C, Rochat de la Vallee E 1990–1991 The practitioner–patient relationship. Journal of Traditional Acupuncture Winter: 14–17, 48–50

Lee M 1992 Insights of a senior acupuncturist. Blue Poppy Press, Boulder, CO

Legge D 1990 Close to the bone. The treatment of musculoskeletal disorder with acupuncture and other Traditional Chinese Medicine. Sydney College Press, Australia

Liu F, Liu YM 1989 Chinese medical terminology. Commercial Press, Hong Kong

Lushang W, Fei X 1997 Improving the complexion by needling Renying ST 9. Journal of Chinese Medicine 54: 19

Maciocia G 1989 The foundations of Chinese medicine. Churchill Livingstone, London

Maciocia G 1993 Lecture notes. Southwest Acupuncture College, Santa Fe, NM

Marcus A 1991 Acute abdominal syndromes. Blue Poppy Press, Boulder, CO

Matsumoto K 1987 Lecture notes. Southwest Acupuncture College, Santa Fe, NM

Matsumoto K, Birch S 1988 Hara diagnosis. Reflections on the sea. Paradigm Publications, Brookline, MA

Nagano K 1991 Immune enhancement through acupuncture and moxibustion: specific treatment for allergic disorders, mild infectious disease and secondary infections. American Journal of Acupuncture 19(4): 329–338

O'Brien T 1994 Learn the patterns of stress. Knight–Ridder, Tribune News Service October 14

Ornstein R 1989 Healthy pleasures. Addison-Wesley, New York

Raloff J 1996 Umbilical clamping affects anemia risk. Science News 149(17): 263

Reich JD, Cazzaniga AL, Mertz PM, Kerdel FA, Eaglstein WH 1991 The effect of electrical stimulation on the number of mast cells on healing wounds. Journal of the American Academy of Dermatology 25: 40–46

Requena Y 1986 Terrains and pathology, vol. 1. Paradigm Publications, Brookline, MA

Rosenfeld I 1986 Modern prevention: the new medicine. Linden Press/Simon and Schuster, New York

Ross J 1984 Zang Fu: the organ systems in traditional Chinese medicine. Churchill Livingstone, London

Ryan S, Travis W 1991 Wellness. Ten Speed Press, Berkeley, CA

Seem MD 1989a TCM versus non-TCM: putting the acupuncture back into Chinese medicine. Journal of the American College of Traditional Chinese Medicine 7(4): 10–11, 45

Seem MD 1989b Body mind energetics. Healing Arts Press, Rochester, VT

Seem MD 1990 Acupuncture imaging: perceiving the energy pathways of the body. Healing Arts Press, Rochester, VT

Seem MD 1992 Integrationist acupuncture: plurality in the practice of American acupuncture. American Journal of Acupuncture 20(3): 231–233

Serizawa K 1988 Clinical acupuncture. Japan Publications, Tokyo

Skardis J 1995 Injection therapy in the practice of Oriental medicine. New Mexico Association of Acupuncture and Oriental Medicine Newsletter 3: 10–16

Smith A 1968 The body. Walker and Company, New York

Stephenson J 1995 Terms of engraftment: umbilical cord blood transplants arouse enthusiasm. Journal of the American Medical Association 272(23): 1813

Sternfeld M, Eliraz A, Fink A et al 1992 Moxibustion therapy for allergic rhinitis. American Journal of Acupuncture 20(2): 151–155

Time, June 2, 1997; 23

Trott A, Trunkey D, Wilson S 1995 Acute abdominal pain: a guide to crisis management. Patient Care 29(13): 104

Unschuld P 1979 Medical ethics in Imperial China. University of California Press, Berkeley, CA

Unschuld P (trans) 1986 Nanching: the classic of difficult issues. University of California Press, Berkeley, CA

Van Nghi N 1987 An exploration of the eight curious vessels. Southwest Acupuncture College, Santa Fe, NM

Verrees M 1996 Touch me. Journal of the American Medical Association 276(16): 1285

Vithoulkas G 1980 The science of homeopathy. Grove Press, New York

Weiss DS, Eaglstein WH, Falanga V 1989 Exogenous electric current can reduce the formation of hypertrophic scars. Journal of Dermatology and Surgical Oncology 15: 1272–1275

Weisman N, Ellis A 1985 Fundamentals of Chinese medicine. Paradigm Publications, Brookline, MA

Ziegler J 1995 Immune system may benefit from the ability to laugh. Journal of the National Cancer Institute 87(5): 342

Appendices

Appendix 1

Energetics of important points in the Japanese acupuncture system by disease

Illness/energetics	Points (treatment, diagnosis and clearance)
A	
Abdomen (drumlike)	LI 10 (Shousanli), KI 14 (Siman)
Abdominal distension	ST 36 (Zusanli), SP 4 (Gongsun)
Abdominal pain	CV 8 (Shenque) – moxa on ginger
Abdominal pain and lumps	KI 6 (Zhaohai) and PC 6 (Neiguan)
Abdominal pain (with fever)	ST 44 (Neiting)
Acne	CV 8 (Shenque) – moxa on salt, cupping
Acute dysmenorrhea	SP 10 (Xuehai)
Acute lumbago (back strain)	SI 6 (Yanglao), BL 63 (Jinmen)
Acute stomachache	LR 8 (Ququan), SP 10 (Xuehai), ST 34 (Liangqiu), ST 44 (Neiting), SP 4 (Gongsun)
Adenoid reflex	TE 16 (Tianyou), Naganos
Adjust blood pressure	KI 1 (Yongquan)
Adrenal exhaustion	GV 14 (Dazhui)
Adrenal reflex	GV 3 (Yaoyangguan)
Adrenal reflex, shock, trauma	KI 6 (Zhaohai)

Illness/energetics	Points (treatment, diagnosis and clearance)
A	
Allergic diseases	CV 8 (Shenque) – indirect moxa, sinus points
Allergic reaction	ST 44 (Neiting)
Allergic rhinitis	CV 8 (Shenque) – indirect moxa, moxa on ginger, sinus points
Allergy point	GV 4 (Mingmen)
Antiinflammatory point, any 'itis'	LR 5 (Ligou), KI 6 (Zhaohai)
Anxiety	KI 25 (Shencang), HT 7 (Shenmen)
Appendicitis reflex	ST 25R (Tianshu)
Appetite, increase	KI 2 (Rangu)
Asthma	KI 25 (Shencang), KI 6 (Zhaohai), LU 5 (Chize) (3 locations)
Atopic dermatitis	CV 8 (Shenque) – cupping
Autonomic nervous system disturbance	SCM muscle tight, wiry, stringy Right = KI Yin Xu Left = KI Yang Xu
B	
Backache	LR 4 (Zhongfeng)
Back pain from Kidney Yang Xu	Eight Needle technique (see points)
Bladder reflex	CV 2 (Qugu)–3 (Zhongji)
Bleeding	SP 4 (Gongsun)
Bleeding gums	ST 44 (Neiting)
Blood pressure	KI 1 (Yongquan)
Blood Stagnation reflex	ST 25L (Tianshu)
Bone Mu	KI 27 (Shufu)
Brachial reflex point	ST 12 (Quepen) releases scalene compression R = right lymphatic duct congestion L = HT Qi Xu

Illness/energetics	Points (treatment, diagnosis and clearance)
B	
Bronchitis	LU 5 (Chize) – three locations, KI 6 (Zhaohai)
C	
Calcium adjustment	KI 27 (Shufu) (Bone Mu)
Carpal tunnel syndrome	LU 7 (Lieque), LU 8 (Jingqu), ST 12 (Quepen), shoulder point under eye, area between LI 6 (Pianli) and 7 (Wenliu)
Chemotherapy effects: nausea accompanying radiation damage	LI 4 (Hegu), ST 36 (Zusanli), PC 6 (Neiguan), SP 6 (Sanyinjiao), CV 12 (Zhongwan)
Chest congestion	PC 6 (Neiguan)
Chest fullness	LU 1 (Zhongfu)
Chest pain	LU 4 (Xiabai), LU 1 (Zhongfu), KI 25 (Shencang)
Chest reflex (inside)	CV 17 (Tanzhong)
Chong mai disturbance, prolapses	ST 30 (Qichong)
Chronic illness	KI 6 (Zhaohai)
Chronic sinusitis	Tonsillar treatment (see points)
Circulation in lower limbs	SP 6 (Sanyinjiao)
Cold (systemic)	CV 8 (Shenque) – moxa on ginger
Cold limbs	CV 8 (Shenque) – moxa on salt
Common cold	Tonsillar treatment (see points)
Congestion in rectal vein	GV 1 (Changqiang), LU 6 (Kongzui)
Constipation	Special point lateral to HT 7 (Shenmen), TE 6 (Zhigou), SP 9 (Yinlingquan), CV 8 (Shenque) – moxa on ginger, ST 44 (Neiting)
Coronary artery (heart reflex)	SI 11 (Tianzong) on left

Illness/energetics	Points (treatment, diagnosis and clearance)
C	
Cough	KI 25 (Shencang)
D	
Dermatitis	CV 8 (Shenque) – cupping
Deviated septum reflex	ST 2 (Sibai)
Diabetes	GV 5 (Xuanshu)
Digestion	Six Flowers: BL 17 (Geshu), 18 (Ganshu), 20 (Pishu)
Digestive disturbances	CV 8 (Shenque) – moxa on salt, SP 6 (Sanyinjiao)
Dripping urine reflex	CV 1.5 (between CV 1 and 2 (Qugu))
Drug detox	KI 9 (Zhubin)
Drug use	KI 6 (Zhaohai)
Dysmenorrhea	SP 8 (Diji)
E	
Eczema	ST 44 (Neiting)
Edema of foot, leg	BL 66 (Zutonggu)
Elimination of toxins	KI 9 (Zhubin)
Emotional problems (stuck energy)	PC 6 (Neiguan)
Enuresis	SP 6 (Sanyinjiao)
Evil Wind reflex	GV 14 (Dazhui)
F	
Fat metabolism reflex, adrenal exhaustion	GV 14 (Dazhui)
Fatigue	CV 8 (Shenque) – 8 needles around navel
Fecal stagnation	LU 10 (Yuji)
Fibrocystic breasts	PC 8 (Laogong)

Illness/energetics	Points (treatment, diagnosis and clearance)
F	
Food poisoning, allergic reaction, toothache, migraines, eczema	ST 44 (Neiting), ST 34R (Liangqiu), GB 41 (Zulinqi), TE 5 (Waiguan)
G	
Gas reflex, sigmoid colon reflex (constipation due to nervous colon)	SP 9 (Yinlingquan)
General immunity points	LI 10 (Shousanli), 11 (Quchi) + Naganos, ST 36 (Zusanli)
Gingivitis	Between LI 6 (Pianli) and 7 (Wenliu), ST 44 (Neiting), GV 26 (Shuigou)
Greater saphenous vein	LR 12 (Jimai)
Goiter	TE 5 (Waiguan)
Gum pain	ST 44 (Neiting)
Gum problems	Between LI 6 (Pianli) and 7 (Wenliu)
H	
Hamstring release	GB 34 (Yanglingquan)
Headache	CV 8 (Shenque) – indirect moxa
Headache accompanying food poisoning	ST 34 (Liangqiu), ST 44 (Neiting)
Heart disease reflex	KI 25, 24, 23 (Shencang, Lingxu, Shenfeng), Huatous of GV 11 (Shendao)
Heart Qi Xu	ST 12L (Quepen)
Heart reflex area	CV 14, 15 (Juque, Jiuwei)
Hemorrhoids	LU 6 (Kongzui)
Herpes (oral)	Between LI 6 (Pianli) and 7 (Wenliu)
Herpes zoster	Tonsillar treatment (see points)
Hip joint pain	GB 1 (Tongziliao)

Illness/energetics	Points (treatment, diagnosis and clearance)
H	
Hives	CV 8 (Shenque) – indirect moxa
Hormonal disturbances	SI 3 (Houxi)
Hot flashes	KI 6 (Zhaohai) and BL 62 (Shenmai)
Hydrochloric acid excess	ST 44 (Neiting) or 36 (Zusanli)
Hydrochloric acid insufficiency	ST 36 (Zusanli) – moxa
I	
Immune deficiency disease	Chinese immunity treatment: CV 4 (Guanyuan), GV 4 (Mingmen), ST 36 (Zusanli), GV 14 (Dazhui), BL 23 (Shenshu)
Immunity	Naganos, ST 13 (Qihu), ST 36 (Zusanli), GV 4 (Mingmen), GV 14 (Dazhui)
Infection reflex	TE 16 (Tianyou), ST 2 (Sibai)
Inflammation	LR 5 (Ligou), KI 6 (Zhaohai), KI 9 (Zhubin)
Inner thigh compression	KI 1 (Yongquan), LR 4 (Zhongfeng), KI 6 (Zhaohai), KI 3 (Taixi), SP 6 (Sanyinjiao)
'Itis' (any)	LR 5 (Ligou)
K	
Kidney deficiency	BL 23 (Shenshu)
Kidney Mu, Spleen reflex	KI 16 (Huangshu) (Manaka)
Kidney organ reflex	KI 7 (Fuliu)
Kidney reflex	CV 4–6 (Guanyuan–Qihai)
Knee, heavy, fluid on knee	ST 35 (Dubi)
Knee pain	ST 31 (Biguan), ST 32 (Futu), ST 33 (Yinshi), ST 34 (Liangqiu), ST 35 (Dubi)

Illness/energetics	Points (treatment, diagnosis and clearance)
L	
Lethargy	CV 8 (Shenque) – moxa on salt
Ligament problems	LR 4 (Zhongfeng)
Liver Fire	LR 2 (Xingjian)
Lumbar region, flat	GB 25 (Jingmen)
Lymphatic duct congestion	ST 12R (Quepen)
Lymphatic glandular exhaustion	TE 16 (Tianyou) area, Naganos, ST 25 (Tianshu)
M	
Menopause	KI 6 (Zhaohai), BL 62 (Shenmai)
Menstrual cramps	SP 10 (Xuehai)
Midline back pain	GB 25 (Jingmen)
Migraine	ST 44 (Neiting), GB 41 (Zulinqi), LR 5 (Ligou)
Miscarriage, habitual	CV 8 (Shenque) – cup
Missing organ Shu (placenta)	KI 16 (Huangshu)
Mouth problems	LI 6 (Pianli)–7 (Wenliu) area
N	
Nasal congestion	CV 8 (Shenque) – indirect moxa, sinus area
Nasal itching	CV 8 (Shenque) – indirect moxa, sinus area
Nausea from chemotherapy	ST 36 (Zusanli), PC 6 (Neiguan)
Neck pain	GV 14 (Dazhui) area, TE 16 (Tianyou) area
Nerve root inflammation	LR 5 (Ligou), KI 9 (Zhubin), SI 3 (Houxi), GV 14 (Dazhui)
Neurovascular compression	ST 12 (Quepen)

Illness/energetics	Points (treatment, diagnosis and clearance)
O	
Ovary reflex	ST 28 (Shuidao)
Oxygen to all areas	PC 4 (Ximen)
P	
Pain, all types	PC 6 (Neiguan), ST 34, (Liangqiu), LI 4 (Hegu), HT 7 (Shenmen)
Pain, abdominal	CV 8 (Shenque) – moxa on ginger
Pain along the iliac crest, posterior iliac spine	TE 16 (Tianyou), Naganos, ST 13 (Qihu)
Pain in chest	KI 25 (Shencang), LU 1 (Zhongfu), LU 4 (Xiabai)
Pain in gums	ST 44 (Neiting)
Pain lateral to spine in the quadratus lumborum muscle or BL channel	KI 1 (Yongquan), LR 4 (Zhongfeng), SP 4 (Gongsun), BL 20 (Pishu), GB 25 (Jingmen), BL 25 (Dachangshu), Shiqizhui, Bl 1 and 2 (Jingming, Zanzhu)
Pain in lumbar area and sacral area	LR 4 (Zhongfeng), GV 14 (Dazhui)
Pain in the mid-back	BL 62 (Shenmai), BL 17, 18, 19 (Geshu, Ganshu, Danshu), LR 2 (Xingjian)
Pain on midline of back	LR 4 (Zhongfeng), SI 3 (Houxi), BL 62 (Shenmai), BL 20 (Pishu), GB 25 (Jingmen), BL 25 (Dachangshu), BL 1 (Jingming) Shiqizhui
Pain in stomach	ST 44 (Neiting)
Pain at tailbone	Beneath tailbone
Painful period	CV 8 (Shenque) – moxa on ginger, SP 8 (Diji), SP 10 (Xuehai), LR 8 (Ququan)
Palpitation reflex	CV 17 (Tanzhong)
Parathyroid Shu, adjusts calcium levels	KI 27 (Shufu)

Illness/energetics	Points (treatment, diagnosis and clearance)
P	
Pericarditis, endocarditis	CV 14, 15 (Juque, Jiuwei)
Periodontitis	Between LI 6 (Pianli) and 7 (Wenliu)
Phlegm anywhere, especially in head	LI 14 (Binao)
Pituitary gland reflex	SI 3 (Houxi), BL 1 (Jingming), Yintang
Portal vein congestion	LR 3 (Taichong), LR 14 (Qimen)
Posttraumatic disorientation	KI 6 (Zhaohai), Ear Shenmen
Profuse daytime sweating	HT 6 (Yinxi)
Prolapses	ST 13 (Qihu)
Prostatitis	LR 5 (Ligou), auricular point – prostate
Prostatomegaly	Tonsillar treatment (see points)
Psychosomatic reflex (autonomic nerve disturbance)	GV 9–14 (Zhiyang–Dazhui)
R	
Radiation damage	SP 6 (Sanyinjiao), CV 12 (Zhongwan), ST 36 (Zusanli), PC 6 (Neiguan), LI 4 (Hegu)
Rashes	CV 8 (Shenque) – cupping and indirect moxa
Rebellious Lung Qi	LU 5 (Chize) – three locations
Rectal and sigmoid vein congestion	ST 25–27 (Tianshu–Daju), LU 6 (Kongzui), GV 13 (Taodao), GV 1 (Changqiang), BL 32–35 (Ciliao–Huiyang)
Ren channel opening	LU 7 (Lieque)
Right lymphatic duct congestion	ST 12R (Quepen)

Illness/energetics	Points (treatment, diagnosis and clearance)
S	
Sacrotuberous ligament	BL 62 (Shenmai), SI 3 (Houxi), GB 34 (Yanglingquan), BL 23 (Shenshu), TE 5 (Waiguan), GB 41 (Zulinqi), KI 6 (Zhaohai)
Sacrum, puffy	GB 25 (Jingmen)
Salivary gland reflex	TE 17 (Yifeng)
Salivary reflex point	GV 15 (Yamen), TE 3 (Zhongdu)
Scalene compression	LU 7, 8 (Lieque, Jingqu), ST 12 (Quepen)
Sciatica	Shoulder area under eye, BL 2 (Zanzhu), GB 1 (Tongziliao)
Shen disturbance	GV 11 (Shendao)
Shock	KI 6 (Zhaohai)
Sigmoid colon, toxin reflex	SP 9 (Yinlingquan)
Sinus problems	BL 1, 2 (Jingming, Zanzhu)
Sinus reflex	ST 2 (Sibai)
Sinusitis	CV 8 (Shenque) – indirect moxa
Skin diseases	CV 8 (Shenque) – moxa on salt or cupping
Sneezing	CV 8 (Shenque) – indirect moxa
Spasm	ST 34 (Liangqiu)
Spine (to straighten)	BL 60–62 (Kunlun–Shenmai)
Spleen reflex	KI 16 (Huangshu), CV 8 (Shenque) – Birth Trauma Mu
Stagnant Qi or Stagnant Blood	PC 6 (Neiguan)
Stagnant Blood in lower abdomen	SP 10 (Xuehai)

Illness/energetics	Points (treatment, diagnosis and clearance)
S	
Stagnation of Blood anywhere, especially in lower abdomen	ST 25L (Tianshu), SP 10 (Xuehai)
Steroid hormone reflex: reduces inflammation	KI 6 (Zhaohai)
Stomach disharmony	PC 6 (Neiguan)
Stomach reflection	CV 12–14 (Zhongwan–Juque)
Stomachache, acute	LR 8 (Ququan), ST 34 (Liangqiu)
Stomatitis	Between LI 6 (Pianli) and 7 (Wenliu), LR 5 (Ligou)
Stool (loose with undigested food)	CV 8 (Shenque) – moxa on salt or ginger
Stool (alternating constipation and loose)	TE 5 (Waiguan), TE 6 (Zhigou), TE 9 (Sidu), GB 40 (Qiuxu), HT 7 (Shenmen), KI 6 (Zhaohai)
Strengthen elimination or detox	LR 5 (Ligou), KI 9 (Zhubin)
Stress	KI 6 (Zhaohai)
Sugar cravings	BL 17, 18, 20 (Geshu, Ganshu, Pishu)
Sugar metabolism problems	LR 2 (Xingjian)
Sugar reflex	BL 18, 19, 20, 21 (Ganshu, Danshu, Pishu, Weishu), SP 2–3 (Dadu–Taibai)
Sympathetic dominance reflex	Top of SCM right side
Sympathetic nervous system disturbance	TE 16 (Tianyou)
T	
Thoracic outlet syndrome	LU 7 (Lieque)
Threatened abortion	CV 8 (Shenque) – cup
Thrush	Between LI 6 (Pianli) and 7 (Wenliu)

Illness/energetics	Points (treatment, diagnosis and clearance)
T	
Thymus Mu	CV 17 (Tanzhong)
Thymus Shu	GV 12 (Shenzhu)
Thyroid cartilage reflex	LI 18 (Futu)
Thyroid Mu	ST 9 (Renying) or height of SCM
Thyroid reflex	KI 3 (Taixi)
Tonsil reflex, three bronchitis points	LU 5 (Chize) (three positions)
Tonsillitis with muscle pain	LU 5 (Chize)
Toothache	ST 44 (Neiting)
Toothache (lower)	LI 11 (Quchi), LI 1 (Shangyang)
Toothache (upper)	LI 4 (Hegu)
Toxicity	LR 5 (Ligou)
Toxin reflex	SP 9 (Yinlingquan)
Trauma	KI 6 (Zhaohai)
U	
Ulcer reflex for stomach	ST 21L (Liangmen)
Ulcer reflex for duodenum	ST 21R (Liangmen)
Umbilical herniation	CV 8 (Shenque) – local needle around

Illness/energetics	Points (treatment, diagnosis and clearance)
U	
Urinary retention	CV 3 (Zhongji)
Urine dripping	CV 1–2 area (Huiyin –Qugu).
Urticaria	CV 8 (Shenque) – cupping
Uterus ligament (reflex)	ST 30 (Qichong)
Uterus reflex	KI 13 (Qixue), ST 30 (Qichong)
V	
Vascular problems	KI 1 (Yongquan)
Venous circulation	SP 6 (Sanyinjiao)
Vomiting	CV 8 (Shenque), PC 6 (Neiguan)
W	
Watery nose and eyes	CV 8 (Shenque) – indirect moxa
Weakness	CV 8 (Shenque) – special treatment of 8 needles around it
White blood cells (to increase)	GV 14 (Dazhui)
Will (lack of will to live)	CV 8 (Shenque) – moxa on salt
Women's disorders	GB 41 (Zulinqi)

Cross-reference by meridian of important point energetics in the Japanese acupuncture system

Lung

1	Clearance point for ST 25R Increases energy of the whole body Chest fullness, chest pain
4	Chest pain
5	Bronchitis Asthma Rebellious Lung Qi Tonsil reflex
6	Rectal vein congestion, i.e. hemorrhoids
7	Opens Ren channel Carpal tunnel syndrome Thoracic outlet syndrome
7–8	Opens scalene compression Carpal tunnel syndrome
10	Fecal stagnation

Large Intestine

1	Toothache in lower quadrant
4	Upper toothache Clearance point for ST 25R All types of pain Chemotherapy effects – nausea, radiation damage
Between 6 & 7	Any mouth problem: Oral herpes Periodontitis Gingivitis Stomatitis Thrush
10	Drumlike abdomen
11 area (Naganos)	General immunity points Adenoid reflex Lymphatic glandular exhaustion

14	Phlegm anywhere in the body, especially the head		Pain along the iliac crest, posterior iliac spine
18	Thyroid reflex	25R	Lung Mu
			Large Intestine Mu
			Triple Warmer Mu

Spleen

2–3	Sugar reflex		Lymphatic glandular exhaustion reflex
	Any spine problem involving the neck (SP 3)		Appendix reflex
			Ileocecal valve reflex
4	Opens Chong channel	25L	Blood Stagnation reflex
	SP Qi Xu syndromes		Rectal and sigmoid vein congestion
	Dampness		
	Removes Excess		
	Clearance point for CV 12	28	Ovary reflex
	(Zhongwan)	30	Chong mai disturbance
	Pain in the quadratus lumborum muscle		Prolapses
			Sea of Blood
	Any spine problem involving the neck	31–35	Knee problems
	Acute stomachache	34R	Headache accompanying food poisoning
	Bleeding		Spasm
6	Circulation, especially lower limb and Blood Stagnation in abdomen due to poor venous circulation		Acute stomachache
			All types of pain
			Clearance point for CV 12
			Food poisoning
	Inner thigh release point	36	Regulates hydrochloric acid
	Nausea accompanying radiation		Immunity
	Damage from chemotherapy		Abdominal distension
	Digestive disturbances		Nausea accompanying radiation
	Enuresis		Damage from chemotherapy
8	Dysmenorrhea	44	Food poisoning
9	Gas reflex		Allergic reaction
	Sigmoid colon reflex		Toothache
	Toxin reflex		Migraine
	Constipation due to nervous sigmoid colon		Eczema
			Hydrochloric acid excess
10	Stagnant Blood anywhere in the body, particularly in lower abdomen		Gum pain, gingivitis
			Stomach pain (acute)
			Constipation
	Acute dysmenorrhea		Abdominal pain with fever
	Acute stomachache		Bleeding gums

Stomach

2	Sinus problems
	Infection
9	Thyroid Mu
12 area	Neurovascular compression
	Right lymphatic duct congestion
	Heart Qi Xu (on left)
	Brachial reflex point
	Carpal tunnel syndrome
13	Primary point for prolapses

Heart

6	Profuse daytime sweating
7	Constipation due to nervousness
	Primary pain point

Small Intestine

3	Pituitary gland reflex
	Hormonal disturbances
	Clearance point for ST 25R
	Nerve root inflammation
	Salivation (insufficiency)

Sacrotuberous ligament problems
Midline back pain

6   Acute lumbago (back strain)

11   Heart Qi Xu reflex, left side

Bladder

1   Pituitary gland reflex
Primary point for sinus problems
Midline back pain
Pain in the quadratus lumborum
or BL channel

2   Primary point for sinus problems
Sciatica
Pain in the quadratus lumborum
or BL channel

17, 18, 20   Digestive problems
Sugar cravings
Mid-back pain

20   Midline back pain
Pain in the quadratus lumborum
or BL channel

23   Kidney Deficiency
Kidney Shu
Sacrotuberous ligament problem
Immune deficiency disease

25   Midline back pain
Pain in the quadratus lumborum
or BL channel

32–35   Rectal vein congestion

60–62   Sacrotuberous ligament release
Straightens spine
Clearance point for CV 4–6 area
Menopause
Mid-back pain
Midline back pain

63   Acute lumbago (back strain)

66   Edema of foot, leg

Kidney

1   Adjusts Blood pressure
Inner thigh release
Any vascular problem
Clearance point for CV 4–6 area

2   Increases appetite

3   Thyroid reflex
Inner thigh release

6   Adrenal reflex
Shock, trauma, stress, drug use
Antiinflammatory point

Increases steroid hormone
production
The point for Yin Xu
Clearance point for CV 14, CV
4–6 area
Chronic illness
Abdominal pain and lumps
Bronchitis, asthma
Alternating stool with
nervousness

7   Strengthens Kidney Yang
Clearance point for CV 4–6 area
Kidney organ reflex

9   Strengthens elimination
Drug point
Steroid hormone production
Nerve root inflammation

13   Uterus reflex point

14   Drumlike abdomen

16   Kidney Mu
Spleen reflex
Missing Organ Shu (placenta)

23–25   Heart disease reflex
Anxiety
Chest pain
Asthma
Cough

27   Parathyroid Shu
Adjusts calcium levels
Bone Mu

Pericardium

4   Sends oxygen to all areas

6   Clearance point for CV 14–15 area
Abdominal pain and lumps
Stuck energy and emotional
problems
All types of pain
Chest congestion
Qi and Blood Stagnation
Nausea accompanying radiation
Damage from chemotherapy
Stomach disharmony
Vomiting
To move Stagnation anywhere in
the body

8   To decrease Heat or Heat Stasis
in the breast and/or Heart area

Triple Warmer

3   Promotes salivation

3–4 area	Clearance point for ST 25R
5	Opens Dai channel
	Clearance point for ST 25
	Ear problems
	Food poisoning
	Goiter
	Alternating stools
6	Constipation
	LR Qi Stagnation
	Chest Stagnation
	Alternating stools
9	Alternating stools
16	Adenoid reflex
	Lymphatic glandular exhaustion reflex
	Sympathetic nervous system reflex
	Infection reflex
	Pain along the iliac crest, posterior iliac spine
17	Salivary gland reflex

Gall Bladder

1	Hip joint pain
	Sciatica
15	Sinus reflex
25	Kidney Mu
	Treatment point for puffy sacrum and flat lumbar area
	Pain on the center line of back
	Pain in the quadratus lumborum muscle
31	Wind reflex
34	Pain
	Leg spasm
	Sacrotuberous ligament problems
40	Source point
	Strengthens Gall Bladder
	Alternating stools
41	LR Yang rising
	Yin Xu
	Clearance point for ST 25L and ST 25R
	Food poisoning
	Women's disorders
	Migraine

Liver

2	Failure of Liver to metabolize sugar
	Mid-back pain
3	Clears portal vein congestion
	Clears ST 25L
4	Backache
	Loosen ligaments
	Inner thigh release point
	Moves Liver Qi Stagnation
5	Antiinflammatory point
	Any 'itis'
	Strengthen detox
	Stomatitis
	Nerve root inflammation
	Prostatitis
	Toxicity
	Migraines
8	Acute stomachache
12	Clears greater saphenous vein
14	Clearance point for portal vein congestion

Conception Vessel

1–2	Dripping urine reflex
2–3	Bladder reflex
4–6	Kidney reflex
	Center of energy of the body
	Immune deficiency disease (CV 4)
7	Reflection of abdominal SP 6 Yin crossing
8	Birth Trauma Mu
	Spleen reflex area
	Gate of Shen
	Digestive disturbances – difficult defecation, loose stools with undigested food, vomiting
	Skin diseases – hives, dermatitis, rashes, acne, itching, urticaria
	Allergic diseases
	Sinusitis
	Allergic rhinitis
	Fatigue
	Lack of will to live
	Threatened abortion, habitual miscarriage
	Abdominal pain
	Headache
9	Water metabolism (SP Yang Xu)
	Heart reflex area
12–14 area	Front Mu of the ST
	ST reflex
	Reflection of stress
	Headache accompanying food poisoning

	Nausea accompanying radiation	5	Diabetes
	Damage from chemotherapy		Insulin
14–15 area	Pericarditis	11	Shen disturbance reflex
	Endocarditis		Excess Heart patterns
	Heart reflex area	12	Thymus Shu
	Emotional release point		
		14	Fat metabolism reflex
17	Chest reflex		Adrenal exhaustion reflex
			Evil Wind reflex

Governing Vessel

			Nerve root inflammation
1	Rectal vein congestion		White Blood cell increase
3–4 area	Adrenal reflex		Immune deficiency disease
	Deficient KI Yang		Neck pain
4	Birth trauma Shu		Pain in the lumbar and sacral area
	Allergies	15	Salivary reflex point
	Immune deficiency disease	26	Gingivitis

Appendix 3

Clinical manifestations of the Extraordinary Meridians

Du

aftereffects of stroke
cold extremities
conjunctivitis
contraction of throat, jaw, neck
cough with mucus
deafness
deep muscle aches
dementia
emotional irritability
epileptic seizures
failure to sweat when needed
febrile disease with continuous high fever
hallucinations
headache (Yang)
headaches due to Cold or Heat
lumbago
mental confusion
motor trouble of extremities
mouth disease
muscle spasms due to tetanus
neuralgia of forehead and eyebrows
night sweats
occipital muscle spasms
overstimulation
pain
  – back
  – eyes
  – knees and thighs due to Cold
  – neck
  – vertebrae
paralysis of the hands and feet
problems of the neck, shoulders, back and inner canthus
redness and swelling of the eyes
rheumatic pain
running eyes
sore throat
spasms
  – hands and feet
  – neck and back muscles
  – spine

sweating and dislike of wind
after giving birth
swelling and pain of the cheek
swelling of the throat
tearing due to wind
tonsillitis
toothache
torticollis
tremors of the hands and feet
vertigo
warm back

Ren

abdominal pain due to Cold in
the intestines
acne
afterpains
aphonia
asthenia
asthma
breast abscess
bronchitis
chest pain
chronic itching
constipation
convulsions
coryza
cough
coughing with sputum
diabetes
diarrhea
difficult labor
difficult urination
difficulty in swallowing
dyspepsia
eczema
emphysema
enuresis
epigastric pain
epilepsy
hay fever
heart disease
hemoptysis
hemorrhoids
hernia
hot flashes
infertility in both men and
women
influenza
irregular menses
laryngitis
leukorrhea
lower abdominal pain with
Blood Stagnation
mouth diseases
nausea
pain

  – epigastric and lower
    abdomen
  – genitals
  – head and neck
  – umbilicus
painful swelling of the throat
periods (not virgins)
pharyngitis
pleurisy
pneumonia
postpartum depression
problems of the throat, chest,
lungs and epigastric region
pulmonary TB
retained placenta
retention of urine
rhinitis
sinusitis
sneezing
toothache with swollen gums
whooping cough

Dai

abdominal fullness and swelling
abdominal pain
aftereffects of stroke
amenorrhea
anemia
arthritis in general
continuous febrile disease
contracture of hands and feet
disease of the mastoid region,
cheek and outer canthus
distension and fullness in
abdomen
dysmenorrhea
fainting in general
flank pain
headaches with dizziness
hot extremities
inflammation of breasts
itchy skin
knee pain
leukorrhea
loins as seated in water
loss of hearing
menstrual disturbance (not in
virgins)
migraines
motor impairment of lower
extremities
motor troubles of extremities
muscular atrophy
pain
  – arms and shoulder together
  – cheeks
  – feet and ankles

  – lower limbs
painful spasms of the hands
and feet
painful swelling
  – ankles
  – knees
  – throat
prolapse of uterus
pruritus
redness of wrists and knees
spasms in general
swelling of the top of the head
thinness
trembling in general
tremor of the hands
vomiting
weakness and general fatigue
weakness and pain of the
lumbar area

Chong

abdominal gas
afterpains
angina pectoris
anorexia
arrhythmias
asthmatic breathing
atonic arthritis
atonic constipation
bad appetite
chest pain
cholecystitis
diarrhea
  – children
  – general
difficult digestion
digestive troubles in general
diseases in the heart, chest,
lungs
dizziness after birth
dysmenorrhea
endocarditis
gastric ulcer
heart pains
hiccough
hyperacidity
infertility in men and women
irregular menstruation
jaundice
lower abdominal pain and
distension
lumbar pains
malaria
myocarditis
painful spasms around the
umbilicus
palpitations

Paludeen fever
severe abdominal pain
spasm and pain in the abdomen
stomach afflictions
superficial pain of abdomen and
flanks
tightness around the heart
vomiting
watery diarrhea
whooping cough

Yangwei

abscess of head
acne
arthritis of fingers and toes
articular pain
chills and fever
deep muscle pain
difficulty in extending the arms
and legs
dislike of wind after childbirth
epistaxis
excessive sweating due to
febrile diseases
fevers in general
frequent nosebleeds
furuncles
general neuralgia
general swelling of the body
after childbirth
headache
headaches and dizziness due to
Cold
hematemesis
hot extremities
incoordination of the
extremities
mumps
muscle spasms due to tetanus
night blindness
night sweats
otitis
pain
 – arms
 – around eyes
 – ears
 – hands and feet
 – lower molars
painful swelling of the back
photophobia
pruritus
swelling of heel
swollen eyes with redness and
pain
tearing due to wind
thinness
tinnitus

tongue disease

Yangqiao

abscesses in general
aphasia
apoplexy
arm pain due to Cold
arthritic pain in the legs
articular pains
articular rheumatism
boils
cerebral congestion
contracture in general
epileptic seizures
excessive sweating
 – dislike of wind after giving
 birth
 – face only
facial paralysis
frequent nosebleeds
furuncles
general swelling of the body
headaches due to febrile
diseases
hemiplegia
incoordination of the hands and
feet
loss of hearing
lumbar pains
monoplegia
muscle spasms due to tetanus
obsessions
pain
 – eye and periorbital areas
 with tearing
 – joints of the arms and legs
painful swelling of the knees
and thighs
paraplegia
sciatica
spasms of the back muscles
around the Kidneys
sweating due to cold
swollen breasts with soreness
torticollis

Yinwei

abdominal Blood Stagnation
abdominal pain
agitation
alternating Hot and Cold
symptoms
amnesia
apprehension
cardiac pain
cardialgia
chest pain

convulsions
delirium
dysmenorrhea
emotional states
epigastric pain
epilepsy
fear
hemorrhoids
hypertension
indigestion
internal fullness
mental depression
nausea
nervous laugh
nightmares
poor digestion
rectal prolapse in infants
spasmodic constipation
tightness in the chest
timidity
ulcers
unquietness
varicose veins
vertical pain on the side of the
abdomen
watery diarrhea

Yinqiao

absence of sexual pleasure
afterpains
albuminuria
anuria
Bladder spasms
chest pains
constipation in women
cystitis
diarrhea with gas
difficult delivery
difficult urination
dizziness during menstruation
dysmenorrhea of virgins
enuresis
epilepsy
fluid retention during
pregnancy
gastrointestinal problems
habitual abortion
hematuria
Hot soles and Cold legs
impotence
inversion of foot
lethargy
leukorrhea
lower abdominal swelling
metritis
metropathia
nephritis

orchitis
ovarities
pain
 – Bladder
 – lower abdomen
 – referring to lumbar region
   and hip
postpartum hemorrhages

postpartum pains
prostatitis
pulmonary TB
retained placenta
seminal loss
somnolence
spasm of lower limbs
sterility

tightness in the chest
toxic pregnancy
urinary retention
urinary trouble
vomiting
weakness in the legs
weakness of women and
elderly

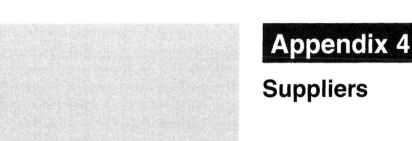

Appendix 4

Suppliers

HERBS
Mayway Corporation
1338 Mandela Parkway
Oakland
California 94607
Tel: 1–510–208–3123
Fax: 1–510–208–3069

ACUPUNCTURE SUPPLIES
OMS (Oriental Medical Supplies Inc.)
1950 Washington Street,
Braintree
Massachusetts 02184
Tel: 1–800–322–1839
Fax: 1–617–335–5779

BOOKS AND CHARTS
Redwing Book Company
44 Linden Avenue,
Brookline
Massachusetts 02146
Tel: 1 800 487 9296
Fax: 1–617–738–4620

REJUVENESS SILICON SCAR SHEETING
RichMark International Corporation
Malta Commons
Suite 47–48, Ballston Spa
New York 12020
Tel: 1–800–588–7455
Fax: 1–518–899–5320

SILICON OCCLUSIVE SHEETING
Selfcare Catalog
104 Challenger Driver
Portland
Tennessee 37148–1716
Tel: 1–800–345–3371

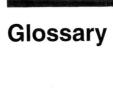

Glossary

Abdominal clearing
The process by which pathology is removed from the abdomen by palpation of points distal to the abdomen, i.e. the clearance points

Ah shi
Literally means 'Oh yes'. These are points that are tender or sensitive when palpated

Alarm points (Front Mu)
Points on the front of the body diagnostic of the Yin and the Yang of a specific Zang-Fu organ. Also known as front collecting points

Ancestral energy
Prenatal Qi, Yuan Qi, the original Qi one acquires from one's parents

Back Shu points
Points on the back of the body diagnostic of the Qi and the Blood of the organ in close proximity. Also known as associated points of the back

Ba guan liao fa
Cupping

Ba hui xue
Influential point

Ba mai jiao hui xue
Confluent point

Bao gong
The 'palace' or the 'envelope of the child', that is, the uterus

Belly bowl
A Korean-style moxa instrument in which moxa is generally burned directly over the navel

Channels and collaterals
The meridians and the Luo vessels respectively that run throughout the body

Ching Wan Hung
A Chinese ointment for burns, scalds and other skin problems

Chong ji
Parasites

Chong mai
One of the Eight Extraordinary Meridians, also known as the Penetrating Vessel and the Sea of Blood

Clarity
Ying or Nutritive Qi

Clearance points
Points that remove pathology from the abdomen

Coalescent points
Points of intersection of a main meridian with an Extra Vessel

Confluent points
The Master points that connect the Eight Extraordinary Meridians with the 12 regular meridians and activate the Curious Vessel

Dai mai
One of the Eight Extraordinary Meridians, the Girdle Vessel or the Belt Channel

Dan tian
The area below the umbilicus, particularly in the CV 4 (Guanyuan)–CV 6 (Qihai) area where the root of the Qi, the energy of the Kidney, resides

Divergent meridian
A branch arising from a main meridian which travels to another part of the body

Du mai
One of the Eight Extraordinary Meridians, the Governing Vessel

Eight Principle pulse categorization
A system of pulse diagnosis which evolved in relation to the Eight Principle diagnosis framework

Endogenous pathogens
The emotions

Essence
Jing, a rarefied form of stored Qi

Essential substances
The building blocks of life according to Chinese medicine – Qi, Blood, Jing, Body Fluids, Shen and Marrow

Evil wetness
The Chinese phrase for the Damp nature of wine

Exogenous pathogens
The external climate or other factors which mimic the internal climates such as Wind, Cold, Damp, Dryness, Heat, Summer-Heat or a combination of these

Fire syndromes
Illnesses characterized by Heat of the excess or deficient variety. They generally have inflammation and its characteristic symptoms of pain, redness, fever and swelling as part of their presentation

Five Preliminaries
The basic area of questioning which includes the major complaint with its accompanying symptoms, the onset and duration of the major complaint, as well as any history of the same or similar complaint and what treatment was sought for it, personal medical history and family medical history

Five Seas
The Seas of Qi, Blood, Marrow, Nourishment and Internal Pollution within the body which are located at specific points

Five viscera
The five Yin organs. The Heart and the Pericardium were considered the same organ

Four Methods of Diagnosis
The four traditional Chinese methods of diagnosis used to gather information about the patient

Front Collecting points
Synonymous with the Front Mu points

Fu organs
The Yang or hollow organs

Gejiang jiufa
Moxa on ginger

Geyen jiufa
Moxa on salt

Group Luo
A point of intersection of the Yin or the Yang meridians of the arms or the legs, such as SP 6

(Sanyinjiao) group, Luo of the Three Leg Yin (SP, LR and KI)

Hara
A Japanese term representing the abdomen which houses the internal organs

He (sea)
One of the five elemental Shu points located in or around the area of the elbow or the knee where the Qi of the channel is the most flourishing

Healing crisis
A temporary exacerbation of symptoms which brings about a change in the course of the illness towards improvement

Healthy Hara examination
The first physical palpatory examination of the abdomen in which the fundamental entities of Yin, Yang, Qi and Blood, Excess and Deficiency are determined

Homeopathic aggravation
The term for a healing crisis in homeopathic medicine

Horary cycle
The Chinese clock or the daily superficial flow of energy through each of the 12 organ–meridian systems

Hot above/Cold below syndromes
An abnormal energetic pattern where the area above the umbilicus is hot and the area below is cold

Huang Di Ba Shi Yi Nan Jing
The Yellow Emperor's classic of 81 difficult problems (the Nanjing)

Huatoujiaji
A group of points on both sides of the spinal column at the lateral borders of the spinous processes of the first thoracic to the fifth lumbar vertebrae

Hun
That part of the spirit which resides in the Liver

Idan
Definitive medicine by Yohimasu Todo

Influential points
A group of points that exert special influence on their associated entities. There are eight influential points for the Zang and the Fu organs, the Qi,

Blood, tendons and muscles, Marrow, bone and the vessels

Injection therapy
A method of treatment in which saline, homeopathic injectables or Chinese herbs are injected into scars or acupoints

Inner thigh compression
Tension of the tissues of the inner thigh

Internal Wind
Liver Yang which creates Wind symptoms

Irregular Vessels
The Eight Extraordinary Meridians

Japanese physical exam
The examination inspecting important areas of the body prone to tension such as the back, thighs, neck, scars and others

Jian jie jiu
Indirect moxa

Jin ye
The pure fluids retained by the body for its own use such as synovial fluid, cerebrospinal fluid, etc.

Jing
Rarefied Essence

Jing (river)
One of the five elemental Shu points on the extremities where the Qi of the channel increases in abundance

Jing (well)
One of the five elemental Shu points. They are the most distal points located on the sides of nails or tips of the fingers and toes, where the Qi of the channel starts to bubble

Jing level
Where the combined prenatal and postnatal Qi resides. It is a deep energetic core level consisting of stored Essence and genetic potential

Jueyin
One of the Six Division levels, 'the terminal Yin' corresponding to the Liver and the Pericardium

Latent points
Healthy acupuncture points of the body which do not exhibit any signs of point pathology. They are not tender when palpated or mechanically accessed

Law of Cure
A maxim in naturalistic medicine that charts the progression of an illness from worse to better as it resolves itself

Li Shi Zhen
The most famous physician of Chinese medicine

Lion Thermie warmer
A metal instrument used to apply moxa

Longitudinal Luo
A vessel which stimulates the organ–meridian complex proper that it is on. For instance, when needling LU 7 (Lieque), the Luo point of the Lung meridian, with a certain technique, it can connect to the organ of the Lung as well as stimulate the meridian

Luo point (Luo Xue)
A special vessel of communication between channels that can be used to drain Excesses from one channel and supplement Deficiency in another; connecting point

Mai
Meridian, Blood vessel

Maijing
The pulse classic, 1564 AD

Master point
Also known as a Confluent point. It activates a Curious Vessel

Meridian acupuncture
A system of therapeutics involving palpation of the meridian systems, including the secondary vessels (Extraordinary Meridians)

Mingmen
Kidney Yin and Yang inextricably bound together manifesting as slightly more Yang

Mini-thread moxa
Very small pieces of moxa, the size of rice grains, which are usually applied directly to an area or point on the skin

Miscellaneous causes of illness
The neither internal nor external causes of diseases such as foods, trauma, and exercise

Modified abdominal examination
A modern modification of classical abdominal maps in which six points corresponding to the internal organ–meridian complexes are palpated to

further diagnose the Yin, Yang, Qi and Blood of the body

Moxa box
A wooden box used to burn moxa over the abdomen or in the lower back area

Naganos
A group of four points located between the Large Intestine and Triple Warmer meridians. They are found at the lateral end of the elbow crease and proceed distally, about one fingerbreadth apart. They are indicative of the condition of the person's immunity

Nanjing
The classic of difficulties, the five element classic, written about the same time as the *Neijing*

Neijing
The Yellow Emperor's classic, The classic of internal medicine, the oldest body of Chinese medical literature, 500–300 BC

Organ–meridian complex
The Chinese concept of organ, that is, not just the gross anatomical organ per se but the entire energetic sphere of function that it encompasses

Pernicious influences
Causative factors of illness

Phlegm
A secondary pathological product

Raw physiological energy
Gu Qi, the Qi derived from food and drink by the action of the Stomach

Ren mai
One of the Curious Vessels, the Conception Vessel channel

Sea of Blood
Points which are matrices of Blood such as SP 10 (Xuehai)

Secondary pathological products
Stagnant Blood and Phlegm, pathological products which are formed within the body itself

Secondary tonification point
The grandmother point or the controlling point. For instance, LU 9 (Taiyuan) is the tonification point of the Lungs because it is the Earth point of the Lungs and Earth is the mother of Metal. The secondary tonification point is the controlling

point. In this case that is Heart 7 which is the Earth point on the Fire meridian. Fire controls Metal and Earth is the mother of Metal. Thus, it is referred to as the secondary tonification point

Shang Han Lun
The treatise of Cold induced disorders

Shaoyang
One of the energetic levels of the Six Divisions, the 'hinge' corresponding to the Gall Bladder and the San Jiao

Shaoyin
One of the levels of the Six Divisions, the 'lesser Yin'

Shen
Spirit

Shi
Excess

Shi wen
The Ten Questions

Shu (stream) point
One of the five elemental points on the extremities where the Qi of the channel flourishes

Si Hai
The Four Seas

Six bowels
The Yang organs

Six Divisions
The diagnostic framework discussed in the *Shang Han Lung* or *Treatise of Cold induced disorders* about 220 CE by Zhong Zhong-jing. It explains the invasion of a Cold or Wind-Cold pathogen into the body and how its manifestations may change if it progresses through six distinct energetic zones of the body

Taiyang
One of the Six Division levels, the 'greater Yang'.

Taiyin
One of the Six Division levels, 'greater Yin', which corresponds to the Lung and the Spleen meridians

Ten Questions
The multitudinous detailed Chinese questions pertaining to body temperature, perspiration, food/drink, appetite, stools and urination, sleep, energy, exercise, reproductive/sexual history and the emotions

TENS machines
Various types of electrical machines used within the practice of Chinese medicine to stimulate areas or points of the body

The clear
Nutritive Qi, Ying Qi

Three Treasures
A particular diagnostic framework referring to Jing, Qi and Shen

Tieh Da Yao Gin
A Chinese herbal liniment used to treat a wide variety of injuries including fractures, sprains, tears to muscles and ligaments and bruising

Tiger Thermie warmer
A metal instrument used to apply moxa

Transverse Luo
A vessel which connects to the Source point of its Coupled meridian. For instance, when needling LU 7 (Lieque) the Luo point of the Lung meridian with a certain technique, it connects to the source point of its couple, LI 4 (Hegu). Transverse Luos are used to establish equilibrium between a husband/wife pair

Vessels, secondary, irregular
The Eight Extraordinary Meridians

Wan Hua
A Chinese herbal liniment for burns and trauma

Wei level
The first and most exterior of the four stages, see theory of the Four Stages (1368–1644), that can be invaded by exogenous Heat. It corresponds essentially to the skin and the muscles

Wu xing
Five Elements

Xi (cleft) points (Xi Xue)
Points of accumulation or blockage within the meridian

Xin bao
The Pericardium

Xu
Deficiency

Yangming
One of the Six Divisions, 'resplendent sunlight', corresponding to the Large Intestine and Stomach energetic level

Yangqiao mai
One of the Eight Extraordinary Meridians, the Yang heel vessel

Yangwei mai
One of the Eight Extraordinary Meridians, the Yang connecting vessel

Yi Zong Jin Jian
The golden mirror of ancestral medicine

Ying (spring)
One of the five elemental points on the extremities in which the Qi of the channel starts to gush

Ying level
The second of the four stages corresponding to the nutritive Qi that is associated with the Blood

Yinqiao mai
One of the Eight Extraordinary Meridians, the Yin heel vessel

Yintang
An extra point at the glabella region

Yinwei mai
One of the Eight Extraordinary Meridians, the Yin connecting vessel

Zhang Jie Bing
Chinese physician who wrote, *The complete book of pulse diagnosis*

Zheng Gu Shui
A Chinese herbal liniment effective for resolving Blood stasis, promoting healing and stopping pain. Effective for a wide variety of traumatic injury

INDEX

Printed and bound by CPI Group (UK) Ltd, Croydon, CR0 4YY

03/10/2024

01040363-0002